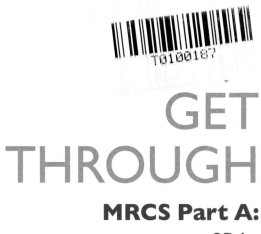

GET
THROUGH

MRCS Part A:
SBAs

GET
THROUGH

MRCS Part A:
SBAs

Edited by

Nikhil Pawa, MD, LLM, MSc, MD, FRCS (Eng)
Higher General Surgical trainee, London, UK

Paul Cathcart, BSc (Hons), LLM, MBBS, MRCS (Eng)
undertaking an MRC-funded PhD, Imperial College London, UK

Howard Tribe, BSc (Hons), MEd, PgCert, MBBS, MRCS (Eng)
specialist trauma and orthopaedics registrar
Wessex Deanery, Winchester, UK

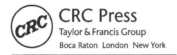

CRC Press
Taylor & Francis Group
Boca Raton London New York

CRC Press is an imprint of the
Taylor & Francis Group, an **informa** business

CRC Press
Taylor & Francis Group
6000 Broken Sound Parkway NW, Suite 300
Boca Raton, FL 33487-2742

© 2016 by Taylor & Francis Group, LLC
CRC Press is an imprint of Taylor & Francis Group, an Informa business

No claim to original U.S. Government works

Printed on acid-free paper
Version Date: 20151214

International Standard Book Number-13: 978-1-4987-2621-4 (Paperback)

Library of Congress Cataloging-in-Publication Data

Names: Pawa, Nikhil, author. | Cathcart, Paul, author. | Tribe, Howard, author.
Title: Get through MRCS part A : SBAs / Nikhil Pawa, Paul Cathcart, Howard Tribe.
Other titles: Get through.
Description: Boca Raton : Taylor & Francis, 2016. | Series: Get through | Includes bibliographical references and index.
Identifiers: LCCN 2015048586| ISBN 9781498726214 (paperback : alk. paper) | ISBN 9781498726221 (ebook)
Subjects: | MESH: General Surgery | Anatomy | Physiological Phenomena | Pathology, Clinical | Examination Questions
Classification: LCC RD37.2 | NLM WO 18.2 | DDC 617.0076--dc23
LC record available at http://lccn.loc.gov/2015048586

Visit the Taylor & Francis Web site at
http://www.taylorandfrancis.com

and the CRC Press Web site at
http://www.crcpress.com

CONTENTS

Acknowledgements   vii

Introduction   ix

Editors   xi

Contributors   xiii

Part I   Applied surgical anatomy

1   Applied surgical anatomy: Questions   3

2   Applied surgical anatomy: Answers   65

Part II   Physiology

3   Physiology: Questions   131

4   Physiology: Answers   171

Part III   Pathology

5   Pathology: Questions   221

6   Pathology: Answers   253

Part IV   System-specific pathology

7   System-specific pathology: Questions   289

8   System-specific pathology: Answers   327

Part V   Practice paper

9   Practice paper: Questions   369

10   Practice paper: Answers   395

Index   425

ACKNOWLEDGEMENTS

This book is dedicated to my wife Jasmin and children Amaya and Anay for their unwavering support and patience, and to my parents who continue to inspire me.

Nikhil Pawa

Writing and editing a book is never an easy task without the support of those close to you, from both personal and working lives. Thank you in particular must go to my parents and partner Nad'a, as well as my dear friends and colleagues.

Paul Cathcart

To my wonderful wife,

Thank you for your support and understanding for all the time I spent away from you during the writing and editing of this book.

Howard Tribe

Finally, we thank all the contributors for their input, the editorial team, especially Amy Rodriguez and Alice Oven at Taylor & Francis, for the opportunity to write this book and Viswanath Prasanna for his close attention to detail during the final edits.

INTRODUCTION

It is always a challenge to know the best way to revise and practice for an exam so that you are as prepared as you can possibly be. Any examination requires careful preparation, background reading and prior self-assessment to ensure success. During our surgical careers, we have found that it is often difficult to dedicate hours on end reading large surgical textbooks in preparation for exams. There is no doubt that these textbooks should form the basis of your quality revision, but often we found that answering revision questions during the working day or during or after a night shift was the best way to increase the amount of quality exam preparation when there are only a few spare minutes. Questions in such format can be a valuable resource in comparison to pay-per-view* internet questions.

Our aim with this book is, therefore, to provide you with a useful revision tool. Each question is accompanied by a detailed answer together with a road map highlighting important topics within the syllabus. The questions may also be used secondarily as a self-assessment tool prior to the exam.

---

* Pay-per-view internet questions are internet websites that essentially rent the use of questions for a set time as part of exam revision. The user is unable to download them. Such sites include www. onexamination.com

EDITORS

Nikhil Pawa qualified in 2002 and expanded his academic interest by successfully completing a Masters in Medical Law (LLM with Merit), MSc in surgical technology and MD (Research) from the University of Kent, Kent, UK, in 2004, and a further MSc in surgical technology from Imperial College London in 2008. Having completed his basic surgical training in Nottingham, Nikhil completed an MD (research) investigating serum-based biomarkers for colorectal cancer. He is currently a higher general surgical trainee on the North West London rotation. Nikhil has a keen interest in medical education and has been regularly involved in courses associated with the Royal College of Surgeons and the Royal Society of Medicine.

Paul Cathcart qualified from Imperial College London in 2006 with a BSc in endocrinology. He successfully completed the MRCS in 2009 and subsequently obtained a general surgical training number in the East of England Deanery. In 2015, Paul successfully completed a master of laws from Northumbria University, Newcastle upon Tyne, UK. He is currently undertaking an MRC-funded PhD research project under Professor Stebbing at Imperial College London. Paul has a keen interest in medical education and regularly teaches medical students at the Royal Society of Medicine in preparation for their OSCE examinations, and also acts as an advanced trauma life support instructor.

Howard Tribe qualified from Imperial College London in 2006. He has been a surgical trainee since 2008 and is currently a specialist trauma and orthopaedics registrar in the Wessex Deanery. Alongside his clinical work, Howard has been awarded several academic qualifications, the latest being a postgraduate certificate in trauma and orthopaedics from Brighton and Sussex University. Howard is particularly enthusiastic about education and has completed a masters in surgical education at Imperial College London. He has been an anatomy demonstrator and is a certified OSCE examiner for medical school examinations. Currently, you will find him most at home teaching anatomy or aspects of orthopaedic examination and management to a group of junior doctors.

CONTRIBUTORS

Darshan Srishail Angadi MBBS, MRCS, PGCE, ST6, trauma and orthopaedics, East of England Deanery

Paul Cathcart BSc (Hons), LLM, MBBS, MRCS (Eng), undertaking MRC-funded PhD, Imperial College London

Cameron Davies-Husband MBBS, BSc (Hons), FRCS (ORL-HNS), DOHNS, PGCME, head and neck surgical oncology TIG Fellow (Training Interface Group), Freeman Hospital, Newcastle upon Tyne

Akan Emin Bsc, Msc, MBBS, MRCS, higher general surgical trainee in the West of Scotland Deanery

Neil Utpal Maitra MBBS, MRCS, higher surgical trainee urology West of Scotland Deanery

Asiya Maula MBBS, BSc, MRCS, MPH (distinction), ACF, GP trainee ST3, East Midlands Deanery

Nikhil Pawa MD, LLM, MSc, MD, FRCS (Eng), higher general surgical trainee on the North West London rotation

Saravanan Royan MRCGP, MRCS, BMBS, BMedSci, general practitioner, Nottingham

Howard Tribe BSc (Hons), MEd, PgCert, MBBS, MRCS (Eng), specialist trauma and orthopaedics registrar in the Wessex Deanery

PART I
APPLIED SURGICAL ANATOMY

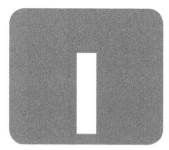

CHAPTER I
APPLIED SURGICAL ANATOMY

Questions

THORAX

1. The lung pleurae meet in the midline and then separate to allow space for the heart. At the level of which costal cartilage does the pleura of the left lung separate from the pleura of the right lung?
   a. 1st
   b. 2nd
   c. 4th
   d. 6th
   e. 8th

2. At which costochondral joint do the oblique fissures of the lung finish?
   a. 4th
   b. 5th
   c. 6th
   d. 7th
   e. 8th

3. When examining a fit young patient you would anticipate to find the apex beat of the heart in the mid-clavicular line of which intercostal space?
   a. 2nd
   b. 3rd
   c. 4th
   d. 5th
   e. 6th

4. At which vertebral level does the aorta pass through the diaphragm?
   a. T9
   b. T10
   c. T11
   d. T12
   e. L1

5. A 52-year-old man with oesophageal carcinoma undergoes an Ivor Lewis oesophagectomy. Two days postoperatively you notice a thick, creamy liquid in the chest drain effluent. It was thought his thoracic duct may have been iatrogenically injured during the procedure. The internal thoracic duct lies laterally to which of the following anatomical structures?
   a. Thoracic aorta
   b. Oesophagus
   c. Left brachiocephalic vein
   d. Vertebral bodies
   e. Azygous vein

6. A 60-year-old woman is seen in the preoperative clinic awaiting a para-umbilical hernia repair. Her past medical history includes rheumatic fever as a child. Clinical examination reveals a rumbling diastolic murmur. Which of the following is the correct anatomical location of the affected cardiac valve?
   a. 2nd intercostal space
   b. 5th costal cartilage
   c. 3rd costal cartilage
   d. 4th intercostal space
   e. 4th costal cartilage

7. A patient with chest pain is found to have an occlusion of his left coronary artery (LCA) on angiogram. Which of the following statements regarding the LCA is false?
   a. The LCA supplies the majority of the left ventricle.
   b. The LCA supplies the left atrium.
   c. The LCA supplies the sinoatrial (SA) node in 40% of hearts.
   d. The LCA supplies the atrioventricular (AV) node in most cases.
   e. The LCA supplies part of the right ventricle.

8. A young man is admitted as an emergency following a road traffic accident suffering injury to his sternum. Reviewing the computed tomography (CT) scan of his chest, which of the following statements regarding the anatomy of the level of the sternal angle is true?
   a. It demonstrates the bifurcation of the brachiocephalic artery.
   b. It demonstrates the bifurcation of the trachea.
   c. It gives a clear section through the left ventricle.
   d. It shows the commencement of the aortic arch.
   e. It demonstrates the T4 vertebral body.

9. Which of the following statements regarding the movements of inspiration is false?
   a. It involves descent of the diaphragm.
   b. It involves an increase in the anteroposterior dimension of the chest.
   c. It involves an upward/forward movement of the first rib.
   d. It involves contraction of the intercostal muscles.
   e. It involves the long thoracic nerve of Bell.

10. Which of the following statements regarding paralysis of the left hemidiaphragm is true?
    a. It may be caused by the transection of the cord below C6.
    b. It may be caused by the section of the left phrenic nerve alone.
    c. It causes flattening of the diaphragm during inspiration.
    d. It increases intrathoracic pressure on the left.
    e. It does not cause paradoxical chest movement.

11. An elderly patient suffers a myocardial infarction after a routine elective anterior resection for rectal cancer. Which of the following statements regarding blood supply to the heart is false?
    a. The right coronary artery has a marginal and posterior branch.
    b. The left coronary artery has a circumflex branch.
    c. The right and left coronaries arise from immediately inferior to the aortic valve.
    d. The anterior interventricular branch supplies the ventricular septum.
    e. Venous drainage of the heart opens into the right atrium via the coronary sinus.

12. Which of the following statements about the anatomy of the diaphragm is correct?
    a. The central portion obtains its sensory supply from the lower six intercostal nerves.
    b. The oesophageal hiatus opens at T12.
    c. The left phrenic nerve pierces the central tendon.
    d. The inferior vena cava opening is at T10.
    e. The sympathetic chain passes through the median arcuate ligament.

13. Concerning the arterial supply and venous drainage, which of the following statements is correct?
    a. The arterial supply to the upper third is derived from the superior thyroid artery.
    b. The arterial supply to the lower third is derived from the left gastric artery.
    c. The thoracic oesophagus drains into the hemiazygous vein.
    d. The abdominal oesophagus drains via the splenic vein.
    e. The arterial supply to the middle third is derived from the inferior thyroid artery.

14. Which of these structures passes through the opening in the diaphragm at the level of T10?
    a. Thoracic duct
    b. Right phrenic nerve
    c. Azygous vein
    d. Inferior vena cava
    e. Left gastric artery

15. Which of the following veins does not drain into the coronary sinus of the heart?
    a. Small cardiac vein
    b. Oblique cardiac vein
    c. Great cardiac vein

d. Anterior cardiac vein
e. Middle cardiac vein

16. During embryological development, there are a series of six paired aortic arches. Which of the following statements about the paired aortic arches is true?
    a. The 1st and 3rd arches disappear.
    b. The 2nd arches become the carotid arteries.
    c. The 4th arch on the left side becomes the definitive aortic arch.
    d. The 5th arch forms the right and left pulmonary arteries.
    e. On the left side the recurrent laryngeal nerve hooks around the 4th arch.

17. Which of the following are the correct relations of the thoracic trachea?
    a. Anterior – left recurrent laryngeal nerve
    b. Posterior – left common carotid artery
    c. Left – left brachiocephalic vein
    d. Right – azygous vein
    e. Posterior – thymus

18. Which of the following statements regarding the thoracic duct is correct?
    a. It commences at the level of T10.
    b. It passes upwards between the vena cava and azygous vein.
    c. It drains into the confluence of the right internal jugular and subclavian veins.
    d. The right lower limb is drained by the right lymphatic trunk.
    e. In adults the thoracic duct transports up to 4 L of lymph per day.

19. Which of the following is the most common site of Bochdalek (diaphragmatic) hernias?
    a. Left anterior
    b. Right posterior
    c. Right anterior
    d. Left posterior
    e. None of the above

20. A 35-year-old man is brought in with severe breathlessness following a road traffic collision. The chest X-ray shows a rib fracture with haemothorax and you are required to insert a chest drain. Which one of the following anatomical landmarks is least useful to you?
    a. Anterior border of latissimus dorsi
    b. The mid-clavicular line
    c. The nipple
    d. The mid-axillary line
    e. Inferolateral border of pectoralis major

21. A 5-year-old boy is about to undergo bronchoscopy for a suspected inhaled peanut. Which of the following is the most likely site for the inhaled peanut?
    a. Right middle lobe bronchus
    b. Left inferior lobe bronchus

    c. Right superior lobe bronchus
    d. Left superior lobe bronchus
    e. Right lower lobe bronchus

22. Which of the following statements is true regarding the anatomy of the oesophagus?
    a. The oesophageal wall comprises inner longitudinal and outer circular muscle layers.
    b. It receives all of its arterial blood supply directly from aortic branches.
    c. All blood drains into the portal venous system.
    d. The oesophagus commences at the level of C6 and enters the abdomen at the level of T12.
    e. Lymph from the abdominal portion of the oesophagus usually drains into the gastric and coeliac lymph nodes.

23. The normal oesophagus has four constrictions where adjacent structures produce impressions, as can be seen on video fluoroscopy. Which of the following structures/sites causes oesophageal indentation only when pathologically enlarged?
    a. Approximately 15 cm from the incisors at the level of the cricopharyngeus muscle
    b. Aortic arch
    c. Left main bronchus
    d. Left atrium
    e. Lower oesophageal sphincter

24. Which of the following arteries is a direct branch of the subclavian artery?
    a. Posterior circumflex humoral
    b. Internal thoracic artery
    c. Thoracoacromial artery
    d. Superior thoracic artery
    e. Lateral thoracic artery

25. The thoracic aorta is described as the thoracic aspect of the descending aorta. Which of the following arteries arises as a direct branch of the thoracic aorta?
    a. Coeliac trunk
    b. Subcostal artery
    c. Inferior phrenic artery
    d. Lumbar arteries
    e. Superior mesenteric artery

26. Which one of the following statements regarding the lungs is correct?
    a. The parietal pleura invests the lung surface.
    b. The right lung has two lobes.
    c. The right main bronchus is longer than the left main bronchus.
    d. The bronchial arteries supply the lung with oxygenated blood.
    e. The left bronchial artery usually arises from the subclavian artery.

27. An 18-year-old is brought into the accident and emergency department with a superficial knife stab wound on the side of his right chest wall. His airway, breathing and circulation are unremarkable. On further assessment he is unable to raise his right arm above the horizontal position. Also, when he presses his hands against a wall, his right scapula protrudes away from the chest wall. Which of the following nerves is most likely damaged in this situation?
    a. Suprascapular nerve
    b. Upper subscapular nerve
    c. Lower subscapular nerve
    d. Long thoracic nerve
    e. Thoracodorsal nerve

28. Regarding the anatomy of the first rib, the following statements are true except:
    a. It is a true rib.
    b. It is an atypical rib.
    c. It articulates with T1 and T2 vertebrae.
    d. The scalenus anterior muscle attaches to it.
    e. It contains a groove for the subclavian vein.

ABDOMEN, PELVIS AND PERINEUM

29. Which of the following structures are found within the spermatic cord?
    a. The testicular artery
    b. The pampiniform plexus
    c. The cremastic artery
    d. All of the above
    e. a and b only

30. Which of the following layers of the anterior abdominal wall is correctly paired with its corresponding layer surrounding the spermatic cord and scrotum?
    a. Transversalis fascia – internal spermatic fascia
    b. External oblique aponeurosis – external spermatic fascia
    c. Fascia of internal oblique muscle – cremasteric fascia
    d. Peritoneum – tunica vaginalis
    e. All of the above

31. Which one of the following structures predominantly forms the posterior border of the inguinal canal?
    a. The inguinal ligament
    b. The conjoint tendon
    c. The pectineal ligament
    d. The transversalis fascia
    e. The external oblique aponeurosis

32. Which of these examples of dilated venous systems are characteristically associated with liver cirrhosis?
    a. Haemorrhoids
    b. The bare area of the liver connections
    c. Retroperitoneal connections
    d. Caput medusae
    e. All of the above

33. You are asked to assist your consultant in theatre with an emergency laparotomy on a 45-year-old man with a bleeding duodenal ulcer. Which of the following arteries is commonly associated with this condition?
    a. The gastroduodenal artery
    b. The left gastric artery
    c. The right gastric artery
    d. The superior mesenteric artery
    e. The common hepatic artery

34. A 26-year-old man is admitted after a road traffic accident. He has sustained a liver laceration and is haemodynamically unstable. Following initial resuscitation he is taken to theatre for a laparotomy. At the beginning of the emergency operation your consultant asks you to perform the Pringle's manoeuvre. Which of the following structures are compressed?
    a. The superior mesenteric artery
    b. The hepatic artery

   c. The portal vein

   d. All of the above

   e. b and c only

35. While reviewing an abdominal CT scan you note the report comments on a possible abnormality at the level of the transpyloric plane. Which of the following structures would you expect to find at this level?

   a. Adrenal glands

   b. The first part of the duodenum

   c. The 10th costal cartilages

   d. The tail of the pancreas

   e. L2 vertebral body

36. During an elective inguinal hernia repair you are asked to define the boundaries of the inguinal canal. Which of the following structures make up the roof of the inguinal canal?

   a. Transversalis fascia and lacunar ligament

   b. External and internal oblique

   c. Lacunar ligament and conjoint tendon

   d. Internal oblique, conjoint tendon and transversus abdominis

   e. Pectineal ligament and inguinal ligament

37. A 23-year-old man is diagnosed with a direct inguinal hernia. The registrar intraoperatively asks you to define Hesselbach's triangle. Which of the following structures makes up the medial boundary of Hesselbach's triangle?

   a. Lacunar ligament

   b. Inferior epigastric artery

   c. Femoral artery

   d. Rectus abdominis

   e. Inguinal ligament

38. A 45-year-old woman undergoes a cholecystectomy several weeks after an episode of acute cholecystitis. During the operation the surgeon correctly identifies Calot's triangle in order to locate the cystic artery. Which of the following anatomical structures form Calot's triangle?

   a. Cystic duct, liver edge and left hepatic duct

   b. Portal vein, liver and common bile duct

   c. Common hepatic duct and inferior border of the liver and cystic duct

   d. Right hepatic artery, cystic duct and common bile duct

   e. Left hepatic duct and inferior border of the liver and cystic duct

39. You are asked to assist your consultant in a routine laparoscopic cholecystectomy. Before dividing any structures he correctly identifies Calot's triangle and the cystic artery. From which of the following arteries does the cystic artery commonly originate?

   a. Left hepatic artery

   b. Superior pancreaticoduodenal artery

   c. Gastroduodenal artery

d. Right gastric artery

e. Right hepatic artery

40. A 62-year-old man undergoes an emergency upper gastrointestinal (GI) endoscopy for a bleeding gastric ulcer. The ulcer is found to be in the lower greater curvature of the stomach. Which of the following arteries supplies this area?
a. Left gastric artery
b. Right gastric artery
c. Superior pancreaticoduodenal artery
d. Short gastric arteries
e. Left gastroepiploic artery

41. An 81-year-old lady presents with peritonitis to the emergency department. She is otherwise well with no previous surgical history. After resuscitation a computed tomography (CT) scan confirms the diagnosis of perforated diverticular disease. She therefore undergoes a Hartmann's procedure. In which region of the abdomen is the stoma most likely to be found?
a. RUQ (right upper quadrant)
b. LUQ (left upper quadrant)
c. RLQ (right lower quadrant)
d. LLQ (left lower quadrant)
e. Umbilical

42. A young 10-year-old boy is taken to theatre for an open appendicectomy. The registrar commences the operation with a Lanz incision. Which of the following structures is not divided during routine dissection?
a. Scarpa's fascia
b. External oblique aponeurosis
c. Internal oblique muscle
d. Transverse abdominal muscle
e. Rectus abdominal muscle

43. An 18-year-old man is involved in a violent assault. He is stabbed in the groin and the abdomen. He recovers from the assault and, following a short stay in hospital, he is discharged. On follow-up 3 months later he reports that he finds standing and walking difficult. These symptoms are attributed to damage to which of the following anatomical structures?
a. Sciatic nerve
b. Femoral nerve
c. Ilioinguinal nerve
d. Quadriceps muscles
e. Hip and knee joints

44. A 57-year-old male presents to his general practitioner (GP) with a swelling of his scrotum. The GP diagnoses a varicocele. This is attributed to a recent open inguinal hernia repair. Damage to which one of the following structures would account for this?
a. Ilioinguinal nerve
b. Vas deferens

c. Testicular artery
d. Pampiniform plexus of veins
e. Lymphatic vessels

45. Which of the following arteries supplies the fundus of the stomach?
   a. Short gastric arteries
   b. Right gastric artery
   c. Left gastric artery
   d. Left and right gastroepiploic arteries
   e. Gastroduodenal artery

46. A patient undergoes a Billroth I operation for treatment of a persistent gastric ulcer. Which of the following does this procedure entail?
   a. Resection of the distal third of the stomach and anastomosis to the duodenum
   b. Resection of the distal two-thirds of the stomach and anastomosis to the jejunum
   c. Total gastrectomy
   d. Roux-en-Y reconstruction
   e. Resection of the distal two-thirds of the stomach and a gastrojejunostomy

47. A 70-year-old man presents to the emergency department with abdominal pain and a pulsatile mass per abdomen. Which of the following statements is true regarding aneurysms?
   a. An aneurysm is defined as abnormal dilatation of a vessel by at least 35%.
   b. Abdominal aneurysms often rupture even when they are less than 5.5 cm in diameter.
   c. Aneurysms of the thoracic aorta do not rupture and therefore rarely require treatment.
   d. Immediate complications of abdominal aortic aneurysm (AAA) surgery include aortoduodenal fistula.
   e. Late complications of AAA surgery include false aneurysm.

48. On a ward round your consultant asks you to examine a patient. On abdominal palpation you find a mass in the left upper quadrant. Which of the following statements is true regarding splenomegaly?
   a. A splenic mass should be ballotable.
   b. The splenic notch is always an obvious landmark.
   c. In massive splenomegaly, the spleen is rarely palpable in the lower abdomen.
   d. Niemann–Pick syndrome is a known cause of splenomegaly.
   e. Traumatic splenic injury is always an indication for splenectomy.

49. Which of the following statements concerning the arterial supply of the stomach is correct?
   a. The right gastric artery is derived from the splenic artery.
   b. The cystic artery is derived from the left gastric artery.
   c. The gastroduodenal branch of the hepatic artery gives off the left gastroepiploic artery.

d. The splenic artery gives off the superior pancreaticoduodenal artery.

e. The short gastric arteries are derived from the splenic artery.

50. Which of the following statements concerning the anatomy of the kidney is correct?

a. There is an inferior opening in Gerota's fascia.

b. The third part of the duodenum is anteriorly related to the right kidney.

c. The right testicular vein drains into the left renal vein.

d. The left testicular vein drains into the inferior vena cava.

e. The hilum medially transmits artery, ureter, vein and artery (in this order) from anterior to posterior.

51. Which of the following statements related to the course of the ureter is correct?

a. Its course is retroperitoneal until it reaches the vesicoureteric junction.

b. It passes under the genitofemoral nerve.

c. It runs over the external iliac artery and vein.

d. It passes over the vas deferens.

e. It enters the bladder superolaterally.

52. Which of the following statements concerning the anatomy of the femoral triangle is correct?

a. It is bound laterally by the lateral border of adductor magnus.

b. It is bound medially by the medial border of adductor longus.

c. The femoral artery lies medial to the femoral nerve at the midpoint of the inguinal ligament.

d. The floor is formed by fascia lata.

e. The roof consists of iliopsoas and pectineus.

53. Which of the following statements concerning the anatomy of the femoral canal is correct?

a. It is bound laterally by the pectineal ligament.

b. It is bound medially by the femoral vein.

c. It is bound posteriorly by the lacunar ligament.

d. It is bound anteriorly by the inguinal ligament.

e. It transmits the spermatic cord.

54. Concerning the branches of the abdominal aorta, the following vertebral levels all correspond correctly except:

a. Inferior mesenteric artery: L3

b. Iliac arteries: L4

c. Renal artery: L1

d. Coeliac trunk: T12

e. Superior mesenteric artery: L1

55. Which of the following features does not distinguish the jejunum from the ileum?

a. Thick valvulae conniventes

b. A tendency to lie at the umbilical region

c. Multiple vascular arcades

    d. A thick mesentery from above downwards, attaching to the left side of the aorta

    e. Absence of Peyer's patches

56. Which of the following structures is found in the transpyloric plane (L1)?
    a. Body of stomach
    b. Ileocaecal junction
    c. Fundus of the gallbladder
    d. Hilum of the spleen
    e. Seventh costal cartilage

57. At laparoscopy the surgeon identifies the median umbilical fold on the anterior abdominal wall. Which of the following structures is present within the fold?
    a. Remains of urachus
    b. Inferior epigastric vessels
    c. Remains of umbilical artery
    d. Remains of umbilical vein
    e. Superior epigastric vessels

58. You are asked to assist the registrar in theatre performing an elective inguinal hernia repair on a 32-year-old man. The surgeon is extremely careful not to injure the spermatic cord. Which of the following structures is not found within the spermatic cord?
    a. Iliohypogastric nerve
    b. Artery of the vas
    c. Pampiniform plexus
    d. Nerve to cremaster
    e. Testicular artery

59. Which of the following statements regarding the renal veins is incorrect?
    a. The renal veins lie in front of the renal arteries.
    b. The renal veins enter the vena cava at the level of L4 vertebra.
    c. The left renal vein is three times longer than the right renal vein.
    d. The left renal vein receives the left gonadal and suprarenal veins.
    e. The left renal vein may sometimes be ligated during aortic aneurysm surgery.

60. A young 10-year-old boy is admitted with lower abdominal pain. After resuscitation he undergoes surgery where a Meckel's diverticulum is found to be the cause. Which of the following statements regarding a Meckel's diverticulum is correct?
    a. It is found in approximately 4% of individuals.
    b. It always lies on the antimesenteric border of the ileum.
    c. It represents a partial persistence of the Mullerian duct from fetal life.
    d. Approximately 20% of cases have heterotopic gastric mucosa.
    e. The diverticulum is supplied by its own ileal branch from the inferior mesenteric artery.

61. Which of the following nerves passes through the greater sciatic notch above the piriformis muscle?
    a. Pudendal nerve
    b. Nerve to obturator internus
    c. Superior gluteal nerve
    d. Inferior gluteal nerve
    e. Posterior femoral cutaneous nerve

62. Which of the following is the correct boundary of the epiploic foramen?
    a. Anteriorly – inferior vena cava
    b. Posteriorly – portal vein
    c. Inferiorly – the lesser curvature of the stomach
    d. Posteriorly – free margin of the lesser omentum
    e. Superiorly – the caudate process of the liver

63. Which of the following is not the correct border of the inguinal canal?
    a. Anteriorly – superficial fascia and external oblique aponeurosis
    b. Posteriorly – inguinal ligament
    c. Superiorly – internal oblique and transversus abdominis
    d. Inferiorly – inguinal ligament
    e. Posteriorly – conjoint tendon

64. Which of the following statements about the anatomy of the anal canal is correct?
    a. Above the dentate line it is lined by squamous epithelium.
    b. The arterial supply below the dentate line is from the superior rectal artery.
    c. Venous drainage above the dentate line is into the internal pudendal vein.
    d. There are anal columns present below the dentate line.
    e. Lymphatic drainage above the dentate line is to the internal iliac nodes.

65. Which of the following statements about the portal vein is correct?
    a. It is formed behind the tail of the pancreas.
    b. It lies anterior to the common bile duct and hepatic artery in the free edge of the epiploic foramen.
    c. It is usually formed by the union of the splenic and inferior mesenteric veins.
    d. Behind the first part of the duodenum the gastroduodenal artery lies anterior to the portal vein.
    e. Normally portal venous blood empties into the systemic circulation via the hepatic artery.

66. Which of the following regarding the relations of the urinary bladder is incorrect?
    a. Anteriorly – pubic symphysis
    b. Superiorly – peritoneum with small intestine and sigmoid colon
    c. Laterally – levator ani and obturator internus
    d. Laterally – puborectalis
    e. Posteriorly – rectum and seminal vesicles in the male and vagina in the female

67. Which statement regarding the rectus abdominis muscle is correct?
    a. The lateral head arises from the front of the pubic symphysis.
    b. Two tendinous intersections are found in the muscle.
    c. The rectus abdominis is the most powerful extensor of the trunk.
    d. The medial head arises from the pubic crest.
    e. The muscle inserts onto the 5th to 7th costal cartilages.

68. Which of the following statements concerning the male urethra is correct?
    a. The total length of the urethra is approximately 30 cm.
    b. The distal urethra develops from the mesonephric ducts.
    c. The distal part of spongy urethra is lined with transitional epithelium.
    d. The narrowest point of the urethra is at the external meatus.
    e. The prostatic portion of the urethra is the narrowest part.

69. Which of the following statements regarding the inferior epigastric artery is correct?
    a. It originates below the inguinal ligament.
    b. It originates from the internal iliac artery.
    c. It enters the rectus sheath above the arcuate line.
    d. It runs deep to the rectus abdominis.
    e. It anastomoses directly with the internal thoracic artery.

70. Which of the following statements regarding the anterior abdominal wall is incorrect?
    a. Inferior to the arcuate line, the rectus muscle lies directly on the transversalis fascia.
    b. The external oblique aponeurosis always lies anterior to the rectus abdominis muscle.
    c. The internal oblique aponeurosis splits around the rectus abdominis below the arcuate line.
    d. The transversus abdominis lies anterior to the rectus muscle below the arcuate line.
    e. Above the costal margin, the rectus sheath consists of only the external oblique aponeurosis.

71. Which of the following statements regarding a spigelian hernia is incorrect?
    a. Medial to the defect lies the rectus abdominis.
    b. It occurs most commonly below the arcuate line.
    c. It can be repaired easily laparoscopically.
    d. It is usually covered by an intact external oblique aponeurosis.
    e. There is a low risk of strangulation.

72. Which of the following statements is incorrect regarding the arterial supply/venous drainage of the spleen?
    a. The splenic vein drains into the portal vein.
    b. The splenic artery derives from the coeliac artery.
    c. The splenic artery gives branches to the pancreas.
    d. The splenic artery supplies all of the greater curvature of the stomach.
    e. Splenic artery aneurysm is the most common visceral artery aneurysm.

73. Which of the following statements regarding the adrenal glands is correct?
    a. Two arteries supply the adrenals.
    b. The left adrenal vein drains into the inferior vena cava.
    c. The right adrenal vein drains into the right renal vein.
    d. The medulla can be divided into the zona glomerulosa, fasciculata and reticularis.
    e. The zona glomerulosa forms the outermost layer of the adrenal gland cortex.

74. Which of the following structures does not drain directly into the portal vein?
    a. Superior mesenteric vein (SMV)
    b. Cystic vein
    c. Right gastric vein
    d. Right gastroepiploic vein
    e. Splenic vein

75. Which of the following statements regarding the portal vein is incorrect?
    a. The portal vein ascends anterior to the inferior vena cava.
    b. The portal vein forms anterior to the neck of the pancreas.
    c. About 75% of hepatic blood flow is derived from the portal vein.
    d. The portal vein empties directly into the liver.
    e. The portal vein does not contain any valves.

76. Which of the following statements regarding the lesser omentum is incorrect?
    a. It connects the lesser curvature of the stomach to the liver.
    b. It attaches to the fissure of the ligamentum venosum of the liver.
    c. The hepatogastric ligament contains the portal triad.
    d. The right and left gastric arteries supply the lesser omentum.
    e. The omental foramen connects the lesser sac to the greater peritoneal sac.

77. Which of the following comments regarding the boundaries of the omental foramen is incorrect?
    a. The portal vein lies anterior.
    b. The inferior vena cava lies posterior.
    c. Superiorly lies the caudate lobe of the liver.
    d. Posteriorly lies the first part of the duodenum.
    e. The right crus of the diaphragm lies posterior.

78. When performing a total abdominal hysterectomy, it is important to identify the ureter because of its close proximity with the uterine artery. Where does the uterine artery lie in relation to the ureter?
    a. Anterior and superior
    b. Posterior and inferior
    c. Medial
    d. Posterior and superior
    e. Lateral

79. A 29-year-old man presents with right-sided loin to groin pain. A diagnosis of renal colic is made. Which of the following statements regarding the nerve supply of the ureter is incorrect?
    a. It receives nerve supply via the inferior hypogastric plexus.
    b. It receives nerve supply via the superior hypogastric plexus.

c. Cutaneous referred pain is in T11–L2 distribution.

d. The ureter is supplied by the obturator nerve.

e. Ureteric nerve supply has sympathetic and parasympathetic innervation.

80. Which of the following statements regarding the anatomy of the ureter is incorrect?

a. The abdominal ureter is completely retroperitoneal.

b. The ureter runs posterior to the internal iliac arteries in the pelvis.

c. The inferior end of the ureter is surrounded by a vesical venous plexus.

d. Blood from the ureter drains mainly into the renal and gonadal veins.

e. The ureter wall is composed of two layers of muscle.

81. A 1-year-old boy is diagnosed with an ectopic testicle. Which of the following is an example of a position for an ectopic testicle?

a. Intra-abdominal

b. Superficial inguinal ring

c. Femoral

d. High in scrotum

e. Inguinal canal

82. Which of the following statements regarding the prostate gland is incorrect?

a. The prostate consists of five lobes.

b. The posterior lobe is felt on digital rectal examination.

c. Females have Skene's glands that are homologous with the male prostate gland.

d. The prostate gland lies between the bladder and urogenital diaphragm.

e. The membranous urethra is contained within the prostate.

83. A 12-year-old boy presents as an emergency with testicular pain. He is taken to theatre immediately for an exploration. When exploring the scrotum for a suspected testicular torsion, which of the following layers covers the testes with a tough fibrous coat?

a. Parietal layer of tunica vaginalis

b. Tunica albuginea

c. Tunica vasculosa

d. Visceral layer of tunica vaginalis

e. Tunica intima

84. When exploring the scrotum, several layers must be dissected before reaching the testicle. Which layer is closely related to the scrotal skin?

a. Dartos

b. Tunica vaginalis

c. Cremasteric muscle

d. External spermatic fascia

e. Internal spermatic fascia

85. The cremasteric reflex is a useful test when examining a patient with suspected torsion. Which nerve innervates the cremasteric muscle?

a. Iliohypogastric

b. Genitofemoral

c. Ilioinguinal
d. Obturator
e. Pudendal

86. Which of the following are not permanent folds of gastrointestinal tract?
   a. Rugae
   b. Plicae semilunaris
   c. Spiral valve of Heister
   d. Transverse rectal
   e. Villae

87. Which one of the following is the terminal group of lymph nodes in colonic drainage?
   a. Pre-aortic
   b. Intermediate
   c. Paracolic
   d. Epicolic
   e. Subpectoral

88. All of the following are features of the trigone area within the urinary bladder except:
   a. It has smooth mucosa.
   b. It is loosely attached to underlying mucosa.
   c. It is lined by transitional epithelium.
   d. It is a remnant of the mesonephric duct opening into post-urogenital sinus.
   e. The two ureters enter the bladder at each of the upper corners.

89. When performing a subcostal flank approach to the kidney, which of the following structures may be incised to increase upward mobility of the 12th rib?
   a. The latissimus dorsi muscle
   b. The lumbodorsal fascia
   c. The quadratus lumborum muscle
   d. The costovertebral ligament
   e. The intercostal muscles between ribs 11 and 12

90. Which one of the following sites represents the narrowest part of the urethra?
   a. The navicular fossa
   b. The site of seminal colliculus
   c. Membranous urethra
   d. The external urethral orifice
   e. The bulbous urethra

91. A 64-year-old man is admitted with a severe haematemesis. Upper gastrointestinal (GI) endoscopy identifies a posterior gastric ulcer. Bleeding is most likely to have occurred from which main vessel?
   a. Splenic artery
   b. Left gastroepiploic artery
   c. Inferior pancreaticoduodenal artery

d. Oesophageal branch of the left gastric artery
e. Gastroduodenal branch of the right gastric artery

92. Which one of the following statements is correct concerning the bony pelvis?
    a. The male pelvis has a larger superior pelvic aperture than the female pelvis.
    b. The obturator foramina are round in the female.
    c. The male sacrum is less curved than that of the female.
    d. The ischial tuberosities are farther apart in the female pelvis.
    e. The male pelvis is shallower than that of the female.

93. Which of the following vessels drain into the inferior vena cava?
    a. Renal veins
    b. Inferior mesenteric vein
    c. Superior mesenteric vein
    d. Splenic vein
    e. All of the above

94. Which of the following is not a site of portosystemic anastomosis?
    a. The spleen
    b. The liver
    c. The gastroesophageal junction
    d. The anorectal junction
    e. None of the above

95. Which of the following statements regarding the arterial blood supply of the stomach is incorrect?
    a. The right gastric artery supplies the lower right part of the stomach.
    b. Short gastric arteries supply the pylorus.
    c. The left gastroepiploic artery supplies the upper part of the greater curvature.
    d. The right gastroepiploic artery supplies the lower part of the greater curvature.
    e. The left gastric artery supplies the upper right part of the stomach.

96. You are performing an elective inguinal hernia repair under supervision. You open the inguinal canal to identify the spermatic cord. Which of the following structures is not contained within the spermatic cord?
    a. Ilioinguinal nerve
    b. Pampiniform plexus
    c. Genital branch of genitofemoral nerve
    d. Cremasteric artery
    e. Testicular artery

97. Inguinal hernias are the most common type of abdominal hernia. Which one of the following statements regarding inguinal hernias is true?
    a. Indirect hernias lie medial to the inferior epigastric artery.
    b. Inguinal hernias commonly lie above and lateral to the pubic tubercle.
    c. The deep inguinal ring lies approximately 1.5 cm above the midpoint of the inguinal ligament.

d. Inguinal hernias are more common in females.

e. Direct hernias commonly extend into the scrotum.

98. Which one of the following arteries is a direct branch arising from the abdominal aorta?

a. Common hepatic

b. Pericardial

c. Splenic

d. Subcostal

e. Median sacral

99. Which one of the following statements regarding the pancreas is incorrect?

a. The pancreas is a retroperitoneal structure.

b. The body of the pancreas lies over L2.

c. The pancreas is supplied in part by branches of the splenic artery.

d. The accessory pancreatic duct drains the uncinate process.

e. The uncinate process lies anterior to the superior mesenteric artery.

100. Which one of the following statements regarding the pancreas is correct?

a. The head of the pancreas is supplied by branches of the splenic artery.

b. The portal vein is formed posterior to the neck of the pancreas.

c. In the majority of people, the bile duct and main pancreatic duct drain separately into the duodenum.

d. The pancreas is formed from the embryonic midgut.

e. The accessory pancreatic duct drains into the duodenum at the major duodenal papilla.

101. Which of the following structures is not retroperitoneal?

a. Aorta

b. Rectum

c. Tail of pancreas

d. Second part of the duodenum

e. Kidneys

102. When performing a laparotomy, there are several structures that lie near to the second part of the duodenum. Which one of the following statements regarding relations to the second part of the duodenum is correct?

a. The transverse colon lies posterior.

b. The pancreatic and bile duct drain on its lateral side.

c. The hilum of the right kidney lies laterally.

d. The right psoas major lies posterior.

e. It is situated at the level of the L4 vertebra.

103. Which one of the following statements regarding the third part of the duodenum is correct?

a. The third part of the duodenum lies vertically within the abdomen.

b. Posterior to the duodenum lies the superior mesenteric vein.

c. Anterior to the duodenum lies the aorta.

d. The ligament of Treitz supports the duodenojejunal junction.

e. The duodenum is a completely retroperitoneal structure.

104. Which one of the following statements regarding the blood supply to the stomach is correct?
    a. The coeliac trunk divides into the left gastric, splenic and right hepatic arteries.
    b. The left gastro-omental (gastroepiploic) artery is a direct branch from the aorta.
    c. The gastroduodenal artery is a direct branch of the splenic artery.
    d. The right gastro-omental (gastroepiploic) artery is a branch of the gastroduodenal artery.
    e. The right gastric artery supplies the distal portion of the oesophagus.

105. During a laparoscopic cholecystectomy, an intraoperative cholangiogram may be performed not only to check for any distal occlusion, but also to identify which one of the following structures prior to it being transected?
    a. Cystic duct
    b. Common bile duct
    c. Common hepatic duct
    d. Right hepatic duct
    e. Pancreatic duct

106. An 80-year-old man requires a right hemicolectomy for caecal carcinoma. Which one of the following statements regarding the blood supply to the area resected is correct?
    a. The ascending colon is supplied by branches of the inferior mesenteric artery.
    b. The ascending colon venous drainage is into the portal vein.
    c. The ascending colon is supplied mainly by the middle colic artery.
    d. The ascending colon is supplied by the left colic artery.
    e. The ascending colon is supplied by the intestinal arteries.

107. Which one of the following statements is correct regarding the blood supply to and from the descending colon?
    a. The main arterial blood supply to the descending colon is from branches of the superior mesenteric artery.
    b. The left colic artery supplies the descending colon.
    c. The sigmoid artery supplies the descending colon.
    d. The inferior mesenteric vein rarely drains into the splenic vein.
    e. The artery of Drummond connects branches of the coeliac trunk with the superior mesenteric artery.

108. During an elective open abdominal aortic aneurysm repair, which of the following structures does not lie anterior to the abdominal aorta?
    a. Body of the pancreas
    b. Splenic vein
    c. Horizontal part of duodenum
    d. Coils of small intestine
    e. Right renal vein

109. When performing an open appendicectomy via a transverse incision, which of the following statements is true?
   a. The ilioinguinal nerve is at risk of damage.
   b. There is increased risk of developing an inguinal.
   c. McBurney's point lies two-thirds of the way from the anterior–superior iliac spine to the umbilicus.
   d. The most common location for the tip of the appendix is retrocaecal followed by pelvic.
   e. The blood supply of the appendix is from the appendicular artery, a branch of the superior rectal artery.

110. You are about to perform a laparoscopic cholecystectomy with your consultant. Which of the following statements is true?
   a. Calot's triangle is bounded by the common hepatic duct, cystic duct and hepatic artery.
   b. The cystic artery is rarely found in Calot's triangle.
   c. The bile duct joins with the pancreatic duct to enter the third part of the duodenum.
   d. Intraoperative cholangiogram can be used before full transection of the cystic duct.
   e. The gallbladder obtains all its arterial blood supply from the cystic artery.

111. Which one of the following comments is incorrect regarding the anatomy of the rectum?
   a. The middle third of the rectum has no peritoneal covering.
   b. The upper third of the rectum has peritoneal covering on the anterior and lateral surfaces.
   c. The lower third of the rectum is covered anteriorly with peritoneum.
   d. There are two transverse folds formed by the mucous membrane in the rectum.
   e. The rectum begins in front of the first sacral vertebra.

112. Which one of the following statements is correct regarding the rectum?
   a. The superior rectal artery is a branch of the internal iliac artery.
   b. The middle rectal artery is a branch of the internal iliac artery.
   c. The inferior rectal artery is a branch of the internal iliac artery.
   d. Lymph drains directly into the inguinal lymph nodes.
   e. The superior rectal vein drains into the internal pudendal vein.

113. Which of the following structures is found outside the spermatic cord?
   a. The testicular artery
   b. The genital branch of the genitofemoral nerve
   c. The ilioinguinal nerve
   d. The vas deferens
   e. Sympathetic nerve fibres

114. Which of the following structures is not transmitted via the greater sciatic foramen?
    a. Sciatic nerve
    b. Superior gluteal artery
    c. Inferior gluteal nerve
    d. Piriformis
    e. Obturator internus

115. Concerning the vasculature of the rectum, the following statements are true except:
    a. The middle rectal vein drains into the portal circulation.
    b. The main blood supply is via the superior rectal artery.
    c. The inferior rectal artery is a branch of the internal pudendal artery.
    d. The superior rectal vein drains into the inferior mesenteric vein.
    e. The median sacral artery comes off directly from the aorta.

116. The following muscles are attached to the perineal body except:
    a. The superficial transverse perineal muscle
    b. The bulbospongiosus
    c. The ischiocavernosus
    d. The external anal sphincter
    e. The levator ani

117. The following statements regarding the vasculature of the testes are true except:
    a. The left testicular vein drains into the inferior vena cava (IVC).
    b. Venous drainage is via the pampiniform plexus.
    c. The testicular artery branches directly off the aorta.
    d. The testicular artery anastomoses with the artery to the vas.
    e. The testicular artery is retroperitoneal.

118. Which of the following statements concerning the anal sphincters is incorrect?
    a. The internal anal sphincter is composed of smooth muscle.
    b. The external anal sphincter blends superiorly with the puborectalis muscle.
    c. The external anal sphincter can be divided into three parts.
    d. The internal anal sphincter surrounds the lower two-thirds of the anal canal.
    e. The external anal sphincter is mainly supplied by S4.

119. The external spermatic fascia of the spermatic cord is derived from which one of the following?
    a. External oblique aponeurosis
    b. Internal oblique
    c. Transversalis fascia
    d. Transverse abdominal
    e. Rectus sheath

UPPER LIMB, BREAST

120. Which of the following muscles is supplied by the median nerve?
    a. Abductor pollicis brevis
    b. Abductor pollicis longus
    c. Flexor pollicis brevis
    d. All of the above
    e. a and c only

121. Which of the following muscles is supplied by the ulnar nerve?
    a. Ulnar half of flexor digitorum profundus
    b. Ulnar half of flexor digitorum superficialis
    c. Opponens pollicis
    d. Radial two lumbricals
    e. a and b only

122. A 20-year-old man is brought into the accident and emergency department after being stabbed in the axilla and you suspect damage to the musculocutaneous nerve. Which of the following clinical findings would you expect?
    a. Paralysis of biceps brachii
    b. Loss of sensation of the ulnar aspect of the forearm
    c. Paralysis of brachioradialis
    d. Paralysis of pronator teres
    e. All of the above

123. A 75-year-old man undergoes an angiogram of his upper limb to investigate symptoms of ischaemia. Which of the following arteries arises from the first part of the axillary artery?
    a. Anterior circumflex humeral
    b. Superior thoracic
    c. Posterior circumflex humeral
    d. Lateral thoracic
    e. Thoracoacromial

124. Which of the following muscles are rotator cuff muscles?
    a. The supraspinatus
    b. The teres minor
    c. The infraspinatus
    d. The subscapularis
    e. All of the above

125. What is the action of the rhomboid major muscle?
    a. Retraction of the scapula
    b. Abduction of the humerus
    c. Adduction of the humerus
    d. Elevation of the scapula
    e. Medial rotation of the humerus

126. Which of the following statements is correct regarding the surface anatomy of the shoulder?
    a. The acromion process forms a sharp bony edge at the medial extremity of the scapular spine.
    b. The deltoid muscle does not cover the greater tuberosity of the humerus.
    c. The coracoid lies immediately below the clavicle.
    d. The medial border of the scapula can be felt but not seen.
    e. The supraclavicular nerves cannot be rolled against the clavicle during palpation of its subcutaneous border.

127. A 25-year-old male attends the accident and emergency department following a fall while ice skating. He is complaining of pain around the left elbow. Clinical examination suggests that he may have sustained a fracture. Which of the following is true concerning fractures around the elbow?
    a. The anterior humeral line is not reliable in the identification of a supracondylar fracture.
    b. Radiological evidence of a posterior fat pad does not imply a fracture.
    c. A hanging cast is first-line management.
    d. Elbow fractures are uncommon in children.
    e. An above-elbow back slab is the preferred method of holding the fracture until definitive treatment.

128. Which one of the following statements is correct regarding hand injuries?
    a. A Bennett fracture dislocation involves the proximal phalanx of the thumb.
    b. Scaphoid injuries may be complicated by avascular necrosis at the distal pole.
    c. Neighbour strapping is an adequate treatment for a mallet finger injury.
    d. Fractures of the scaphoid bone are almost always immediately visible on X-ray.
    e. Gamekeeper's thumb is an injury to the ulnar collateral ligament complex of the metacarpophalangeal (MCP) joint of the thumb.

129. Which of the following statements is true regarding upper limb nerve injuries?
    a. Axonal regeneration occurs at the speed of 1 cm/day.
    b. Axonotmesis has a worse prognosis than neurotmesis.
    c. Ulnar nerve entrapment does not occur in Guyon's canal.
    d. Saturday night palsy is caused by neurotmesis.
    e. Froment's sign may be associated with ulnar nerve injury.

130. In total, how many branches of the axillary artery are there?
    a. Six
    b. Three
    c. Eight
    d. Five
    e. Eleven

131. An 84-year-old woman falls over onto an outstretched arm. She presents with a 'dinner fork deformity', immense pain and a swollen left wrist. Which of the following carpal bones may also be fractured?
    a. Triquetral
    b. Lunate
    c. Scaphoid
    d. Hamate
    e. Pisiform

132. A 65-year-old osteoporotic woman presents to the emergency department after having an epileptic seizure on the street lasting 5 minutes. An X-ray is reviewed by the orthopaedic Foundation Year 2 on call, who feels there may be a fractured surgical neck of humerus. The patient is examined for loss of damage to a nerve which passes through the quadrangular space. Which other anatomical structure passes with this nerve?
    a. Circumflex scapular artery
    b. Deep brachial artery
    c. Recurrent radial artery
    d. Subscapular artery
    e. Posterior circumflex humeral artery

133. A 42-year-old woman undergoes a right total mastectomy with axillary lymph node clearance for breast cancer. Two days postoperatively it was noted that she had winging of her right scapula, thought to be due to a commonly damaged nerve intraoperatively. Which of the following best describes the insertion of the muscle this nerve supplies?
    a. Inferior surface of clavicle, at the middle third
    b. Coracoid process of scapula
    c. Anteromedial scapular border
    d. Lateral lip of intertubercular groove of humerus
    e. Medial lip of intertubercular groove of humerus

134. A 47-year-old woman has been referred to the one-stop breast clinic with a suspicious lump in her left breast. On clinical examination you note she has axillary lymphadenopathy. Which of the following anatomical structures comprise the posterior border of the axilla?
    a. Axillary fascia from serratus anterior to deep fascia of the arm
    b. Upper part of serratus anterior
    c. Pectoralis major and minor
    d. Subscapularis, teres major and latissimus dorsi
    e. Clavicle, 1st rib and upper border of scapula

135. A middle-aged man presents with a history of shoulder pain. The patient is normally quite active and plays tennis regularly. On examination he has a full range of active, strong movement but a 'painful arc'. Which of the following is the most likely diagnosis?
    a. Adhesive capsulitis
    b. Rotator cuff tear

    c. Glenohumeral joint degeneration

    d. Subluxation of the acromioclavicular joint

    e. Supraspinatus tendonitis

136. During a routine mastectomy, your consultant asks you about the blood supply and lymphatic drainage of the breast. Which of the following statements is untrue regarding the anatomy of the breast?

    a. Axillary lymph nodes form approximately 75% of the lymphatic drainage.

    b. The intercostal perforating branches are part of the blood supply.

    c. The pectoral branches of the thoracoacromial artery supply the lower breast.

    d. The lateral thoracic artery is a main part of the blood supply.

    e. Parasternal lymph nodes are important in the lymphatic drainage of the breast.

137. A 33-year-old male falls onto an outstretched hand while skiing. He complains of wrist pain, particularly within the anatomical snuffbox. Which of the following statements regarding the anatomical snuffbox is true?

    a. The radial artery runs along its floor.

    b. The abductor pollicis longus forms its ulnar border.

    c. The extensor pollicis brevis forms its ulnar border.

    d. Tenderness in the snuffbox is characteristic of a fractured radius.

    e. The extensor pollicis longus forms its radial border.

138. Concerning the ulnar artery, which of the following statements is correct?

    a. It is smaller than the radial artery.

    b. The ulnar nerve lies radial to it at the flexor retinaculum.

    c. It crosses the ulnar nerve superficially in the proximal forearm.

    d. It forms the deep palmar arch with the radial artery at the wrist.

    e. It becomes superficial in the distal forearm between the flexor digitorum superficialis and flexor carpi ulnaris.

139. When describing metastatic axillary lymph node spread, surgeons and pathologists refer to levels. Which of the following statements regarding the levels of axillary nodes is correct?

    a. Level II nodes lie above pectoralis minor.

    b. Level III nodes lie behind pectoralis minor.

    c. Level I nodes lie above pectoralis minor.

    d. Level III nodes lie above pectoralis minor.

    e. Level II nodes lie behind pectoralis minor.

140. From which part of the brachial plexus does the suprascapular nerve arise?

    a. The medial cord

    b. The C7 nerve root

    c. The posterior cord

    d. The upper trunk

    e. The lateral cord

141. Which of the following ligaments are not attached to the scapula?

    a. Coracohumeral ligament

    b. Coracoacromial ligament

c. Suprascapular ligament

d. Spinoglenoid ligament

e. Costoclavicular ligament

142. Which are the correct boundaries of the triangular/quadrangular spaces in the upper limb?
    a. Triangular space – teres minor, teres major and biceps
    b. Quadrangular space – subscapularis, teres minor, triceps and supraspinatus
    c. Quadrangular space – teres minor, teres major, neck of humerus and supraspinatus
    d. Quadrangular space – teres major, subscapularis, long head of triceps and neck of humerus
    e. Triangular space – subscapularis, supraspinatus and biceps

143. What is the correct nerve supply of the intrinsic muscles of the hand?
    a. The thenar eminence is supplied by the recurrent branch of the median nerve.
    b. The hypothenar eminence is supplied by the median nerve.
    c. The palmar interossei are supplied by the radial nerve.
    d. All the lumbrical muscles are supplied by the ulnar nerve.
    e. The dorsal interossei are supplied by the median nerve.

144. All of the following structures are present within the carpal tunnel except:
    a. Median nerve
    b. Flexor pollicis longus
    c. Flexor digitorum profundus
    d. Flexor digitorum superficialis
    e. Palmaris longus

145. You are asked by your registrar to assist in a subclavian artery thrombectomy. The occlusion is located at the outer border of the first rib. Which of the following arteries does not help maintain circulation to the upper limb?
    a. Thyrocervical trunk
    b. Suprascapular
    c. Subscapular
    d. Superior thoracic
    e. None of the above

146. The nerves of the brachial plexus are surrounded by a fascia which originates from which of the following?
    a. Prevertebral fascia (PVF)
    b. Clavipectoral fascia
    c. Deep cervical fascia
    d. Pectoral fascia
    e. Fascia lata

147. A 79-year-old woman suffers a displaced transverse fracture of her left olecranon. The fracture is treated conservatively in a cast. Which of the following functions is she most likely to have difficulty with?
    a. Brushing her hair
    b. Fastening buttons

    c. Pouring a kettle

    d. Pushing to standing from an armchair

    e. Reaching into a high cupboard

148. The first compartment under the extensor retinaculum of the wrist contains which of the following tendons?

    a. Extensor carpi radialis longus and extensor carpi radialis brevis

    b. Extensor pollicis longus

    c. Extensor pollicis brevis and abductor pollicis longus

    d. Extensor carpi ulnaris

    e. Extensor digiti minimi

149. A structure which passes under the brachioradialis muscle emerges distally on the ulnar side to become superficial in the forearm lying over the radius being covered by skin and deep fascia. This statement describes the course of:

    a. Ulnar artery

    b. Radial artery

    c. Median nerve

    d. Profunda brachii artery

    e. The superficial branch of the radial nerve

150. A 49-year-old woman has been complaining of a tingling feeling in her right hand at night and is under the impression that her hand is swollen, although there is no obvious oedema. In the last few days she has noticed numbness in her right index finger and the tip of her thumb, especially while working. Which nerve is most likely to be responsible for her symptoms?

    a. Ulnar nerve

    b. Median nerve

    c. Radial nerve

    d. Nerve root C7

    e. Nerve root C8

151. A man attends the emergency department with an anterior dislocation of his right shoulder. He is in obvious pain and is unable to move his right arm. On further assessment, there is loss of sensation of the skin overlying his deltoid muscle. Which one of the following nerves is affected in this case?

    a. Musculocutaneous nerve

    b. Long thoracic nerve

    c. Axillary nerve

    d. Suprascapular nerve

    e. Medial cutaneous nerve of arm

152. A 24-year-old man is brought to the emergency department after falling and landing on his right arm while skiing. There is obvious deformity of the right arm. X-rays show a transverse fracture of the middle third of the humerus with displacement. Which nerve is most likely to be affected in this injury?

    a. Axillary nerve

    b. Radial nerve

c. Median nerve

d. Ulnar nerve

e. Musculocutaneous nerve

153. Which one of the following muscles is responsible for the function of internal rotation of the humerus?

a. Subscapularis

b. Supraspinatus

c. Infraspinatus

d. Teres minor

e. Levator scapulae

154. Which of the following muscles does not arise from the medial epicondyle of the humerus?

a. Flexor carpi ulnaris

b. Flexor digitorum profundus

c. Flexor digitorum superficialis

d. Palmaris longus

e. Pronator teres

LOWER LIMB

155. A 25-year-old gentleman sustains an injury to the common peroneal nerve while playing rugby. Which area of the foot would you touch to test the deep peroneal nerve?
    a. The posterolateral aspect of the calf and foot
    b. The medial aspect of the sole
    c. The lateral aspect of the sole
    d. The anterolateral aspect of the calf and most of the dorsum of the foot
    e. None of the above

156. A 67-year-old man walks into your orthopaedic clinic after his total hip replacement and you notice he has a Trendelenburg gait. Which muscles are most likely to have been damaged to cause this type of gait?
    a. The iliopsoas
    b. The quadriceps muscles
    c. The gluteus maximus
    d. The gluteus minimus and medius
    e. The short external rotators

157. Which one of the following structures forms the medial border of the femoral ring?
    a. The pectineal ligament
    b. The lacunar ligament
    c. The inguinal ligament
    d. The femoral vein
    e. None of the above

158. Which of the following muscles form part of Hunter's canal?
    a. The adductor longus
    b. The adductor magnus
    c. The sartorius
    d. All of the above
    e. b and c only

159. A 21-year-old man undergoes an emergency fasciotomy after being diagnosed with lower extremity compartment syndrome. The patient was noted to have a decreased dorsiflexion of the ankle, extension of the toe and loss of sensation in the first dorsal web space. Which of the following compartments had raised pressure?
    a. Anterior compartment
    b. Deep posterior compartment
    c. Superficial posterior compartment
    d. Lateral compartment
    e. Medial compartment

160. A 25-year-old woman is involved in a road traffic accident where her pelvis has fractured. It is thought her sciatic nerve has been injured as it exits the pelvis. Which of the following muscles will lose its innervation?
    a. Sartorius
    b. Adductor longus
    c. Semimembranosus
    d. Adductor brevis
    e. Pectineus

161. When using ultrasound guidance to insert a central venous catheter into the femoral vein, it is noted there are several fascial planes surrounding the various anatomical structures. In which compartment of the femoral sheath does the femoral vein lie in?
    a. Intermediate compartment
    b. Medial compartment
    c. Lateral compartment
    d. Anterior compartment
    e. Posterior compartment

162. A 50-year-old man is undergoing a total hip replacement. The operating surgeon takes a lateral approach to the joint. Which of the following anatomical structures does not attach to the greater trochanter?
    a. Obturator internus
    b. Gluteus minimus
    c. Iliacus
    d. Piriformis
    e. Obturator externus

163. Which of the following statements regarding the adductor canal is not correct?
    a. It is bounded posteriorly by the adductor longus proximally.
    b. It is bounded posteriorly by the adductor magnus distally.
    c. It is bounded anteromedially by the vastus medialis.
    d. The femoral artery leaves the canal via the adductor hiatus in the adductor magnus.
    e. The adductor canal represents the most common site for atherosclerosis in the lower limb.

164. An elderly woman presents with a fall and a tender right hip. Which of the following is true regarding the hip and neck of femur (NOF) fractures?
    a. Limb shortening in NOF fracture is uncommon.
    b. The lateral circumflex artery supplies the majority of blood to the femoral head.
    c. Metaphyseal blood supply arises from the extracapsular arterial ring.
    d. Extracapsular fractures commonly compromise the blood supply.
    e. The artery of ligamentum teres is the main blood supply to the hip joint.

165. An obese 15-year-old boy presents with pain in the hip. He walks with an antalgic gait with some shortening of the affected limb. Which of the following is the most likely diagnosis?
    a. Perthes disease
    b. Congenital hip dysplasia
    c. Septic arthritis
    d. Neck of femur fracture
    e. Slipped upper femoral epiphysis (SUFE)

166. If concerned about compartment syndrome following reperfusion of the lower leg, what action would you perform in order to test the deep part of the posterior compartment of the lower leg?
    a. Plantarflexion of the foot
    b. Eversion of the foot
    c. Extension of the great toe
    d. Dorsiflexion of the foot
    e. Flexion of the 2nd to 5th toes

167. Which of the following statements regarding the hamstring muscles is incorrect?
    a. The hamstring muscles arise from the ischial tuberosity.
    b. Semimembranosus inserts on the medial condyle of the tibia.
    c. The short head of biceps femoris originates from the linea aspera.
    d. All three muscles are supplied by the sciatic nerve.
    e. The hamstring compartment receives its blood supply from the femoral artery.

168. Concerning the blood supply to the femoral head, which of the following statements is correct?
    a. The arterial supply from the ligamentum teres contributes more significantly in adulthood.
    b. The main blood supply is derived from the obturator artery in the adult.
    c. Lateral and medial circumflex femoral arteries supply the femoral head via retinacula.
    d. Vessels from the diaphysis of cancellous bone provide a negligible arterial blood supply in adulthood.
    e. Fractures that are extracapsular have a high risk of resulting in avascular necrosis.

169. Which of the following statements regarding the popliteal fossa is correct?
    a. The superior and medial boundary is the biceps femoris.
    b. The roof contains the terminal branch of the posterior cutaneous nerve.
    c. The floor contains the oblique popliteal ligament.
    d. The capsule of the knee joint is found in the roof of the fossa.
    e. The small saphenous vein is found in the floor of the fossa.

170. The lower limb below the knee is divided into four compartments. Which of the following statements regarding these compartments is incorrect?
    a. The lateral compartment contains the peroneus longus, brevis and tibialis anterior muscles.
    b. The superficial posterior compartment contains the plantaris muscle and soleus.
    c. The anterior compartment contains the anterior tibial vessels and tibial nerve.
    d. The lateral compartment contains the deep peroneal nerve.
    e. The deep posterior compartment contains the flexor hallucis longus, flexor digitorum longus and peroneus tertius.

171. A middle-aged woman undergoes surgery for varicose veins.
    A saphenofemoral junction ligation is performed. Which of the following tributaries does not commonly join the long saphenous vein at the opening?
    a. Superficial epigastric vein
    b. Superficial external pudendal vein
    c. Superficial circumflex iliac vein
    d. Inferior epigastric vein
    e. Deep external pudendal vein

172. Which of the following statements regarding the tibial nerve is correct?
    a. Cutaneous supply within the popliteal fossa is via a branch of the sural nerve.
    b. The roots of the tibial nerve are L3, L4, L5, S1, S2.
    c. The nerve descends superficial to soleus in the calf.
    d. The nerve divides into the medial and lateral tibial nerves in the foot.
    e. It does not supply the extrinsic muscles of the foot.

173. Which of the following muscles in the sole of the foot is not supplied by the medial plantar nerve?
    a. Flexor digitorum brevis
    b. Flexor digiti minimi brevis
    c. Flexor hallucis longus
    d. Abductor hallucis
    e. Flexor hallucis brevis

174. Which of the following statements regarding the posterior cruciate ligament is correct?
    a. It is attached to the lateral femoral condyle.
    b. It is made up of three separate bundles.
    c. It prevents posterior dislocation of the tibia.
    d. It plays no role in resisting hyperextension.
    e. It is intrasynovial.

175. Which one of the following is the main function of the psoas major muscle?
    a. Flexes the thigh at the hip joint
    b. Extends the thigh at the hip joint

c. Adducts the thigh at the hip joint
d. Abducts the thigh at the hip joint
e. Assists in the full contraction of the diaphragm

176. A 31-year-old patient develops a common peroneal nerve palsy after treatment with a below-knee cast for 6 weeks for an undisplaced ankle fracture following a fall. Which one of the following statements regarding clinical examination is true?
a. The patient is unable to stand on tiptoe.
b. There would be complete sensory loss below the knee.
c. There would be no dorsiflexion of the foot.
d. The patient would complain of complete sensory loss on the sole of the foot.
e. Sensation would be normal on the dorsum of the foot.

177. Moving from lateral to medial, which of the following describes the order of the structures in the femoral triangle?
a. Femoral vein, femoral artery, femoral nerve
b. Femoral nerve, femoral vein, femoral artery
c. Femoral nerve, femoral artery, femoral vein, long saphenous vein
d. Long saphenous vein, femoral vein, femoral artery, femoral nerve
e. Short saphenous vein, femoral vein, femoral artery, femoral nerve

178. Which of the following muscles is not present in the anterior compartment of the leg?
a. Tibialis anterior
b. Extensor hallucis longus
c. Extensor digitorum longus
d. Peroneus tertius
e. Peroneus brevis

179. Following open reduction and internal fixation of both the distal tibia and the distal fibula, a patient complains of numbness along the lateral side of the foot. Which nerve is likely to have been injured?
a. Sural nerve
b. Saphenous nerve
c. Deep peroneal nerve
d. Superficial peroneal nerve
e. Tibial nerve

180. Multiple structures are contained within or pass through the popliteal fossa. Which one of the following statements is correct?
a. The popliteal vein becomes the femoral vein at the adductor hiatus.
b. The short saphenous vein is the deepest structure within the fossa.
c. The popliteal artery is initially lateral to the tibial nerve, then moves medially when travelling distally though the popliteal fossa.
d. The short saphenous vein drains into the femoral vein.
e. The popliteal artery is formed from the profunda femoris.

181. Which of the following structures does not enter the adductor canal?
    a. Femoral artery
    b. Femoral vein
    c. Nerve to adductor longus
    d. Nerve to vastus medialis
    e. Saphenous nerve

182. The following structures are contained within the femoral sheath except:
    a. The femoral nerve
    b. The femoral artery
    c. The femoral vein
    d. The femoral canal
    e. Lymphatics

183. Which of the following muscles does not insert into the greater trochanter of the femur?
    a. Superior gemellus
    b. Inferior gemellus
    c. Quadratus femoris
    d. Piriformis
    e. Gluteus minimus

184. Which of the following muscles act together to invert the foot?
    a. Peroneus brevis and peroneus longus
    b. Peroneus brevis and peroneus tertius
    c. Peroneus tertius and tibialis anterior
    d. Peroneus longus and tibialis posterior
    e. Tibialis anterior and tibialis posterior

185. Which of the following structures is not found within the popliteal fossa?
    a. Saphenous nerve
    b. Popliteal vein
    c. Common peroneal nerve
    d. Posterior cutaneous nerve of thigh
    e. Small saphenous vein

186. Which of the following muscles is not found within the posterior compartment of the leg?
    a. Tibialis posterior
    b. Peroneus tertius
    c. Flexor digitorum longus
    d. Soleus
    e. Plantaris

187. Which of the following structures does not travel under the flexor retinaculum behind the medial malleolus?
    a. The posterior tibial artery
    b. The tibial nerve
    c. The tibialis posterior

d. The flexor digitorum longus

e. The deep peroneal nerve

188. Which of the following statements regarding the iliopsoas muscle is correct?
    a. It attaches to the greater trochanter of the femur.
    b. It extends the thigh at the hip joint.
    c. It is formed by iliacus and the psoas minor muscle.
    d. It passes deep to the inguinal ligament.
    e. It is innervated by the superior gluteal nerve.

189. Which of the following muscles acts as a flexor for both the knee joint and the hip joint?
    a. Biceps femoris
    b. Sartorius
    c. Semimembranosus
    d. Rectus femoris
    e. Adductor brevis

HEAD, NECK AND SPINE

190. Which of the following structures are contained within the scalp?
    a. Connective tissue
    b. Investing fascia
    c. Loose areolar tissue
    d. All of the above
    e. a and c only

191. Which of these arteries is a primary branch of the external carotid artery?
    a. The inferior thyroid artery
    b. The facial artery
    c. The occipital artery
    d. All of the above artery
    e. b and c only artery

192. Which one of the following cranial nerves (CNs) exits the skull via the stylomastoid foramen?
    a. VII
    b. VIII
    c. IX
    d. X
    e. XI

193. Through which foramen in the base of the skull does the maxillary nerve exit?
    a. The foramen caecum
    b. The foramen ovale
    c. The foramen spinosum
    d. The foramen rotundum
    e. The foramen lacerum

194. Which of the following structures pass through the foramen magnum in the base of the skull?
    a. The dural veins
    b. The anterior spinal arteries
    c. The posterior spinal arteries
    d. The spinal roots of CN XI
    e. All of the above

195. When performing a neck dissection, your consultant points out the muscular triangle. Which of the following structures are you likely to find within it?
    a. The carotid body
    b. The accessory nerve
    c. The external jugular vein
    d. The parathyroid glands
    e. The hypoglossal nerve

196. Which of the following fascial layers would you find in the neck?
    a. The carotid sheath
    b. The pretracheal fascia

    c. The investing fascia

    d. All of the above

    e. a and b only

197. While performing a neck dissection your consultant aims to preserve the accessory nerve. Within which anatomical triangle would you find this structure?

    a. The submental

    b. The muscular

    c. The submandibular

    d. The occipital

    e. The supraclavicular

198. Which of the following bones of the skull form the pterion?

    a. The zygoma

    b. The occipital

    c. The zygomatic

    d. All of the above

    e. a and c only

199. When performing a procedurally correct lumbar puncture, which of the following structures should you pass through?

    a. The ligamentum flavum

    b. The interspinous ligament

    c. The supraspinous ligament

    d. All of the above

    e. a and b only

200. You are asked to review a patient in the accident and emergency department who is believed to have cavernous sinus thrombosis on a recent computed tomography (CT) scan. Which of the following structures would be at risk?

    a. The internal carotid artery

    b. CN III

    c. CN IV

    d. CN VI

    e. All of the above

201. Which of the following are branches of the first part of the subclavian artery?

    a. Vertebral, internal thoracic and thyrocervical arteries

    b. Common carotid and vertebral arteries

    c. External carotid and internal carotid arteries

    d. Dorsal scapular and thyrocervical arteries

    e. Posterior intercostal, costocervical trunk and internal thoracic arteries

202. Which of the following bony processes makes up part of the zygomatic arch?

    a. Frontal

    b. Mandible

    c. Lacrimal

    d. Maxilla

    e. Ethmoid

203. Which of the following structures makes up the pterion together with the squamous temporal bone, greater wing of the sphenoid and frontal bone?
    a. Lesser wing of the sphenoid
    b. Parietal
    c. Zygomatic
    d. Nasal
    e. Lacrimal

204. Which of the following is not a sign of a longitudinal temporal bone fracture?
    a. Tear of the tympanic membrane
    b. Cerebrospinal fluid otorrhoea
    c. Facial nerve palsy
    d. Conductive hearing loss
    e. Cranial nerve IX palsy

205. Which one of the following is not a sign of a transverse temporal bone fracture?
    a. Facial nerve palsy
    b. Vertigo
    c. Sensorineural hearing loss
    d. Hemotympanum
    e. Abducens nerve injury

206. A 3-year-old boy is seen in surgical outpatients with a neck lump. The non-fluctuant lump is present in the anterior triangle and has only been present for 2 weeks. Which of the following diagnoses is most likely to represent the lump?
    a. Cystic hygroma
    b. Sebaceous cyst
    c. Lipoma
    d. Branchial cyst
    e. Lymph node

207. A 47-year-old man presents to the accident and emergency department with a head injury and neck laceration. The attending surgeon requests a CT scan, which shows an injury to the external jugular vein. Which demonstrates a laceration of the external jugular vein is false?
    a. It has no valves.
    b. It does not pierce the deep fascia.
    c. It receives a branch from the retromandibular vein.
    d. It joins the subclavian vein.
    e. It is anterior the scalenus anterior.

208. A 23-year-old man presents to the accident and emergency department after a fall from height. He is immobilized on a spinal board and you are the first surgical doctor to see the patient. You request C-spine views of his neck. Which of the following statements regarding C-spine injuries is correct?
    a. A clay shoveler's fracture is a fracture of C1.
    b. A hangman's fracture is a fracture of C1.
    c. A Jefferson fracture is a burst fracture of C1.

d. Flexion and extension views should be taken under the supervision of a radiographer.

e. The most common site of fracture is C2/C3.

209. A 72-year-old man presents with acute urinary retention and back pain. You diagnose cauda equina syndrome. Which of the following statements regarding cauda equina syndrome is true?

a. The cauda equina begins at L2.

b. A common feature of cauda equina syndrome is bilateral leg pain.

c. A positive Babinski sign is a common finding when injured.

d. It contains mainly motor fibres.

e. It begins at the subcostal plane.

210. A 36-year-old man presents to the accident and emergency department following a blow to the side of his head. Which of the following statements regarding bleeding from the middle meningeal artery is true?

a. It mainly affects the posterior branch.

b. It results in a subdural haematoma.

c. It may produce ipsilateral pupillary constriction.

d. It typically causes a biconvex-shaped lesion.

e. It is usually caused by a soft blow to the occiput.

211. Which of the following statements regarding the anatomy of the parotid gland is correct?

a. It is related superiorly to the mylohyoid.

b. The retromandibular vein lies superficial to the gland.

c. It is enclosed in the superficial layer of cervical fascia.

d. The parotid duct arises from the inferior part of the gland.

e. The external carotid artery traverses the gland.

212. Which of these statements regarding the relations of the sublingual gland is correct?

a. It is related anteriorly to the hyoglossus.

b. It is related posteriorly to the deep lobe of the submandibular gland.

c. It is related laterally to the genioglossus.

d. It is related medially to the styloglossus.

e. It is related inferiorly to the lingual nerve.

213. Which of the following statements regarding the anatomy of the thyroid gland is correct?

a. It is surrounded by superficial cervical fascia.

b. It is superficial to platysma.

c. It is supplied by a branch of the internal carotid artery.

d. It is supplied by a branch of the ascending pharyngeal artery.

e. It is supplied by a branch of the thyrocervical trunk.

214. Concerning anatomical triangles of the neck, which of the following statements is correct?

a. The floor of the posterior triangle is formed from deep cervical fascia.

b. The submental triangle is formed in part by the posterior belly of the digastric muscle.

    c. The muscular triangle is formed in part by the superior belly of the omohyoid.

    d. The cervical plexus lies in the anterior triangle.

    e. The brachial plexus lies in the muscular triangle.

215. Which of the following boundaries of the infratemporal fossa is correct?

    a. It is related medially to the masseter.

    b. It is related laterally to the styloid process.

    c. It is related superiorly to the greater wing of the sphenoid bone.

    d. It is related anteriorly to the zygomatic process.

    e. It is related inferiorly to the temporal bone.

216. Concerning the fascial layers of the neck, which of the following statements is correct?

    a. The pretracheal fascia lies superficial to the deep investing layer of cervical fascia.

    b. The floor of the posterior triangle is formed by prevertebral fascia.

    c. The superficial cervical fascia encloses the trapezius.

    d. The carotid sheath encloses the vagus nerve, external jugular vein and carotid arteries.

    e. The prevertebral fascia extends from the skull base to the fibrous pericardium.

217. Which of the following arteries is a branch of the external carotid artery?

    a. Descending pharyngeal artery

    b. Deep temporal artery

    c. Inferior thyroid artery

    d. Maxillary artery

    e. Transverse cervical artery

218. Which statement concerning the internal carotid artery is correct?

    a. It receives a rich nerve supply from the vagus nerve.

    b. It enters the base of the skull at the foramen spinosum.

    c. Its terminal branches include anterior and middle cerebral arteries.

    d. It passes superficial to the posterior belly of the digastric muscle.

    e. It gives off the facial artery before entering the stylomastoid foramen.

219. Which of the following statements regarding the relations of the thyroid gland is correct?

    a. The isthmus overlies the 4th and 5th tracheal rings.

    b. The lateral lobes extend from the thyroid cartilage to the 6th tracheal ring.

    c. A pyramidal lobe is most commonly found projecting from the left thyroid lobe.

    d. The isthmus is superficial to the anterior jugular veins.

    e. The internal branch of the superior laryngeal nerve lies deep to the upper pole of the gland.

220. Concerning the lymphatic drainage of the tongue, which of the following statements is correct?

    a. The tip drains to submandibular nodes.

    b. The anterior two-thirds drains to submandibular and anterior cervical nodes.

c. The posterior third has poor lymphatic drainage.
d. Involvement of contralateral nodes is more likely with carcinoma affecting the anterior two-thirds.
e. The posterior third drains to the deep cervical chain of nodes.

221. Which of the following statements concerning the nerve supply to the ear is correct?
   a. The lower half of the pinna is supplied by the auriculotemporal nerve.
   b. The upper medial half of the pinna is supplied by the great auricular nerve.
   c. The lateral tympanic membrane is supplied by Arnold's nerve.
   d. The medial tympanic membrane is supplied by the auriculotemporal nerve.
   e. The upper lateral half of the pinna is supplied by C3.

222. Which of the following statements concerning the laryngopharynx is correct?
   a. It extends from the tip of the epiglottis to the termination of the pharynx at the vertebral level of T1.
   b. The piriform fossae form deep recesses posteriorly.
   c. The cricopharyngeus is tonically relaxed at rest.
   d. Killian's dehiscence refers to an anatomical area of weakness between the two components of the superior constrictor muscle.
   e. The laryngeal inlet comprises the arytenoids, aryepiglottic folds and epiglottis.

223. Concerning the superficial veins of the head and neck, which of the following statements is correct?
   a. The retromandibular vein is formed from the superficial temporal and maxillary veins.
   b. The retromandibular vein is formed from the posterior auricular and facial veins.
   c. The anterior jugular vein passes laterally from the midline of the neck to drain into the internal jugular vein, deep to the sternocleidomastoid.
   d. The external jugular vein crosses under the sternocleidomastoid in deep cervical fascia.
   e. The posterior division of the external jugular vein joins the facial vein to become the common facial vein.

224. Concerning the drainage of the paranasal sinuses, which of the following statements is correct?
   a. The frontal sinus drains into the superior meatus.
   b. The sphenoid sinus drains into the inferior meatus.
   c. The maxillary sinus drains into the middle meatus in the hiatus semilunaris.
   d. The ethmoid sinus drains into the nasal cavity above the superior turbinate.
   e. The nasolacrimal duct drains into the nasal cavity below the inferior turbinate.

225. Concerning the temporomandibular joint and movements, which of the following statements is correct?
    a. The lateral pterygoid elevates the lower jaw.
    b. The geniohyoid depresses the lower jaw.
    c. The articular surface of the joint is composed of hyaline cartilage.
    d. Sensory innervation of the joint is derived from the maxillary branch of the trigeminal nerve (VII).
    e. Temporalis protracts the lower jaw.

226. Concerning the anatomy of the vertebrae, which of the following statements is correct?
    a. There are 34 in total.
    b. The axis has no body.
    c. C1 is known as *vertebrae prominens*.
    d. C1 bears the dens.
    e. Cervical vertebrae are characterized by the presence of foramen transversarium.

227. Which of the following statements regarding the embryology and anatomy of the parathyroid glands is correct?
    a. Approximately 30% are aberrant.
    b. The upper parathyroid glands are 4th branchial arch derivatives.
    c. The upper parathyroid glands are supplied by the superior thyroid artery.
    d. The lower parathyroid glands are 2nd branchial arch derivatives.
    e. The upper parathyroid glands develop in company with the thymus gland.

228. Which of the following nerves does not pass through the superior orbital fissure?
    a. Lacrimal nerve
    b. Frontal nerve
    c. Trochlear nerve
    d. Supraorbital nerve
    e. Nasociliary nerve

229. Concerning blood supply to the orbit, which of the following statements is correct?
    a. The ophthalmic artery enters the orbit above the optic nerve.
    b. The ophthalmic artery spirals around the optic nerve to lie medially to it.
    c. Anterior and posterior ethmoidal arteries accompany branches of the nasociliary nerve.
    d. Valves of orbital veins prevent retrograde flow to the cavernous sinus.
    e. Occlusion of the central retinal artery results in loss of colour vision.

230. Concerning the anatomy of the tympanic cavity, which of the following statements is correct?
    a. Tensor tympani arises from the anterior wall.
    b. The mucous membrane of the Eustachian tube is supplied by branches of the maxillary nerve.

c. The mastoid antrum lies between the aditus and the epitympanic recess.

d. The roof is formed by part of the squamous temporal bone.

e. The external jugular vein is related to the floor of the cavity.

231. Concerning ossicles of the middle ear, which of the following statements is correct?

a. They are united by fibrocartilaginous joints.

b. The handle of the malleus lies in the hypotympanium.

c. The stapes footplate lies adherent to the round window.

d. The long process of the incus is adherent to the tympanic membrane.

e. The head of the malleus lies in the epitympanic recess.

232. Concerning the mastoid antrum and process, which of the following statements is correct?

a. The antrum lies within the tympanic part of the temporal bone.

b. The antrum is well developed at birth.

c. The medial wall of the antrum is related to the lateral semicircular canal.

d. The mucosa of the mastoid air cells is supplied in part by the maxillary nerve.

e. The antrum lies within the squamous part of the temporal bone.

233. Which of the following muscles is not referred to as an infrahyoid strap muscle?

a. Sternohyoid

b. Sternothyroid

c. Mylohyoid

d. Thyrohyoid

e. Omohyoid

234. Which of the following lists correctly defines the anatomical layers encountered when performing a tracheostomy (from superficial to deep)?

a. Skin, superficial fascia, platysma, investing fascia, strap muscles, pretracheal fascia, thyroid isthmus, trachea

b. Skin, superficial fascia, investing fascia, platysma, strap muscles, pretracheal fascia, thyroid isthmus, trachea

c. Skin, superficial fascia, platysma, strap muscles, investing fascia, pretracheal fascia, thyroid isthmus, trachea

d. Skin, superficial fascia, platysma, investing fascia, strap muscles, thyroid isthmus, pretracheal fascia, trachea

e. Skin, platysma, superficial fascia, investing fascia, strap muscles, pretracheal fascia, thyroid isthmus, trachea

235. Which of the following anatomical landmarks related to the larynx is correctly paired with the corresponding vertebral level?

a. The hyoid bone lies at C3.

b. The upper limit of the thyroid cartilage lies at C3.

c. The cricoid cartilage lies at C5.

d. The epiglottis lies at C2.

e. The arytenoid cartilages lie at C3.

236. Which of the following vessels is present in the posterior triangle of the neck?
    a. Ascending cervical artery
    b. Axillary artery
    c. Transverse cervical artery
    d. Inferior thyroid artery
    e. Internal jugular vein

237. Which of the following cutaneous nerves is not a branch of the ophthalmic division of the trigeminal nerve?
    a. Supraorbital nerve
    b. Supratrochlear nerve
    c. Infraorbital nerve
    d. Infratrochlear nerve
    e. Lacrimal nerve

238. Which of the following branches of the maxillary artery passes through the foramen spinosum in the base of the skull?
    a. Inferior alveolar artery
    b. Anterior tympanic artery
    c. Sphenopalatine artery
    d. Accessory meningeal artery
    e. Middle meningeal artery

239. An elderly man presents to hospital with a history of dysphagia, cachexia and repeated respiratory infections. Investigations confirm the presence of a pharyngeal pouch through a weak area in the pharyngeal wall – Killian's dehiscence. Between which muscles does this potential weak area exist?
    a. Middle constrictor and superior constrictor
    b. Thyropharyngeus and cricopharyngeus
    c. Thyropharyngeus and palatopharyngeus
    d. Stylopharyngeus and cricopharyngeus
    e. Stylopharyngeus and palatopharyngeus

240. Which of the following arteries is a branch of the external carotid artery?
    a. Ascending pharyngeal artery
    b. Middle meningeal artery
    c. Ophthalmic artery
    d. Inferior thyroid artery
    e. Axillary artery

241. An elderly man is admitted to hospital with exophthalmus and ophthalmoplegia following a superficial infection of the face. An obstruction within the cavernous sinus secondary to sepsis is diagnosed. Which of the following cranial nerves does not traverse the cavernous venous sinus?
    a. Trochlear nerve
    b. Oculomotor nerve
    c. Abducens nerve
    d. Ophthalmic division of trigeminal nerve
    e. Mandibular division of trigeminal nerve

242. The common and internal carotid arteries are derived from which branchial arch?
    a. I
    b. II
    c. III
    d. IV
    e. VI

243. Which of the following layers is involved in the dissection when performing a tracheostomy?
    a. Prevertebral fascia
    b. Digastric muscle
    c. Thyroid isthmus
    d. Carotid sheath
    e. Sternocleidomastoid muscle

244. A 42-year-old man undergoes a parotidectomy for a tumour. Which of the following statements regarding the surgical relations of the parotid gland is correct?
    a. Inferior to the gland lies the external auditory meatus.
    b. Laterally lies the styloid process.
    c. Medial to the gland is the superficial fascia and skin.
    d. Inferiorly it overflows the posterior belly of the digastric muscle.
    e. Anteriorly it overflows the mandible with overlying buccinators.

245. Which of the following statements regarding the anatomy of the posterior cranial fossa is correct?
    a. The occipital bone forms the roof of the fossa.
    b. The fossa contains the internal acoustic meatus.
    c. Fractures in the fossa can lead to damage to the facial nerve.
    d. External occipital protuberance lies in the midline on the posterior wall.
    e. The fossa contains the foramen lacerum.

246. Which of the following characteristics are helpful in differentiating between cervical and lumbar vertebra?
    a. Foramen transverserium
    b. Transverse process
    c. Shape of spinous process
    d. Heavy vertebral body
    e. All of the above

247. A young man sustains a skull base fracture at the middle cranial fossa that injures his right abducens (VI) nerve. Which of the following signs is most likely to be present on clinical examination?
    a. There is ptosis on the right side.
    b. The pupil on the right side is constricted and fails to respond to light.
    c. The right eyelid is numb.
    d. The patient is unable to deviate his right eye medially.
    e. The patient is unable to deviate his right eye laterally.

248. A 70-year-old man has been diagnosed with a fast-growing pituitary adenoma. Magnetic resonance image (MRI) scanning reveals suprasellar extension. Which one of the following structures is most likely to be affected?
    a. Abducens nerve
    b. Hypothalamus
    c. Oculomotor nerve
    d. Third ventricle
    e. Optic nerve

249. A 45-year-old man presents with a history of back pain that developed 3 months ago when he got up suddenly from a seated position. The pain radiates down the leg to the ankle. On examination he has weakness of the quadriceps, reduced knee jerk reflex and reduced sensation over the patella. Where is the lesion likely to be?
    a. Sciatic nerve
    b. Ilioinguinal nerve
    c. L3 nerve root
    d. L5 nerve root
    e. Femoral nerve at the inguinal ligament

250. Which of the following structures does not pass through the superior orbital fissure?
    a. The oculomotor nerve
    b. The trochlear nerve
    c. The abducens nerve
    d. The ophthalmic vein
    e. The lesser petrosal nerve

251. Which of the following structures is found in the posterior cranial fossa?
    a. The foramen magnum
    b. The condylar canal
    c. The internal acoustic meatus
    d. The hypoglossal canal
    e. The foramen spinosum

252. From which of the following arteries does the posterior communicating artery arise?
    a. External carotid artery
    b. Internal carotid artery
    c. Ophthalmic artery
    d. Middle cerebral artery
    e. None of the above

253. Which of the following is not the correct border of the posterior triangle of the neck?
    a. Anterior – posterior edge of the sternocleidomastoid muscle
    b. Posterior – anterior edge of the trapezius muscle
    c. Base – lateral one-third of the clavicle
    d. Apex – occipital bone just posterior to the mastoid process
    e. None of the above

254. During a thyroidectomy, which of the following layers is not transected when approaching the thyroid gland?
    a. Platysma
    b. Pretracheal fascia
    c. Prevertebral fascia
    d. Strap muscles (sternohyoid)
    e. Superficial investing layer of the deep cervical fascia

255. The neck can be divided into triangles, most commonly the anterior and posterior triangles. Which one of the following structures is contained within the posterior triangle?
    a. Submandibular gland
    b. Hypoglossal nerve
    c. Thyroid gland
    d. Vagus nerve
    e. Accessory nerve

256. The posterior triangle of the neck contains a selection of arteries, veins, nerves and lymphatics. Which of the following structures lies outside the posterior triangle?
    a. Virchow's node
    b. First part of the subclavian artery
    c. Three trunks of the brachial plexus
    d. Accessory nerve crossing beneath the investing fascial layer
    e. Suprascapular artery

257. The subclavian artery can be divided into three parts depending on its relation to surrounding anatomical structures. Which of the following branches of the subclavian artery lies in the second part behind the scalenus anterior?
    a. Vertebral artery
    b. Thyrocervical trunk
    c. Costocervical trunk
    d. Dorsal scapula artery
    e. Internal thoracic artery

258. All but one of the following vessels either supply or drain the thyroid gland. Which of the following vessels is incorrect?
    a. Superior thyroid artery
    b. Middle thyroid artery
    c. Middle thyroid vein
    d. Inferior thyroid vein
    e. Thyroid ima artery

259. Which of the following statements regarding the vasculature of the thyroid gland is true?
    a. The thyroid ima artery is found in approximately 30% of the population.
    b. The superior thyroid artery is a branch of the internal carotid artery.
    c. The inferior thyroid artery is a direct branch of the subclavian artery.

d. The middle thyroid vein drains into the internal jugular vein.
e. The inferior thyroid vein drains into the internal jugular vein.

260. With regard to the thyroid gland, which of the following statements
is correct?
a. During thyroid surgery, the inferior thyroid artery is ligated next
to the gland.
b. The gland originates in the floor of the embryonic pharynx in the foramen
magnum.
c. When ligating the superior pole of the thyroid, there is risk of damage to
the external laryngeal nerve.
d. The gland lies superficial to the pretracheal fascia.
e. The gland overlies the 2nd and 6th tracheal rings.

261. When performing a parotidectomy, there is risk of damage to several
structures within the gland. Which of the following structures is not
contained or does not pass through the parotid gland?
a. Facial nerve
b. Retromandibular vein
c. External carotid artery
d. Parotid lymph node
e. Facial vein

262. Which one of the following statements regarding the anatomy of the parotid
gland is correct?
a. The parotid capsule is supplied by the facial nerve.
b. The parotid duct pierces the masseter muscle and exits through a small
orifice opposite the 2nd upper molar.
c. The parotid capsule is derived from layers of prevertebral fascia.
d. Parotidectomy may be complicated by Frey's syndrome.
e. The facial nerve arises from the foramen spinosum before passing
through the parotid gland.

263. A 23-year-old man sustains a blow to the side of the head with a baseball
bat. He was unconscious at the scene but subsequently has improved to a
Glasgow Coma Scale (GCS) of 14/15. However, you notice that his ipsilateral
pupil has become dilated in comparison with when he first arrived in the
emergency department and that his consciousness level is beginning to
decrease. Which one of the following statements is correct?
a. The patient may have sustained a fractured pterion with such an impact.
b. The middle meningeal artery is unlikely to be involved.
c. Such clinical findings are consistent with a subdural haematoma.
d. Such clinical findings are consistent with a subarachnoid haemorrhage.
e. The autonomic fibres of CN III lie deep within the nerve.

264. Which of the following statements regarding the foramina of the cranial
fossae is correct?
a. The facial nerve passes through the foramen ovale.
b. The maxillary nerve exits the skull through the foramen rotundum.

c. The mandibular nerve passes through the foramen rotundum.

d. The hypoglossal nerve exits through the foramen ovale.

e. The middle meningeal artery passes through the foramen lacerum.

265. During thyroid surgery, there is risk to nearby nerves supplying the larynx. Which one of the following statements is incorrect?

a. The recurrent laryngeal nerve is closely related to the inferior thyroid artery near the inferior pole.

b. The recurrent laryngeal nerve supplies the cricothyroid muscle in the larynx.

c. The internal branch of the superior laryngeal nerve supplies sensation to the laryngeal mucous membrane superior to the vocal folds.

d. The left recurrent laryngeal nerve is more prone to injury during cardiac surgery.

e. Fine nasoendoscopy of the vocal cords is recommended prior to performing thyroidectomy surgery.

266. Which of the following statements regarding the musculature of the vocal cords and sensory innervation of the larynx is correct?

a. The posterior cricoarytenoid muscle adducts the vocal cord.

b. The lateral cricoarytenoid muscle abducts the vocal cord.

c. The cricothyroid muscle stretches and tenses the vocal cord.

d. The thyroarytenoid muscle is supplied by the superior laryngeal nerve.

e. Injury to the recurrent laryngeal nerve causes anaesthesia of the superior laryngeal mucosa increasing aspiration risk.

267. Which of the following statements is correct regarding the anatomy of the pharynx?

a. The pharynx extends from the base of the skull to the level of C4.

b. The oropharynx is the most proximal aspect of the pharynx.

c. The posterior wall of the pharynx lies against the pretracheal layer of the deep cervical fascia.

d. The inferior border of the cricoid cartilage marks the distal aspect of the pharynx.

e. Killian's dehiscence lies between the cricopharyngeus and stylopharyngeus.

268. Tonsillectomy and adenoidectomy are commonly performed procedures in ear, nose and throat surgery. Which one of the following statements regarding the applied anatomy of these procedures is correct?

a. There is no risk of damage to the teeth during a tonsillectomy.

b. The palatine tonsils are derived from the first pharyngeal pouch.

c. Damage to the facial artery during tonsillectomy is the most common cause of post-tonsillectomy bleeding.

d. The palatine tonsils lie between the palatoglossal and palatopharyngeal arches in adults.

e. The adenoids lie in the mucous membrane of the roof and posterior wall of the oropharynx.

269. The pterion is made up of the following bone structures except:
    a. Frontal
    b. Parietal
    c. Temporal
    d. Zygomatic
    e. Sphenoid

270. Which of the following vessels does not originate from the external carotid artery?
    a. Posterior auricular artery
    b. Inferior thyroid artery
    c. Lingual artery
    d. Superficial temporal artery
    e. Ascending pharyngeal artery

271. Which of the following arteries is a branch of the internal carotid artery?
    a. Middle meningeal artery
    b. Middle cerebral artery
    c. Occipital artery
    d. Superficial temporal artery
    e. Posterior auricular artery

272. Which of the following structures is not found within the parotid gland?
    a. External carotid artery
    b. Maxillary nerve
    c. Retromandibular vein
    d. Lymph nodes
    e. Facial nerve

273. Which of the following muscles would not be affected by damage to the recurrent laryngeal nerve?
    a. The posterior cricoarytenoid
    b. The lateral cricoarytenoid
    c. The cricothyroid
    d. The thyroarytenoid
    e. The vocalis

274. Which of the following statements is correct concerning the applied anatomy and pathology of the thyroid gland?
    a. It has its isthmus between the 5th and 6th tracheal rings.
    b. It receives blood supply from the first part of the subclavian artery.
    c. Follicular carcinomas are the most common type of malignancy.
    d. The superior thyroid artery is closely related to the recurrent laryngeal nerve.
    e. Malignancy is commonly associated with Hashimoto's thyroiditis.

275. Which of the following arteries are branches of the first part of the subclavian artery?
    a. Vertebral, internal thoracic and thyrocervical arteries
    b. Common carotid and vertebral arteries
    c. External carotid and internal carotid arteries
    d. Dorsal scapular and thyrocervical arteries
    e. Posterior intercostal, costocervical trunk and internal thoracic arteries

CENTRAL, PERIPHERAL AND AUTONOMIC NERVOUS SYSTEMS

276. Which of the following is the correct order of nerves within the brachial plexus?
    a. Divisions, trunks, cords, branches, roots
    b. Roots, trunks, divisions, cords, branches
    c. Cords, trunks, branches, roots, divisions
    d. Branches, trunks, divisions, roots, cords
    e. None of the above

277. When a patient has a divided thoracodorsal nerve, which of the following muscles would you expect to be paralyzed?
    a. The latissimus dorsi
    b. The teres major
    c. The supraspinatus
    d. The deltoid
    e. The rhomboid major

278. A middle-aged gentleman walks into your clinic with a high stepping gait following a recent trauma. Which of the following nerves has most likely been damaged?
    a. The tibial nerve
    b. The femoral nerve
    c. The sural nerve
    d. The deep peroneal nerve
    e. The saphenous nerve

279. Which of the following nerves form(s) part of the lumbar plexus?
    a. The subcostal nerve
    b. The genitofemoral nerve
    c. The iliohypogastric nerve
    d. All of the above
    e. b and c only

280. A 34-year-old man has sustained an injury to the common peroneal nerve while playing football. Which area of the foot would you touch to test the cutaneous sensation function of the deep peroneal nerve?
    a. The posterolateral aspect of the calf and foot
    b. The medial aspect of the sole
    c. The lateral aspect of the sole
    d. The anterolateral aspect of the calf and most of the dorsum of the foot
    e. None of the above

281. The saphenous nerve is a terminal branch of which nerve in the leg?
    a. The femoral nerve
    b. The tibial nerve
    c. The common peroneal nerve
    d. The obturator nerve
    e. The posterior cutaneous nerve of the thigh

282. Which one of the following cranial nerves exits the skull via the stylomastoid foramen?
    a. VII
    b. VIII
    c. IX
    d. X
    e. XI

283. Through which foramen in the base of the skull does the maxillary nerve exit?
    a. The foramen caecum
    b. The foramen ovale
    c. The foramen spinosum
    d. The foramen rotundum
    e. The foramen lacerum

284. Which of the following nerves is a major branch of the facial nerve in the face?
    a. The supraorbital nerve
    b. The zygomatic nerve
    c. The buccal nerve
    d. All of the above
    e. b and c only

285. Which of the following nerves supply sensation to the auricle and external acoustic meatus?
    a. C1
    b. C2
    c. Cranial nerve V
    d. All of the above
    e. b and c only

286. A 32-year-old male professional cyclist has been brought to hospital after being hit by a car. He has severe pelvic injuries which require angiography and embolization to stem the bleeding. An magnetic resonance image (MRI) of the pelvis done some time later is reported as showing some bruising of the nerve passing through the lesser sciatic foramen. Which of the following nerves is the report referring to?
    a. Superior gluteal nerve
    b. Sciatic nerve
    c. Pudendal nerve
    d. Inferior gluteal nerve
    e. Posterior femoral cutaneous nerve

287. A 48-year-old woman attends fracture clinic for removal of a below-knee plaster of Paris. The cast is removed and it is noted that she has a foot drop. Which branch of the sciatic nerve is injured?
    a. Deep peroneal nerve
    b. Common peroneal nerve

c. Anterior tibial nerve
d. Posterior tibial nerve
e. Femoral nerve

288. A 32-year-old man presents to the emergency department with a right-sided direct inguinal hernia. His past medical history includes an emergency appendicectomy over a year ago. Iatrogenic injury at the time of the appendicectomy was thought to be the cause of the subsequent hernia. Which of the following structures was likely to have been damaged?
a. Femoral branch of the genitofemoral nerve
b. Ilioinguinal nerve
c. Obturator nerve
d. Subcostal nerve
e. Superior gluteal nerve

289. A 25-year-old homeless man was brought into the emergency department after having been stabbed in his thigh. The surgical senior house officer described the wound to be lying over the medial compartment of the thigh. Which of the following nerves supplies the medial compartment of the thigh?
a. Tibial nerve
b. Sciatic nerve
c. Superficial peroneal nerve
d. Sural nerve
e. Obturator nerve

290. A 27-year-old man was brought into the emergency department after having fallen out of a tree. He states that he grabbed onto a branch with his right arm to try and break his fall. Clinical examination reveals that he has suffered brachial plexus nervous damage affecting the lateral cord. Which of the following nerve roots has he damaged?
a. C5 and C6
b. C5, C6 and C7
c. C8 and T1
d. C5, C6, C7, C8 and T1
e. C6 and C7

291. A 15-year-old girl attended the accident and emergency department after having walked over glass barefoot. Clinic examination reveals a shard of glass embedded in the sole of her foot. She is reviewed by the orthopaedic team who state she has paralysis of her flexor digitorum brevis. Which of the following nerves has been injured?
a. Sural nerve
b. Deep peroneal nerve
c. Saphenous nerve
d. Lateral plantar nerve
e. Medial plantar nerve

292. Which of the following peripheral nerves supplies sensation to the lateral area of the forearm?
   a. Axillary nerve
   b. Median nerve
   c. Musculocutaneous nerve
   d. Radial nerve
   e. Ulnar nerve

293. Which of the following peripheral nerves supplies the sensation to the palmar aspect of the index finger?
   a. Axillary nerve
   b. Median nerve
   c. Musculocutaneous nerve
   d. Radial nerve
   e. Ulnar nerve

294. Which of the following peripheral nerves supplies sensation to the little finger?
   a. Axillary nerve
   b. Median nerve
   c. Musculocutaneous nerve
   d. Radial nerve
   e. Ulnar nerve

295. Which is the predominate spinal nerve root which extends the elbow?
   a. C5
   b. C6
   c. C7
   d. C8
   e. T1

296. Which is the predominate spinal nerve root which extends the wrist?
   a. C5
   b. C6
   c. C7
   d. C8
   e. T1

297. Which the predominate spinal nerve root which flexes the fingers?
   a. C5
   b. C6
   c. C7
   d. C8
   e. T1

298. A patient has been diagnosed with a facial nerve lesion proximal to the internal acoustic meatus. Which of the following features are not associated with such a lesion?
   a. Unilateral facial paralysis
   b. Increased salivation

    c. Unilateral hyperacusis

    d. Unilateral loss of taste in the anterior two-thirds of the tongue

    e. Bell's palsy

299. A woman presents to the accident and emergency department with backache. After a clinical examination you diagnose sciatica and send her home with an orthopaedic outpatient appointment. Which of the following statements regarding the sciatic nerve is false?

    a. The roots of the sciatic nerve are L4, L5, S1 and S2.

    b. It passes over the obturator internus and quadratus femoris.

    c. It divides into the common peroneal nerve and tibial nerve.

    d. The lateral aspect of the nerve is the side of relative safety for exposure.

    e. Damage to the nerve may present with foot drop.

300. A patient suffered a stabbing to his back in the midline at the level of L4. Which of the following clinical presentations are associated with stabbings at this level?

    a. Reduced sensation at the knee

    b. Reduced sensation over the shin

    c. Reduced motor in the perianal region

    d. Trendelenburg gait

    e. Reduced hip flexion

301. A 34-year-old male cyclist is hit by a car travelling at 40 mph. On arrival in the emergency department it is noted that the patient has left-sided wrist drop. Further examination reveals weakness of brachioradialis and sensory loss over the dorsal radial part of the hand and posterior part of the forearm. The triceps reflex is preserved. This has occurred secondary to damage at which point along the course of this nerve?

    a. Spiral groove of humerus

    b. Axilla

    c. Wrist

    d. Forearm

    e. Elbow

302. Which of the following statements regarding the course of the vagus nerve is correct?

    a. It exits the cranium via the foramen magnum.

    b. It descends in the neck lateral to the oesophagus.

    c. It gives off a superior laryngeal branch, which supplies the superior constrictor muscles.

    d. On the right side, it gives off the recurrent laryngeal branch as it crosses the subclavian artery.

    e. On the left side, the recurrent laryngeal branch crosses under the ligamentum teres.

303. Which of the following statements regarding the anatomy of the radial nerve is correct?

    a. It arises from nerve roots C5–T1.

    b. It arises from the medial cord of the brachial plexus.

c. It passes between the medial and lateral heads of the triceps.

d. It gives off the lateral cutaneous nerve of the forearm.

e. It lies in contact with the humerus anteriorly in the spiral groove.

304. Which of the following statements regarding the anatomy of the ulnar nerve is correct?

   a. It originates from C7–T1 nerve roots.

   b. It is formed from the lateral cord of the brachial plexus.

   c. It lies deep to the coracobrachialis.

   d. It lies medial to the brachial artery.

   e. It passes medial to the median nerve in the carpal tunnel.

305. Which of the following statements regarding the anatomy of the median nerve is correct?

   a. It arises from spinal nerve roots C6, C7 and C8.

   b. It is separated from the ulnar artery by the deep head of pronator teres.

   c. It enters the forearm between the heads of pronator quadratus.

   d. It gives off an anterior interosseous branch at the mid-humerus.

   e. It lies radial to the flexor carpi radialis at the wrist.

306. Which of the following statements regarding the cervical sympathetic trunk is correct?

   a. The middle ganglion lies at vertebral level C4.

   b. The superior ganglion lies at vertebral level C2.

   c. The inferior ganglion lies at vertebral level C6.

   d. Grey rami pass from the inferior ganglion to cranial nerves VII, IX, XI and XII.

   e. Grey rami pass from the superior ganglion to cranial nerves III, VII, IX and X.

307. Which of the following statements regarding the course of the phrenic nerve is correct?

   a. It arises from posterior cervical rami C3, 4 and 5.

   b. It travels anterior to the vagus nerve.

   c. The right branch passes through the caval orifice of the diaphragm.

   d. It runs on the scalenus medius muscle in the neck.

   e. The left branch courses posterior to the left pulmonary artery in the mediastinum.

308. Which of the following statements regarding the anatomy of the trochlear nerve is correct?

   a. It arises from the anterior midbrain and runs over the free edge of the tentorium.

   b. It enters the dura of the lateral wall of the cavernous sinus inferior and lateral to the oculomotor nerve.

   c. It passes through the superior orbital fissure inside the tendinous ring.

   d. Its action can be tested by asking the patient to look upward and laterally.

   e. It passes medially from the superior orbital fissure to supply the inferior oblique.

309. Which ganglion receives preganglionic parasympathetic fibres from the Edinger–Westphal nucleus?
    a. Ciliary ganglion
    b. Submandibular ganglion
    c. Pterygopalatine ganglion
    d. Otic ganglion
    e. Trigeminal ganglion

310. Which of the following statements regarding the course of the vagus nerve is correct?
    a. Fibres for the vagus nerve originate from the pons.
    b. The vagus nerve enters the abdomen through the caval opening in the diaphragm (T8).
    c. The left recurrent laryngeal nerve hooks behind the subclavian artery in the root of the neck.
    d. The vagus nerve gives off the superior, internal and external laryngeal branches within the neck.
    e. The left vagus nerve travels on the posterior surface of the oesophagus.

311. Which of the following statements regarding the stellate ganglion is incorrect?
    a. It is a sympathetic ganglion.
    b. It lies anterior to the transverse process of C7.
    c. It lies below the subclavian artery.
    d. Damage to the stellate ganglion produces Raynaud's phenomenon.
    e. It is formed from fusion of the inferior cervical ganglion with the first thoracic ganglion.

312. The cremasteric reflex is a useful test when examining a patient with suspected torsion of the testis. Which nerve root innervates the cremasteric muscle?
    a. T11–T12
    b. L1–L2
    c. L3–L4
    d. L5–S1
    e. S1–S2

313. Meralgia paraesthetica results from the involvement of which of the following nerves?
    a. The medial cutaneous nerve of the thigh
    b. The lateral cutaneous nerve of the thigh
    c. The sural nerve
    d. The femoral nerve
    e. The common peroneal nerve

314. The blade of a retractor has rested on the psoas muscle during a lengthy operative procedure. This has resulted in femoral nerve palsy. In the postoperative period the patient will experience which one of the following?
    a. Inability to flex the knee only
    b. Inability to flex the knee and numbness over the thigh

c. Numbness over the anterior thigh only

d. Inability to extend the knee and numbness over the anterior thigh

e. Inability to flex the hip and numbness over the anterior thigh

315. A 40-year-old man presents with pins and needles on the lateral and anterior aspect of his left thigh. On examination, there is no motor deficit. There is no history of trauma. Which of the following is likely to be causing the problem?

a. Lateral cutaneous nerve of the thigh lesion

b. L2 root lesion

c. L3 root lesion

d. Femoral nerve lesion

e. Saphenous nerve lesion

316. A 35-year-old woman attends clinic complaining of pins and needles affecting the radial (lateral) three digits of her hand. The symptoms are worse at night, and after driving long distances. Which of the following motor signs would confirm the likely diagnosis?

a. Inability to flex the radial three digits

b. Inability to adduct all the fingers of her hand

c. Inability to abduct all the fingers of her hand

d. Weakness of abduction of the thumb

e. There will be no motor deficit

317. A 20-year-old motorcyclist is involved in a road traffic accident. He is found to have weakness of right shoulder abduction and forearm flexion, as well as some sensory loss over the lateral aspect of his upper arm. The right biceps and brachioradialis reflexes are absent. Which of the following is the likely level of maximal plexus injury?

a. C4, 5 roots

b. C5, 6 roots

c. C6, 7 roots

d. C7, 8 roots

e. C8, T1 roots

318. A dental surgeon carries out a block of the inferior alveolar nerve by infiltrating local anaesthetic at the mandibular foramen. Which clinical feature may result from this procedure?

a. Numbness of the lower lip on the injected side

b. Ineffective block for the incisor teeth

c. Numbness of the side of the tongue

d. Inability of the patient to clench the jaw

e. Transient weakness of the facial muscles on the injected side

319. During an inguinal hernia repair in a 54-year-old man, the ilioinguinal nerve is injured in the inguinal canal. This will most likely result in which one of the following?

a. Paraesthesia over the dorsum of the penis

b. Paraesthesia over the pubis and scrotum, and loss of cremasteric contraction

    c. Paraesthesia over the pubis and anterior scrotum only

    d. Paraesthesia over the anterior and medial thigh

    e. Paraesthesia over the pubis only

320. Which one of the following signs is consistent with femoral nerve damage in a patient with pelvic trauma?

    a. Preserved knee reflex

    b. Loss of sensation over the anterior femur

    c. Loss of power in the biceps femoris muscle

    d. Loss of power in the peroneus muscle

    e. Reduced power on adduction

321. Morton's neuroma is related to which of the following nerves?

    a. The sural nerve

    b. The common peroneal nerve

    c. The common plantar nerve

    d. The tibial nerve

    e. None of the above

322. Which of the following statements is true regarding the trunks of the brachial plexus?

    a. The anterior rami of C5 and C6 form the upper trunk.

    b. The anterior ramus of C7 forms the middle trunk.

    c. The anterior rami of C8 and T1 form the lower trunk.

    d. All of the above.

    e. None of the above.

323. The following statements about the vagus nerve are true except:

    a. It passes through the diaphragm at the level of T12.

    b. It exits the cranium via the jugular foramen.

    c. It provides sensorimotor supply to the larynx.

    d. It provides parasympathetic innervation to the oesophagus.

    e. It travels within the carotid sheath.

324. Which of the following hand muscles is supplied by the median nerve?

    a. Abductor digiti minimi

    b. Abductor pollicis brevis

    c. Flexor digiti minimi

    d. The 1st dorsal interosseous

    e. Palmar interosseous

325. The nucleus of which of the following cranial nerves is located in the pons?

    a. CN III

    b. CN IV

    c. CN VI

    d. CN X

    e. CN XI

326. The following cranial nerves all give off parasympathetic nervous supply except:

    a. CN III

    b. CN V

c. CN VII
d. CN IX
e. CN X

327. Parasympathetic nervous supply for the parotid gland originates from which one of the following?
a. Vagus nerve
b. Facial nerve
c. Glossopharyngeal nerve
d. Vestibulocochlear nerve
e. Trigeminal nerve

328. The following statements regarding the anatomy of the common peroneal nerve are true except:
a. It is a branch of the sciatic nerve.
b. It provides motor and sensory supply.
c. It gives off superficial and deep branches.
d. It supplies the tibialis posterior muscle.
e. Injury may cause a foot drop.

329. The following statements concerning the anatomy of the radial nerve are true except:
a. It lies between the brachialis and the brachioradialis.
b. It crosses from lateral to medial of the brachial artery at the mid-humeral level.
c. The posterior interosseous nerve can be damaged in fracture of the radial head.
d. Damage to the posterior interosseous nerve still allows wrist extension.
e. It supplies the brachioradialis muscle.

CHAPTER 2
APPLIED SURGICAL ANATOMY

Answers

THORAX

1. c. The lung is invested by and enclosed in a serous pleural sac consisting of two continuous membranes: the visceral pleura investing all surfaces of the lungs and the parietal pleura lining the pulmonary cavities.

The pleurae start approximately 2.5 cm above the border between the medial and middle third of the clavicle. They then run obliquely to meet in the midline at the 2nd costal cartilage. At the 4th costal cartilage the left pleura leaves the midline to make room for the heart. At the 6th costal cartilage the right pleura leaves the midline. Both pleurae cross the mid-clavicular line at the 8th rib. At the 10th rib both pleurae cross the mid-axillary line. Both pleurae then come to the midline in the back at the 12th.

2. c. The horizontal and oblique fissures divide the lungs into lobes, three on the right side and two on the left. The right lung is larger and heavier than the left, but shorter and wider due to the raised right dome of the diaphragm and the heart bulging more to the left.

The oblique fissures start from the level of the tip of the 3rd spinous process. Both fissures then run obliquely along the medial border of the rotated scapula, continuing until the 6th costochondral joint on the anterior chest wall. For the right lung, the horizontal fissure runs medially from the oblique fissure at the mid-axillary line (rib 5) along the lower border of the 4th rib to the midline.

3. d. The apex beat represents the bottom left corner of the heart. The four corners of the heart can be found in the following locations:

- *Bottom left* – fifth intercostal space mid-clavicular line. In this position you will find the apex beat in a fit patient. Conditions such as cardiac failure can lead to cardiomegaly resulting in a laterally displaced apex beat.
- *Bottom right* – overlying the sixth costal cartilage just right-lateral to the sternum.
- *Top right* – overlying the third costal cartilage just right-lateral to the sternum.
- *Top left* – second intercostal space approximately 2 cm left-lateral to the sternum.

4. d.   The aorta crosses the diaphragm at the level of T12. Note that the aorta does not pierce the diaphragm but it passes posteriorly to it. However, questions on this point may say structures 'pass through' the diaphragm. As the aorta does not pierce the diaphragm, movements of the diaphragm during respiration do not affect blood flow. Other structures crossing at this level include the thoracic duct, the greater splanchnic nerve, the lesser splanchnic nerve, the hemiazygos vein and the azygos vein.

5. e.   The thoracic duct originates from the chyle cisterns in the abdomen and ascends through the aortic hiatus in the diaphragm (T12), coursing its way in between the thoracic aorta which lies lateral to it, and the azygous vein medially. The oesophagus lies anteriorly with the vertebral bodes posteriorly until it crosses to the left at the level of T4, T5 or T6. As the thoracic duct is thin walled and sometimes appears colourless, it may not be easily identified during surgical procedures involving the posterior mediastinum. Laceration of this duct leads to chyle escaping into the thoracic cavity, and it may also enter the pleural cavity leading to the formation of a chylothorax.

6. e.   The patient has mitral stenosis. All the heart valves are retrosternal. The mitral valve is at the level of the 4th costal cartilage; the aortic valve is at the 3rd intercostal space and the tricuspid at the 4th intercostal space. The pulmonary valve is at the level of the left 3rd costal cartilage.

7. d.   The left coronary artery (LCA) arises from the left posterior aortic sinus of the ascending aorta, passing between the left auricle and left side of the pulmonary trunk, running in the coronary groove. It divides into the left anterior descending and the circumflex arteries. The left anterior descending runs along the interventricular groove to the apex, anastomosing with the posterior descending branch of the right coronary artery (RCA). The left anterior descending supplies adjacent areas of both ventricles and the anterior interventricular septum. The circumflex branch of LCA follows the coronary groove around the left border to the posterior surface of the heart. About 60% of hearts have the RCA supplying the sinoatrial (SA) node and 40% of hearts have a LCA supply. The LCA supplies the vast majority of the left atrium and ventricle and part of the right ventricle through a conus branch. The atrioventricular node is supplied in 90% of cases by the RCA, the rest by the left circumflex artery.

8. e.   The sternal angle is at the level of T4. At this level, the aortic arch is terminating, the azygos vein enters the superior vena cava, the left recurrent laryngeal loops around the ligamentum venosum and the bifurcation of the pulmonary trunk may be seen.

9. c.   Inspiration involves descent of the diaphragm and elevation of the ribs, increasing the anteroposterior dimensions of the chest. The ribs move upwards and outwards; however, the first rib does not move during respiration. The long thoracic nerve supplies the serratus anterior, which aids lifting the ribs in inspiration.

10. b.   The phrenic nerve has sensory and motor supply to the diaphragm. Each dome has a separate nerve supply. The main motor root is C5 and injury to the phrenic nerve causes paralysis of the corresponding hemidiaphragm. Detection is made by noting the paradoxical movements. Rather than descending during inspiration due to diaphragmatic contraction, the paralyzed dome is pushed superiorly. Similarly in expiration the paralyzed dome descends due to positive pressure in the lungs. X-ray findings may reveal a raised hemidiaphragm.

11. c. The origin of the coronary arteries is immediately superior to the aortic valve. There are two main arteries: the right coronary artery (RCA), dividing into the marginal and posterior interventricular branches, and the left coronary artery, dividing into the anterior interventricular and circumflex branches. The supply territories of the arteries are variable and the artery which supplies the posterior descending artery defines heart dominance. Seventy percent of hearts are right dominant, 20% are co-dominant and 10% are left dominant. The posterior interventricular artery supplies both ventricles and so if the heart is right dominant, then the RCA will supply the right side of the heart as well as a portion of the left ventricle.

12. c. The diaphragm's motor innervation is obtained from the phrenic nerve (C3, 4, 5) – this nerve also conveys sensation to the central portion of the diaphragm, but the lower six intercostal nerves supply sensation to the periphery. The following relate to structures passing through the diaphragm at specific vertebral levels:

- T12: Azygous vein, aorta, thoracic duct
- T10: Vagus nerve, left gastric vein/artery, oesophagus
- T8: Right phrenic nerve, inferior vena cava

The left phrenic nerve pierces the central tendon and the sympathetic chain crosses behind the medial arcuate ligament with the psoas muscle.

13. b. The arterial supply to the oesophagus is as follows:

- Cervical portion: Inferior thyroid artery, a branch of the thyrocervical trunk from the subclavian artery
- Thoracic portion: Descending aorta
- Abdominal portion: Left gastric artery, a branch of the coeliac artery and the left inferior phrenic artery

The venous drainage of the oesophagus is as follows:

- Cervical portion: Inferior thyroid vein
- Thoracic portion: Azygous vein
- Abdominal portion: Left gastric vein (and part of the azygous vein)

14. e. There are three main openings in the diaphragm:

1. T8 – in the central tendon. This transmits the inferior vena cava and the right phrenic nerve.
2. T10 – between the muscular fibres of the right crus. This transmits the oesophagus, the left gastric artery and vein and the two vagi.
3. T12 – this transmits the abdominal aorta, the thoracic duct and the azygous vein.

15. d.   The coronary sinus lies in the posterior atrioventricular groove opening into the right atrium. It receives venous drainage from:

- The small cardiac vein – accompanies the marginal artery along the inferior border of the heart.
- The middle cardiac vein via the inferior interventricular groove.
- The great cardiac vein in the anterior interventricular groove.
- The oblique cardiac vein which lies on the posterior aspect of the left atrium.
- The anterior cardiac veins drain much of the anterior surface of the heart and drain directly into the right atrium.

16. c.   The six pairs of aortic arches arise from the truncus arteriosus. The 1st and 2nd arches disappear. The 3rd arches become the carotid arteries. On the right side the 4th arch becomes the brachiocephalic and subclavian arteries; on the left the 4th arch develops into the definitive aortic arch. The 5th arch is rudimentary and disappears. The truncus arteriosus splits to the ascending aorta and pulmonary trunk with the 6th arch forming the left and right pulmonary arteries.

17. d.   The trachea extends from the lower border of the cricoid cartilage (C6) to its termination into two main bronchi (T5). The relations within the thorax are:

- Anterior – brachiocephalic artery and left common carotid artery, thymus and left brachiocephalic vein
- Posterior – oesophagus, recurrent laryngeal nerves
- Right – vagus nerve, azygous vein
- Left – arch of the aorta, left subclavian vein, left recurrent laryngeal nerve and left common carotid artery

18. e.   The thoracic duct commences at the end of cisterna chyli at the level of T12. It passes upward between the aorta and azygous vein between the crurae of the diaphragm. At the level of T5 it turns to the left passing behind the oesophagus. Travelling upwards vertically it finally arches over the dome of the left pleura entering the point of confluence of the left internal jugular and subclavian veins. Up to 4 L of lymph is drained per day. The right lymphatic trunk drains the right arm, right head and neck and trunk.

19. d.   Diaphragmatic hernias may result from failure of fusion of the component parts or from a primary defect. The majority (85–90%) arise from posterolateral defects (Bochdalek hernia). The left side is most commonly affected (80%). Hernias between the costal and sternal origins (Morgagni hernia) are rare (1–2%). These hernias are noted in neonates and require surgical repair to prevent morbidity and mortality.

20. b.   The 'safe triangle' for the insertion of an intercostal drain is bounded anteriorly by the inferolateral border of pectoralis major, posteriorly by the anterior border of latissimus dorsi and inferiorly by the axial plane at the level of the nipple. The mid-axillary line at the level of the 5th intercostal space may be used within this triangle to help guide placement of the incision. The mid-clavicular line should not be used for placement of an intercostal tube drain. The mid-clavicular line is used when performing needle thoracocentesis for a tension pneumothorax.

21. e. The right main bronchus is wider, shorter and runs more vertically than the left main bronchus. Consequently, foreign bodies small enough to be inhaled more commonly enter the right lung. As a result of gravity, the right lower lobe is more likely to receive such foreign bodies.

22. e. Lymph from the abdominal portion of the oesophagus drains into the gastric and coeliac lymph nodes. Lymphatic drainage from the upper two-thirds of the oesophagus is usually cephalad. The cervical oesophagus drains via the internal jugular nodes, and the thoracic oesophagus drains via the mediastinal nodes. The oesophageal wall has inner circular and outer longitudinal muscular layers. Its blood supply is from the inferior thyroid artery (thyrocervical trunk) in the upper third, oesophageal branches directly from the aorta in the middle third and the left gastric artery in the lower third. Blood from the proximal half of the oesophagus drains into the oesophageal veins leading to the azygous vein. The distal half drains into the left gastric vein leading to the portal venous system. The oesophagus commences at C6 and enters the diaphragm at T10 through the oesophageal hiatus.

23. d. The normal oesophagus is not indented by the left atrium unless there is left atrial dilatation. The indentations occur at the cricopharyngeus muscle (15 cm from incisors), aortic arch (22.5 cm), left main bronchus (27.5 cm) and lower oesophageal sphincter (40 cm). The narrowest constriction is at the cricopharyngeal muscle.

24. b. The left subclavian artery arises at the aortic arch behind the origin of the left common carotid artery. It ascends with the lung and pleura laterally and the trachea and oesophagus medially to lie behind the left sternoclavicular joint. The right subclavian artery forms behind the right sternoclavicular joint. The branches of the subclavian artery can be defined using the mnemonic 'vitamin C and D' (vertebral artery, internal thoracic artery, thyrocervical trunk, costocervical trunk, dorsal scapula artery). The posterior circumflex humoral, thoracoacromial, superior thoracic and lateral thoracic arteries are branches of the axillary artery.

25. b. The branches of the thoracic aorta include bronchial, pericardial, posterior intercostal, superior phrenic, oesophageal, mediastinal and subcostal arteries. Branches of the abdominal aorta can be divided into paired and unpaired. Paired branches include the suprarenal, renal, gonadal, inferior phrenic and lumbar arteries. The origin of the inferior phrenic arteries varies and can arise either from the aorta directly or from the coeliac trunk. Unpaired branches include the coeliac trunk, superior and inferior mesenteric arteries and median sacral artery.

26. d. The right lung has three main lobes, whereas the left lung has only two. The right main bronchus is wider, shorter and travels more vertically than the left. The lungs are invested in visceral pleura, with parietal pleura coating the chest wall. Both apices pass into the supraclavicular fossae. The arterial blood supply is mainly via the bronchial arteries, with a small amount of oxygenation occurring from the pulmonary artery. The left bronchial artery usually arises from the thoracic aorta; the right bronchial artery arises from a number of positions, including the thoracic aorta.

27. d. The nerve injured is most likely to be the long thoracic nerve, which supplies the serratus anterior muscle. This nerve courses superficially over the serratus anterior muscle; hence it is vulnerable to injury especially when the limbs are elevated. The arm cannot be completely abducted above the horizontal position because the serratus anterior is unable to rotate the glenoid cavity superiorly. Also, if the patient were to press his hands against a wall, the scapula would move medially and posteriorly, a condition termed 'winged scapula', whenever the long thoracic nerve is damaged.

28. c. The first rib is a true rib as it attaches directly to the sternum with its own costal cartilage. It is, however, not a typical rib as it has distinctive characteristics. It is broad, short and very sharply curved. It has two grooves on its superior surface where the subclavian vein and artery pass. Between these two grooves is the scalene tubercle where the scalenus anterior attaches. The subclavian vein is anterior and the subclavian artery is posterior to the scalenus anterior muscle. The first rib only articulates with the T1 vertebra.

ABDOMEN, PELVIS AND PERINEUM

29. d.   The spermatic cord consists of the structures running to and then from the testis. It runs from the deep ring of the inguinal canal, through the superficial ring and then to the posterior border of the testis. The main structures within the spermatic cord are:

- The ductus deferens
- *Arteries* – testicular and cremastic arteries and the artery of the ductus deferens
- *Veins* – pampiniform plexus (a large collection of veins arising from the posterior surface of the testis ending in the testicular vein)
- *Nerves* – sympathetic fibres for the arteries and sympathetic and parasympathetic nerves for the ductus deferens; genitofemoral nerve, which supplies the cremaster muscle
- Lymph vessels

The ilioinguinal nerve is within the inguinal canal, but not the spermatic cord. It supplies the anterior surface of the scrotum.

30. e.   The spermatic cord is covered by three layers that originate from the anterior abdominal wall: the external spermatic fascia, the cremastic muscle and the internal spermatic fascia. During an inguinal hernia repair, these layers are not easy to identify separately.

The innermost layer, named the internal spermatic fascia, is made from the transversalis fascia as the processus vaginalis of the peritoneum evaginates through it, forming the deep inguinal ring. As the processus vaginalis continues its journey through the anterior abdominal wall, it gains a few muscle fibres from the internal oblique muscle and its accompanying fascia; this forms the middle layer (the cremaster muscle and cremasteric fascia). The outermost layer, the external spermatic fascia, is made from the external oblique aponeurosis as the processus vaginalis continues its evagination and forms the superficial inguinal ring at the same time. The processus vaginalis surrounds the testis and is, at this point, known as the tunica vaginalis.

31. d.   In adults, the inguinal canal runs for 4-6 cm inferomedially from just superior to the midpoint of the inguinal ligament (the deep ring) to just lateral to the pubic tubercle (the superficial ring). The function of the canal is to allow the spermatic cord in males and the round ligament in females to travel into the peritoneal cavity.

Its borders are posteriorly, the transversalis fascia, reinforced medially by the conjoint tendon; anteriorly, the external oblique aponeurosis, reinforced laterally by the fibres of internal oblique; the floor, the inguinal ligament; and the roof, the conjoint tendon (common tendon of the internal oblique and the transverse abdominis muscles). The pectineal ligament forms the posterior border of the femoral canal.

32. e. Liver cirrhosis leads to venous congestion and portal hypertension, which results in venous enlargement. To decrease the pressure within the portal system the body is able to open channels between the portal and the systemic circulation. There are five anastomoses:

- *Haemorrhoids* – anastomosis between the veins supplying the inferior rectum and the anal canal
- *Oesophageal varices* – anastomosis between the portal and systemic circulation around the inferior oesophagus
- *Caput medusae* – anastomosis between the portal system and the superficial veins around the umbilicus as a result of recanalization of the ligamentum teres
- Swollen venous connection between the portal and systemic circulations at the bare area of the liver
- Swollen venous connection between veins of the retroperitoneal structures of the GI tract and the body wall

33. a. Ulcers within the duodenum commonly lie within the 1st (superior) part of the duodenum. Ulcers that lie posteriorly erode into the gastroduodenal artery and those that lie anteriorly erode into the peritoneal cavity, causing peritonitis. Bleeding occurs in 20% of peptic ulcers and carries a high mortality in patients aged over 55 years. The duodenum is supplied by arteries from the embryonic foregut and midgut. The superior and inferior pancreaticoduodenal arteries directly supply the duodenum and these are branches of the gastroduodenal and superior mesenteric arteries, respectively. The gastroduodenal artery (a branch of common hepatic artery) runs intimately posterior to the duodenum before turning into the superior pancreaticoduodenal artery.

34. e. Pringle's manoeuvre involves grasping the free edge of the lesser omentum during a laparotomy. The manoeuvre is performed to control life-threatening bleeding in a liver laceration. Within the free edge of the lesser omentum lie the hepatic artery, the portal vein and the cystic duct. By compressing these vessels you stop blood reaching the liver, allowing you to control the haemorrhage. This manoeuvre can also be used to control haemorrhage from the cystic artery. The superior mesenteric artery supplies the midgut and therefore does not supply the liver.

35. b. The transpyloric plane of the abdomen is an important anatomical plane as many abdominal viscera are related to it. The plane is defined as being at the midpoint between the suprasternal notch and the pubic symphysis. During an abdominal examination, it is possible to estimate its position by identifying the midpoint between the xiphisternum and the umbilicus.

The plane runs through the inferior part of L1 and the pylorus of the stomach. Other structures include the hila of the kidneys, the gastroduodenal junction and first part of the duodenum, the duodenojejunal junction, the neck of the pancreas and the anterior aspect of the ninth costal cartilages. The adrenal glands lie at the level of T12 and are therefore above the transpyloric plane.

36. d.   The inguinal canal is an oblique 4–6 cm intermuscular slit that lies above the medial half of the inguinal ligament. It is a natural point of weakness in the abdominal wall, but the components of its boundaries help to reduce this weakness. The boundaries of the inguinal canal are:

- Anteriorly: Internal and external oblique
- Posteriorly: Conjoint tendon and transversalis fascia
- Roof: Internal oblique, conjoint tendon and transversus abdominis
- Floor: Inguinal and lacunar ligaments

37. d.   Direct inguinal hernias arise through Hesselbach's triangle, which is bordered by the inferior epigastric artery superiorly and laterally, the inguinal ligament inferiorly and the lateral border of the rectus abdominis medially.

38. c.   There are many variations in biliary tree anatomy, and that is why it is important to correctly identify the structures forming Calot's triangle before starting dissection. The gallbladder is supplied by the cystic artery, which is a branch of the right hepatic artery. The cystic artery lies in Calot's triangle, which is bordered by the inferior border of the liver, the cystic duct and the common hepatic duct.

39. e.   The cystic artery is usually a branch of the right hepatic artery and lies in Calot's triangle. The artery produces three or four small branches known as Calot's arteries and then divides into two main branches. The superficial branch passes over to the left side of the gallbladder, while the deep branch runs between the gallbladder and gallbladder fossa. Anatomical variations include a double cystic artery where the superficial and deep branches do not originate from a common origin, or in 1% of cases the cystic artery can originate from the left hepatic artery. Even if the artery becomes thrombosed, there is a rich secondary supply from the liver bed supplying the gallbladder; therefore gangrene of the gallbladder is rare.

40. e.   The left and right gastroepiploic arteries supply the lower greater curvature and are the most likely source of bleeding. The left gastroepiploic artery originates from the splenic artery, while the right gastroepiploic artery is a terminal branch of the gastroduodenal artery. The fundus and upper left side of the greater curvature is supplied by the short gastric arteries. The lesser curvature is supplied from branches of the left and right gastric arteries, which originate from the coeliac trunk and hepatic artery, respectively.

41. d.   In a Hartmann's procedure the sigmoid colon is resected and the rectum is sewn shut and left as a stump, or in certain cases brought out of the wound as a mucus fistula. The descending colon/proximal sigmoid colon is brought out as a stoma in the left lower quadrant (LLQ); the perforation and associated contamination have made it unsafe to join the remaining pieces together. This can later potentially be reversed in certain circumstances. A permanent end colostomy can also be brought out in the LLQ after abdominoperineal resection. Stomas in the right lower quadrant are normally ileostomies (loop or end depending on circumstances). If present in the right upper quadrant the stoma is most likely a defunctioning transverse colostomy.

42. e. The Lanz incision is a transverse incision across McBurney's point (1/3 distance from anterior superior iliac spine to umbilicus) and is deemed cosmetically better. The rectus abdominal muscle is in the centre of the abdomen; your Lanz incision is lateral to this. The layers of the abdominal wall you will cut through from superficial to deep are:

- Skin
- Superficial fascia – Scarpa's fascia
- Deep fascia – Camper's fascia
- Muscles and fascia – external oblique, internal oblique and transverse abdominis muscles
- Peritoneum

43. b. The femoral nerve is the largest branch of the lumbar plexus originating from the posterior roots of L2, 3 and 4. The nerve traverses behind the inguinal ligament after sending a motor branch to the iliacus muscle. It lies lateral to the femoral sheath within the femoral triangle. The nerve is divided into a superficial and deep branch by the lateral femoral circumflex artery. The superficial branch supplies the sartorius muscle together with cutaneous supply of the thigh (medial and intermediate cutaneous branches). The deep branch supplies the quadratus femoris muscle, and the terminal cutaneous branch continues on as the saphenous nerve supplying the medial aspect of the leg and foot.

Damage to the femoral nerve caused by penetrating trauma classically causes wasting and loss of function of the quadriceps muscles. The patient has difficulty standing and walking and in particular finds it difficult to climb stairs. Severe sciatic nerve damage is normally associated with dislocations of the hip joint; the resulting manifestations are complete anaesthesia below the knee.

44. d. A varicocele is an abnormal enlargement of the pampiniform venous plexus within the scrotum. Symptoms include a dragging discomfort or heaviness within the scrotum. Varicoceles may be idiopathic due to a valvular disorder within the plexus or secondary due to compression of the venous drainage system of the testicle. An abdominal or pelvic malignancy should always be excluded in men presenting with a new onset unilateral varicocele. Common causes include renal cell carcinoma and retroperitoneal fibrosis.

If the ilioinguinal nerve is cut, one suffers with sensory loss in the scrotum. Damage to the vas deferens results in reduced fertility, so patients who plan on having further children should be made aware of this when consenting for the procedure. Testicular artery damage results in ischaemia of the testicles.

45. a. The splenic artery runs in the gastrosplenic ligament; this gives rise to the short gastric arteries which supply the fundus in addition to the superior part of the greater curvature. Branches of the left and right gastric arteries supply the lesser curvature of the stomach. The gastroduodenal artery gives rise to the right gastroepiploic artery and the splenic artery gives rise to the left gastroepiploic artery. Both the right and left gastroepiploic arteries supply the inferior portion of the greater curvature of the stomach.

46. a. Billroth I involves removal of the distal third of the stomach (pylorus) with an end-to-end or end-to-side anastomosis of the proximal stomach to the duodenum. This technique was previously used for the management of peptic ulcer disease and is still used today for malignancy.

Resection of the distal two-thirds of stomach and anastomosis to the jejunum is known as a Billroth II procedure; this leaves a blind-ended duodenal loop. This procedure again is performed for refractory peptic ulcer disease or malignancy. A Roux-en-Y reconstruction involves performing a subtotal gastrectomy while restoring intestinal continuity. This can be performed as part of a resection for malignancy or part of a gastric bypass for obesity.

47. e. An abdominal aortic aneurysm is a localized dilatation of the abdominal aorta to a diameter of greater than 3 cm or more than 50% larger than normal. Symptoms of rupture include abdominal/back pain and a loss of consciousness. Risk factors for developing aneurysms include smoking, hypertension, atherosclerosis and certain genetic conditions. The UK small aneurysms trial (Schermerhorn and Cronenwett, *J Vasc Surg.* 2001;33(2):443.) showed a benefit in repair of abdominal aortic aneurysm (AAA) when it becomes larger than 5.5 cm. It is unlikely that an aneurysm will rupture if smaller than this. Repair of AAAs can be performed open or via an endovascular approach. Early complications include limb/intestinal ischaemia, myocardial infarction with false aneurysms and aortoduodenal fistulae late complications following open repair.

Thoracic aortic aneurysms make up approximately 25% of all aortic aneurysms. Thoracic aortic aneurysms do rupture and often are a cause of sudden death in patients with mortality rates of between 50 and 80% reported.

48. d. A spleen, if palpable, can sometimes be palpated in the lower abdomen, hence the reason why examination for the spleen should begin with palpation in the right iliac fossa. The splenic notch is not always palpable, and it is sometimes difficult to distinguish between a spleen and a large kidney. You should be unable to get above a spleen and it should not be ballotable. The kidney should also be resonant to percussion due to the overlying colon, while the spleen should be dull.

Niemann–Pick syndrome is a lysosomal storage disease known for hypersplenism, defined as splenomegaly plus reduced levels of one or more blood cell elements plus correction of the cytopenia following splenectomy. Trauma is not always an indication for splenectomy.

49. e. The blood supply to the stomach may be summarized as follows:

- Coeliac plexus
  - Left gastric artery
  - Splenic artery
    - Short gastric arteries
    - Left gastroepiploic artery
  - Hepatic artery
    - Right gastric artery
    - Cystic artery
    - Gastroduodenal artery
      - Superior pancreaticoduodenal artery
      - Right gastroepiploic artery

50. a. The kidneys are retroperitoneal organs, the right lying lower than the left; posterior relations include the psoas and quadratus lumborum muscles, the subcostal, ilioinguinal and iliohypogastric nerves and the 11th and 12th ribs. Gerota's fascia encloses the perinephric fat, which itself encloses the fibrous renal capsule; it is deficient inferiorly, which is significant in the spread of infection.

Anterior relations of the right kidney include the 2nd part of the duodenum (D2), the liver and the hepatic flexure of the colon. Anterior relations of the left kidney include the stomach, the pancreas, the splenic flexure of the colon and the spleen. The structures of the hilum comprise the renal vein, artery, ureter and artery (in this order) from anterior to posterior. The left testicular vein drains into the left renal vein (which accounts for the increased incidence of varicocele on the left). The right testicular vein drains directly into the inferior vena cava.

51. c. The ureters are retroperitoneal along their entire course. They descend on psoas major, *over* the genitofemoral nerve, *under* the gonadal vessels. There is a point of narrowing as the ureters cross the pelvic brim at the pelviureteric junction. The ureters run *over* the external iliac artery/vein and *under* the vas deferens. There are three distinct points of narrowing of the ureter during its course: the ureteropelvic junction, the crossing of the iliac vessels and the ureterovesical junction.

52. b. The boundaries of the femoral triangle can be summarized as follows:

- Lateral: Medial border sartorial muscle
- Medial: Medial border adductor longus muscle
- Superior: Inguinal ligament
- Floor: Iliopsoas, pectineus and adductor longus muscles
- Roof: Fascia lata

The femoral artery lies at the *mid-inguinal point* (i.e. midway between the superior anterior iliac spine and the pubic symphysis). Contents of the femoral triangle include:

- Femoral nerve, artery, vein (lateral to medial, in the femoral sheath)
- Great saphenous vein
- Deep inguinal lymph nodes

53. d. The boundaries of the femoral canal, which is a small gap at the medial aspect of the femoral sheath, can be summarized as follows:

- Anterior – inguinal ligament
- Posterior – pectineal ligament
- Medial – lacunar ligament
- Lateral – femoral vein

The canal contains fat and Cloquet's lymph node; the canal has two primary functions:

1. A lymphatic drainage for the lower limb
2. A space to accommodate for femoral vein distension

54. c.   The levels of the abdominal aorta arterial branches are as follows:

- Inferior mesenteric artery: L3
- Iliac arteries: L4
- Renal artery: L2
- Coeliac trunk: T12
- Superior mesenteric artery: L1
- Adrenal artery: T12
- Gonadal artery: L2/3

55. c.   Characteristics of the jejunum:

- Represents two-fifths of the small bowel
- Tendency to lie at the umbilical region
- Comparatively redder
- Wider bore
- Thick wall
- Valvulae conniventes
- Plicae circularis
- Fewer arcades in mesentery
- Mesentery lies relatively superiorly, attached to left aorta
- Tall villi, with tall crypts

Characteristics of the ileum:

- Represents three-fifths of the small bowel
- Tendency to lie at the suprapubic region
- Comparatively pinker
- Thin bore
- Peyer's patches (aggregates of lymphoid tissue)
- Mesentery lies relatively inferiorly, attached to right aorta
- Villi short, with short crypts

56. c.   The transpyloric plane of Addison (L1) lies halfway between the suprasternal notch and the pubis. The plane passes through the pancreatic neck, duodenojejunal junction, pylorus, fundus of the gallbladder, hila of the kidneys, origin of the superior mesenteric artery from the abdominal aorta, root of the transverse mesocolon and tip of the 9th costal cartilage. This level also corresponds to the termination of the spinal cord.

57. a.   The centrally lying median umbilical fold contains the median umbilical ligament (remains of the urachus). On each side are the medial umbilical ligaments containing the remains of the umbilical artery, with the further laterally placed lateral umbilical folds containing the inferior epigastric vessels which enter the rectus sheath.

58. a.   The spermatic cord is comprised of:

- *Three fascia* – external spermatic (from external oblique), cremasteric (from internal oblique) and internal spermatic (from transversalis fascia)
- *Three arteries* – testicular (from aorta), cremasteric (from inferior epigastric artery) and artery of the vas (from inferior vesical artery)

- *Three nerves* – nerve to the cremaster (from genitofemoral nerve), sympathetic fibres and ilioinguinal nerve (on the cord)
- *Three other structures* – the pampiniform plexus, the vas deferens and lymphatics draining the testis to aortic lymph nodes

59. b.   The renal veins lie behind the pancreas and in front of the renal arteries. They join the vena cava at right angles at the level of L2 vertebra. The left renal vein is approximately three times longer than the right crossing anterior to the aorta. The left renal vein receives both the left suprarenal and gonadal veins and occasionally the inferior phrenic vein together with the left 2nd lumbar vein. The right renal vein usually only drains the right kidney with the above branches draining directly into the inferior vena cava. Each renal vein also often has a branch draining the ureter.

60. b.   A Meckel's diverticulum is a vestigial remnant of the vitello-intestinal duct. It is a true diverticulum involving all three layers of the small bowel. Generally it is found in 2% of individuals and is often approximately 2 in. long. It always arises on the antimesenteric border of the ileum and a majority are found within 100 cm of the ileocaecal valve. Heterotopic gastric mucosa or less often heterotopic pancreatic tissue may be present. Blood supply is derived from an ileal branch from the superior mesenteric artery. The risk of complications varies from 4% to 25% including haemorrhage, ulceration, small bowel obstruction (intussusception or volvulus) or diverticulitis.

61. c.   The greater sciatic notch lies between the posterior inferior iliac spine and ischial spine. The foramen is created by the sacrospinous ligament. The notch provides passage to the piriformis muscle, the superior and inferior gluteal nerves and vessels, the sciatic and posterior femoral cutaneous nerve, the internal pudendal vessels and the pudendal nerve.

The superior gluteal nerve (L4, L5, S1) passes through the greater sciatic notch together with the superior gluteal vessels and supplies both gluteus medius and minimus ending in the tensor fasciae latae. Only the superior gluteal nerve and vessels pass through the notch above piriformis; the remaining structures pass below the muscle.

The inferior gluteal nerve (L5, S1, S2) supplies gluteus maximus. The nerve to obturator internus (L5, S1, S2) supplies the superior gamellus. The pudendal nerve (S2, S3, S4) supplies the pelvic floor and perineum. The posterior femoral cutaneous nerve (S1, S2, S3) on the sciatic nerve supplies deep fascia and skin from the buttock to midcalf.

62. e.   The epiploic foramen of Winslow is a vertical slit at the right border of the lesser sac, representing the communication between the greater and lesser sacs. The boundaries are as follows:

- Superiorly – caudate process of the liver
- Inferiorly – first part of the duodenum
- Anteriorly – free edge of the lesser omentum containing the common bile duct, the hepatic artery and the portal vein
- Posteriorly – the inferior vena cava

63. b. The inguinal canal represents the passage taken through the lower abdominal wall by the testis and cord or round ligament. It is 4–6 cm in length, passing inferiorly and medially from the deep to the superficial inguinal rings, lying above the inguinal ligament.

- Anterior – skin, superficial fascia, external oblique aponeurosis
- Posterior – conjoint tendon
- Superior – internal oblique and transversus abdominis
- Inferior – inguinal ligament

64. e. The anal canal is an extraperitoneal structure of between 3 and 5 cm in length, with 2/3 above the dentate line and 1/3 below. The dentate line represents the junction between the embryonic hindgut and the proctodeum.

Above dentate line:

- Lined by columnar epithelium
- Arterial supply – superior rectal artery (branch of inferior mesenteric)
- Venous drainage – inferior mesenteric vein
- Autonomic sensory nerve supply – sympathetic (pelvic plexus) and parasympathetic (pelvic splanchnic nerves)
- Lymphatic drainage to the internal iliac nodes
- Anal columns present

Below dentate line:

- Lined by squamous epithelium
- Arterial supply – inferior rectal artery (branch of internal pudendal)
- Venous drainage – internal pudendal vein
- Somatic innervation – inferior rectal branch of pudendal nerve
- Lymphatic drainage into superficial inguinal nodes
- No anal columns present

65. d. The portal venous system drains blood to the liver emptying into the systemic venous circulation via the hepatic vein. It is formed behind the neck of the pancreas in the transpyloric plane by the joining of the splenic and superior mesenteric veins. The inferior mesenteric vein drains into the splenic vein. The portal vein ascends behind the first part of the duodenum into the anterior wall of the foramen of Winslow and to the porta hepatis. Here it divides into right and left branches and capillaries. The capillaries drain into the radicles of the hepatic vein, emptying into the inferior vena cava.

66. d. The adult bladder in located in the anterior pelvis. It is separated from the pubic symphysis by the prevesical space (retropubic). The dome is covered by peritoneum and the neck is fixed by the pelvic fascia and true pelvic ligaments.

The bladder lies in the true pelvis acting as a distensible reservoir with muscular walls. In males the seminal vesicles, vas deferens, ureters and rectum lie inferoposteriorly to the bladder, with the retropubic space anteriorly. In females the posterior peritoneal reflection is continuous with the uterus and vagina making the vesicouterine pouch. The lateral relations of the bladder are the levator ani and obturator internus muscles.

67. e. Rectus abdominis arises by two heads: a medial head from the front of the pubic symphysis and a lateral head from the upper border of the pubic crest. The two muscles are separated from each other by the linea alba. They insert onto the front of the fifth to seventh costal cartilages. There are typically three tendinous insertions found in the muscle – at the xiphisternum, the umbilicus and in between. Blood supply is from the superior and inferior epigastric arteries together with the lower intercostal. The muscles are innervated by the thoracoabdominal nerves. Actions of the rectus muscle include flexing the trunk and depressing the ribs.

68. d. The male urethra consists of prostatic, membranous and spongy parts. The total length is approximately 20 cm. The proximal urethra and trigone of the bladder develop from the lower ends of the mesonephric ducts with the rest from the urogenital sinus. The urethra is narrowest at the external meatus with dilatations present in the prostatic part, bulb and navicular fossa. The distal part of the spongy urethra is lined with stratified squamous epithelium.

69. d. The inferior epigastric artery arises from the external iliac artery above the inguinal ligament. It runs obliquely, medial to the deep inguinal ring, piercing the transversalis fascia. It runs superiorly entering the rectus sheath below the arcuate line, running deep to rectus abdominis. It supplies the rectus abdominis muscle and the medial aspect of the anterolateral abdominal wall. Superiorly, it anastomoses with the superior epigastric artery, a branch of the internal thoracic artery, above the umbilicus. The inferior epigastric artery is a landmark in distinguishing between inguinal hernias, with indirect hernias originating lateral to the vessel, and direct hernias originating medially to the artery.

Care must be taken during port placement in laparoscopic surgery as the vessel can easily be punctured.

70. c. The rectus sheath enveloping rectus abdominis can be divided into anterior and posterior layers consisting of the external and internal oblique aponeurosis and the transversus abdominis aponeurosis. The composition of the anterior and posterior layer varies in the abdominal wall. Above the costal margin, there is only an anterior sheath of the external oblique aponeurosis. Below the costal margin, the anterior sheath consists of the external oblique aponeurosis. The internal oblique aponeurosis splits to wrap the rectus abdominis, and the transversus abdominis aponeurosis lies posteriorly. The arcuate line demarcates where the internal oblique and transversus abdominis aponeurosis both lie anterior to the rectus abdominis.

71. e. Spigelian hernias occur between the rectus abdominis muscle medially and the semilunar line laterally. The semilunar line is formed by the internal and external oblique aponeurosis, and the transversus abdominis aponeurosis. The hernia most commonly occurs below the arcuate line as this demarcates where the internal oblique and transversus abdominis aponeurosis both lie – anterior to the rectus abdominis – and is therefore an area of weakness. They make up 0.12% of abdominal wall hernias. They are more often seen on the right side commonly between the 5th and 7th decades of life. Diagnosis can often be difficult and an ultrasound or a computed tomography scan may be required. The hernia can be repaired open or laparoscopically, the latter having the benefit of a better view and the ability to place an extraperitoneal mesh. The hernia is usually small with a high risk of strangulation.

72. d.　The splenic vein drains into the portal vein. The splenic artery derives from the coeliac artery and gives rise to branches to the greater curvature of the stomach and the pancreas. The splenic artery gives rise to the short gastric artery, which supplies the upper part of the greater curvature of the stomach. The splenic artery also gives rise to the left gastroepiploic artery, which supplies the upper part of the greater curvature. This vessel anastomoses with the right gastroepiploic artery, which arises from the gastroduodenal artery. Splenic artery aneurysm is the most common visceral artery aneurysm.

73. e.　The adrenal gland is usually supplied by three adrenal arteries: superior, middle and inferior. These are derived from the inferior phrenic artery, abdominal aorta and renal artery, respectively. The adrenal gland drains into one adrenal vein. On the left, the adrenal vein empties into the left renal vein, and on the right, it empties into the inferior vena cava. The adrenal gland consists of the cortex and medulla. The cortex can be divided into the zona glomerulosa (mineralocorticoids), fasciculate (glucocorticoids) and reticularis (gonadocorticoids), where the zona glomerulosa forms the outer and the zona reticularis the inner layer.

74. d.　The portal vein is approximately 8 cm long which travels toward the liver dividing into left (supplies segments II, III and IV) and right branches, the latter dividing into anterior (supplies segments V and VIII) and posterior (supplies segments VI and VII) branches. It is formed by the joining of the superior mesenteric vein and the splenic vein posterior to the neck of the pancreas. Occasionally the portal vein directly communicates with the inferior mesenteric vein, although rare. The cystic vein and right and left gastric veins drain into the portal vein. The short gastric veins and the left gastroepiploic vein drain into the splenic vein. The right gastroepiploic vein drains into the superior mesenteric vein.

75. b.　The portal vein is approximately 8 cm long which ascends anterior to the inferior vena cava toward the liver dividing into left (supplies segments II, III and IV) and right branches, the latter dividing into anterior (supplies segments V and VIII) and posterior (supplies segments VI and VII) branches. It is formed by the joining of the superior mesenteric vein and the splenic vein posterior to the neck of the pancreas. The portal vein does not contain any valves. About 75% of hepatic blood flow is derived from the portal vein and the remainder is from the hepatic arteries.

76. c.　The lesser omentum connects the lesser curvature of the stomach and the proximal part of the duodenum to the fissure of the ligamentum venosum of the liver. It forms the hepatoduodenal ligament laterally containing the portal triad (hepatic artery, portal vein and bile duct). The lesser sac (omental bursa) lies posterior to the stomach and joins the greater peritoneal sac via the omental foramen. This opens posterior to the hepatoduodenal ligament. Compression of this area during liver/biliary surgery is useful to stem bleeding and is known as Pringle's manoeuvre. The lesser omentum is supplied by the right and left gastric arteries.

77. d. The lesser sac (omental bursa) lies posterior to the stomach and joins the greater peritoneal sac via the omental foramen. The boundaries of the omental foramen are as follows:

- Anteriorly: Portal vein, hepatic artery, bile duct
- Posteriorly: Inferior vena cava, right crus of diaphragm covered with parietal peritoneum (retroperitoneal)
- Superiorly: Caudate lobe of liver covered with visceral peritoneum
- Inferiorly: First part of duodenum, portal vein, hepatic artery and bile duct

78. a. The uterine artery is derived from the anterior division of the internal iliac artery and descends on the lateral wall of the pelvis, anterior to the internal iliac artery. It gives off branches to the uterus, vagina, ovary and fallopian tube. The uterine artery lies anterior and superior to the ureter near the lateral part of the vaginal fornix. It commonly anastomoses with the ovarian artery.

79. d. The ureter has an internal pacemaker controlling peristalsis but also receives supply from the autonomic system. Thoracolumbar preganglionic nerves synapse with both the aorticorenal and inferior/superior hypogastric sympathetic plexuses before innervating the ureter. Parasympathetic supply is derived from S2–4 segments. Pain referred to the cutaneous area innervated by spinal cord segments T11–L2. The obturator nerve is responsible for sensory innervation of the skin of the medial aspect of the thigh.

80. b. The ureter is a retroperitoneal structure. In the pelvis, the ureter runs anterior to the internal iliac arteries and passes into the bladder at an oblique angle. The inferior end of the ureters is surrounded by the vesical venous plexus. Its arterial supply is derived from the abdominal aorta and renal and gonadal arteries. Venous drainage is via the renal and gonadal veins. The testicular artery lies anterior to the ureter. The ductus deferens crosses superior to the ureter near the posterolateral angle of the bladder. There are two layers of spiral muscle in the ureter wall.

81. c. Normal testicular development begins in utero at the mesodermal ridge on the posterior abdominal wall. At 7 months the testes reach the inguinal canal and by 9 months descend within the scrotum. The testicles can fail to descend into the scrotum and may have stopped along their line of descent, or be completely ectopic. In maldescended testes, they may be intra-abdominal, within the inguinal canal, within the superficial inguinal ring or on top of the scrotum. Testes are deemed ectopic if they deviate from the normal path. They may lie in the superficial inguinal pouch, perineal, abdominal or femoral region or be positioned at the base of the penis.

82. e. The prostate gland lies between the bladder and urogenital diaphragm. It consists of five lobes: two lateral, anterior, posterior and middle. The urethra can be divided into three sections: prostatic, membranous and cavernous. The membranous urethra is the shortest section lying between the prostatic apex and bulb of the urethra, perforating the urogenital diaphragm. Females have Skene's glands that are homologous with the male prostate gland, and some describe them as the female prostate.

83. b. The tunica vasculosa is a vascular layer that forms the innermost layer adjacent to the testes. The tunica albuginea is a dense fibrous membrane that covers the testes. The tunica vaginalis is a closed peritoneal sac partially surrounding the testicle. The visceral layer is closely applied to the testes, epididymis and inferior part of the ductus deferens. The parietal layer is adhered to the internal spermatic fascia and is separated from the visceral layer by a small amount of fluid.

84. a. The layers of the scrotum and testicular covering, from superficial to deep, are skin, dartos fascia and dartos muscle, external spermatic fascia, cremaster muscle, cremasteric fascia, internal spermatic fascia and tunica vaginalis. The dartos fascia and muscle are closely related to the skin. Contraction of the dartos muscle and fascia causes the scrotal skin to wrinkle.

85. b. The cremasteric muscle is dependent on nerve roots L1 and L2. It is innervated by the genital branch of the genitofemoral nerve. The reflex is elicited by stroking the superior and medial aspect of the thigh causing the cremaster to retract the testes. The cremaster muscle covers the spermatic cord and testes and is derived from the internal oblique muscle.

86. a. Rugae are the mucosal folds present in the stomach, which disappear on distension, and hence are not permanent. Plicae circularis are circular folds of mucous membrane and are permanent (not obliterated by distension). The spiral valve of Heister is formed by the mucosal folds at the terminal opening of cystic duct into the common hepatic duct to form the common bile duct. It is not a true valve but is permanent and narrows down the lumen of cystic duct at the terminal end. When the duct is distended, the spaces between the folds become dilated making the folds more obvious. Transverse rectal folds are permanent mucosal folds and are more marked during rectal distension. They are also called Houston's valves or plicae transversalis.

87. a. Colonic lymphatic drainage terminally reaches superior and inferior mesenteric lymph nodes, which belong to the pre-aortic lymph nodes. Lymph from colon passes through four sets of lymph nodes: epicolic (lie on the serosal wall of gut) → paracolic (on medial side of ascending/descending colon and mesenteric border of transverse/sigmoid colon) → intermediate (on named branches of colonic vessels) → preterminal/pre-aortic (on inferior/superior mesenteric vessels). The efferents from the pre-aortic lymph nodes drain into the coeliac lymph nodes (terminal), which also belong to the pre-aortic category. Coeliac lymph nodes then drain into the intestinal trunks, which ultimately join the cisterna chyli.

88. b. The mucosal lining on the base of the bladder is smooth and firmly attached to the underlying smooth muscle coat of the wall, unlike elsewhere in the bladder where the mucosa is folded and loosely attached to the wall.

89. d. The costovertebral ligament is a strong fascial attachment between the transverse process of the first and second lumbar vertebrae and the inferior margin of the 12th rib. It is encountered only in posterior approaches to the kidney and it can be incised to produce a greater degree of mobility of the 12th rib, thus providing greater exposure and access to the structures that reside within the upper portion of the retroperitoneum.

90. d.   The male urethra is approximately 20 cm long and the narrowest parts are the external urethral orifice, bladder neck and just proximal to the navicular fossa. The seminal colliculus are present in the prostatic urethra at the verumontanum. The prostatic urethra is the widest and most dilatable part of the entire male urethra.

91. a.   A posterior gastric ulcer may adhere to and ulcerate the splenic artery as this runs along the upper border of the pancreas, resulting in a significant haemorrhage. A lesser curve gastric ulcer may implicate the left gastric artery – the gastroepiploic vessels lie along the greater curve of the stomach. A posterior duodenal ulcer may erode the gastroduodenal branch of the right gastric artery – 'the ulcer of duodenal haemorrhage'. The inferior pancreaticoduodenal artery supplies the lower part of the second part of the duodenum, well clear of the site of ulceration. Oesophageal varices commonly extend into the upper stomach and are venous in origin.

92. d.   The general structure of the male pelvis is heavier and thicker than the female pelvis and has more prominent bone markings. The female pelvis is wider, shallower and has both a larger superior and inferior pelvic aperture. The ischial tuberosities are farther apart in the female pelvis because of the wider pubic arch, and the sacrum is less curved in the female pelvis. In addition to this, the obturator foramina are round in the male and oval in the female.

93. a.   The renal veins drain into the inferior vena cava (remember the renal vein is longer on the left). The superior and inferior mesenteric veins, along with the splenic vein, join to form the portal vein and drain proximally into the liver rather than directly into the inferior vena cava.

94. a.   Portosystemic anastomosis refers to the portal venous system draining the liver and spleen and systemic venous circulation. The sites of collaterals between portal and systemic circulation occur at:

- The gastroesophageal junction around the cardia of the stomach, where the left gastric vein and its tributaries form a portosystemic anastomosis with tributaries to the azygos system of veins of the caval system
- The anus – the superior rectal vein of the portal system anastomoses with the middle and inferior rectal veins of the systemic venous system
- The anterior abdominal wall around the umbilicus – the para-umbilical veins anastomose with veins on the anterior abdominal wall.

95. b.   The arterial supply to the stomach comes predominantly from the coeliac axis. The left gastric artery arises directly from the coeliac axis. The splenic artery gives origin to the short gastric arteries as well as the left gastroepiploic artery and may occasionally give origin to a posterior gastric artery. The hepatic artery gives origin to the right gastric artery and the gastroduodenal artery, which in turn gives origin to the right gastroepiploic artery. The short gastric arteries arise from the splenic artery at the hilum of the spleen and pass forward in the gastrosplenic ligament to supply the fundus.

96. a.   Contents of the spermatic cord include the vas deferens, artery to the vas, testicle and cremasteric muscle, and pampiniform plexus. Lymph drainage is to the para-aortic lymph nodes. The sympathetic nerves and the genital branch of the genitofemoral nerve supplying the cremaster muscle are also contained within the spermatic cord. The ilioinguinal nerve, which supplies the skin at the root of the penis, does not run within the spermatic cord.

97. c. Direct hernias lie medial to the inferior epigastric artery. Femoral hernias are below and lateral to the pubic tubercle, whereas inguinal hernias lie above and medial to it. The midpoint of the inguinal ligament lies halfway between the anterior–superior iliac spine and the pubic tubercle. The deep inguinal ring typically lies 1.5 cm above this. Of note, the mid-inguinal point lies halfway from the pubic symphysis to the anterior–superior iliac spine and is a useful landmark for the femoral artery. Indirect hernias are more likely to extend into the scrotum because of their close relation with the spermatic cord and can be the result of a patent processus vaginalis.

98. e. Branches of the abdominal aorta can be divided into paired and unpaired. Paired branches include the suprarenal, renal, gonadal, inferior phrenic and lumbar arteries. The origin of the inferior phrenic arteries varies and can either arise from the aorta directly or from the coeliac trunk. Unpaired branches include the coeliac trunk, superior and inferior mesenteric arteries and the median sacral artery. The branches of the thoracic aorta include bronchial, pericardial, posterior intercostal, superior phrenic, oesophageal, mediastinal and subcostal arteries. The coeliac trunk is part of the abdominal aorta, branching into the common hepatic, left gastric and splenic arteries.

99. e. The pancreas is a retroperitoneal structure, the body of which lies over L2, and forms from the embryonic foregut. The uncinate process extends medially from the left of the pancreatic head posterior to the superior mesenteric artery. The arterial blood supply to the body and tail is derived from the splenic artery, whereas the head is supplied by the gastroduodenal arteries and branches of the superior mesenteric artery. The splenic vein joins the superior mesenteric vein posterior to the neck of the pancreas to form the portal vein. The main pancreatic duct begins in the tail and joins with the bile duct to drain into the duodenum. In 5% of the population they drain separately. The accessory pancreatic duct drains the uncinate process and inferior part of the head opening into the duodenum at the minor duodenal papilla.

100. b. The pancreas is a retroperitoneal structure, the body of which lies over L2, and forms from the embryonic foregut. The uncinate process extends medially from the left of the pancreatic head posterior to the superior mesenteric artery. The arterial blood supply to the body and tail is derived from the splenic artery, whereas the head is supplied by the gastroduodenal arteries and branches of the superior mesenteric artery. The splenic vein joins the superior mesenteric vein posterior to the neck of the pancreas to form the portal vein. The main pancreatic duct begins in the tail and joins with the bile duct to drain into the duodenum. In 5% of the population they drain separately. The accessory pancreatic duct drains the uncinate process and inferior part of the head opening into the duodenum at the minor duodenal papilla.

101. c. The pancreatic tail and the first part of the duodenum are intraperitoneal structures. The remainder of the pancreas is described as retroperitoneal.

Other retroperitoneal structures include the aorta, second and third segments of the duodenum, ureters, bladder and kidneys, rectum and inferior vena cava.

102. d. The second part of the duodenum is situated at the L2–L3 vertebrae. The pancreatic and bile ducts drain into the medial side of the second part of the duodenum. The hilum of the right kidney lies posteriorly with the renal vessels and ureter, and the right psoas major muscle. The transverse colon lies anteriorly to the second part of the duodenum.

103. d. The third part of the duodenum is a retroperitoneal structure that lies horizontally. Anterior to the duodenum lies the superior mesenteric artery and vein. Posteriorly lies the right psoas major muscle, inferior vena cava, aorta and right ureter. Superiorly lies the head and uncinate process of the pancreas, and the superior mesenteric vessels. The ligament of Treitz supports the duodenojejunal flexure and attaches at the third and fourth parts of the duodenum.

104. d. The coeliac trunk divides into the left gastric, splenic and common hepatic arteries. The splenic artery branches into the left gastro-omental artery and short gastric arteries. The right gastro-omental artery is a branch of the gastroduodenal artery which arises, like the right gastric artery, from the common hepatic artery. The left gastric artery also supplies the distal portion of the oesophagus.

105. a. Intraoperative cholangiograms are used after the surgeon has successfully dissected out Calot's triangle and identified the cystic duct and artery. A small incision is made in the cystic duct through which a catheter is introduced. Radio-opaque dye is flushed through the catheter to highlight the biliary tree. Intraoperative cholangiograms are useful to identify any bile leak, distal occlusion and normal biliary tree anatomy and to ensure that the cystic duct has been correctly identified before it is fully transected.

106. b. The ascending colon is supplied by the ileocolic and right colic arteries, which are branches of the superior mesenteric artery. Other branches of the superior mesenteric artery include the middle colic artery supplying the transverse colon, intestinal arteries for the ileum and jejunum and inferior pancreatoduodenal artery. The venous drainage is into the portal vein.

107. b. The descending colon is the part of the colon from the splenic flexure to the brim of the pelvis, where it becomes the sigmoid colon. The sigmoid colon is supplied by several branches of the sigmoid artery. The inferior mesenteric artery terminates into the superior rectal artery. The marginal artery of Drummond is an anastomosis of the middle colic artery (a branch of the superior mesenteric artery) and the left colic artery (a branch of the inferior mesenteric artery). Venous drainage is via the inferior mesenteric vein, which most commonly drains into the splenic vein.

108. e. Anterior relations of the abdominal aorta include the body of the pancreas, splenic and left renal vein, the horizontal part of the duodenum, coils of the small intestine, the coeliac plexus and the ganglion. The left renal vein crosses the abdominal aorta anteriorly into the inferior vena cava. The right renal vein enters the inferior vena cava without crossing the aorta.

109. d. McBurney's point lies one-third of the way from the anterior–superior iliac spine and the umbilicus. At this point an incision can be made on the right side of the abdomen to perform an appendicectomy. There is risk of damage to the iliohypogastric nerve. If damaged, this increases the risk for a direct inguinal hernia owing to lack of innervation of the lower abdominal muscles resulting in weakness. The appendix usually lies retrocaecally. The mesoappendix containing the appendicular artery, a branch of the posterior caecal artery, is tied and ligated.

110. d. Calot's triangle was classically described as the common hepatic duct, cystic duct and cystic artery. Surgeons now use a modified version of this, the hepatobiliary triangle, to identify the cystic artery. The boundaries of this are the common bile duct, common hepatic duct and border of the liver. Correct identification of the cystic duct before full transection is required to prevent significant postoperative complications. Intraoperative cholangiogram has been used to show any damage to the common bile duct, distal blockage or bile leak. The gallbladder is mainly supplied arterially by the cystic artery, but it can also gain some blood supply from the liver bed.

111. b. The rectum is approximately 15 cm long and commences at the level of the third sacral vertebra. It passes through the pelvic diaphragm and is continuous with the anus. Peritoneum does not cover the lower third of the rectum; the middle third only has anterior peritoneal covering, whereas the upper third has anterior and lateral peritoneal coverings. The mucous membrane forms three transverse folds.

112. b. The rectum has a good blood supply from the superior, middle and inferior rectal arteries, which are branches of the inferior mesenteric, internal iliac and internal pudendal arteries, respectively. Venous drainage corresponds exactly to the arterial supply. For example, the superior rectal vein drains to the inferior mesenteric vein. Lymph drains to the pararectal nodes.

113. c. Contents of the spermatic cord can be remembered by classifying them into the following categories:

- *Three arteries:* Testicular artery, cremasteric artery and artery to the vas deferens
- *Three other vessels:* Pampiniform plexus, vas deferens and lymphatics
- *Three layers of fascia:* External spermatic fascia from external oblique aponeurosis, cremasteric fascia from the internal oblique aponeurosis and internal spermatic fascia from the transversalis fascia
- *Two nerves:* Genital branch of the genitofemoral nerve and sympathetic nerve fibres

The ilioinguinal nerve travels alongside the spermatic cord but not within it.

114. e. Several structures are transmitted via the greater sciatic foramen, including the sciatic nerve and the piriformis muscle. The superior and inferior gluteal nerves and vessels are transmitted above and below the piriformis muscle, respectively. Other structures include the posterior cutaneous nerve of the thigh, nerve to the obturator internus, nerve to the quadratus femoris, and pudendal nerve and vessels (which then enter the perineum via the lesser sciatic foramen).

115. a. The arterial supply to the rectum is the superior rectal artery (branch of inferior mesenteric artery), middle rectal artery (branch of internal iliac artery), inferior rectal artery (branch of internal pudendal artery) and median sacral artery (branch of the aorta). Venous drainage of the rectum is into either the portal or systemic circulation. The superior rectal vein drains into the inferior mesenteric vein (portal circulation). The middle rectal vein drains into the internal iliac vein, and the inferior rectal vein drains into the internal pudendal vein (systemic circulation).

116. c. The perineal body is an irregular fibromuscular mass and lies in the midline between the anterior and posterior perineum. It attaches to the posterior border of the perineal membrane. The perineal body is the site of convergence of several muscles. They are the transverse perineal muscle (superficial and deep), bulbospongiosus, external anal sphincter and levator ani. The perineal body is especially important in women as it supports the pelvic viscera. Tearing or damage to the perineal body weakens the floor of the levator ani and may result in a prolapsed vagina.

117. a. The testicular arteries branch directly off the aorta inferior to the renal arteries. They pass retroperitoneally, crossing over the ureters and the external iliac arteries, and enter the inguinal canal, becoming part of the spermatic cord. The testicular artery anastomoses with the artery to the vas (which arises from the inferior vesical branch of the internal iliac artery). Owing to this anastomosis, ligation of the testicular artery does not lead to testicular atrophy. The testicular venules emerge from the testes and join to form a venous network called the pampiniform plexus. This plexus surrounds the testicular artery within the spermatic cord, and the cooler venous blood absorbs heat from arterial blood, keeping the temperature of the testes 1° lower than the trunk. The pampiniform plexus drains into the testicular vein at the deep inguinal ring. The right testicular vein drains directly into the IVC, whereas the left testicular vein drains into the left renal vein.

118. d. The anal canal is surrounded by a complex arrangement of muscles, including the internal and external anal sphincters. The internal anal sphincter is a thickening of the circular muscles of the rectum, composed of smooth muscle, and surrounds the upper two-thirds of the anal canal. It is an involuntary muscle supplied by the autonomic nervous system. The external anal sphincter surrounds the internal anal sphincter but extends further distally. It can be divided into three parts: deep, superficial and subcutaneous. The deep part blends superiorly with the puborectalis part of the levator ani. It has voluntary control and is supplied by the pudendal nerve (S2, S3) and the perineal branch of S4.

119. a. The spermatic cord gains its covering fascia as it penetrates the deep inguinal ring and enters the scrotum via the superficial inguinal ring. This occurs during development of the male foetus. The external spermatic fascia is derived from the external oblique aponeurosis. The middle cremasteric fascia is derived from the internal oblique, and the internal spermatic fascia is derived from the transversalis fascia.

UPPER LIMB, BREAST

120. e.   The intrinsic muscles of the hand supplied by the median nerve (C5–C7 lateral cord, C8, T1 medial cord) are the lateral two lumbricals, the opponens pollicis, the abductor pollicis brevis and the flexor pollicis brevis (these muscles are remembered by the acronym LOAF). The flexor pollicis longus is an extrinsic muscle of the hand supplied by the median nerve. Abductor pollicis longus is an extrinsic muscle of the hand supplied by the radial nerve. The median nerve supplies all the extrinsic flexor muscles of the hand and wrist except for the flexor carpi ulnaris and the ulnar half of the flexor digitorum profundus.

121. a.   The ulnar nerve (C8, T1) in the forearm supplies the flexor carpi ulnaris and the ulnar half of the flexor digitorum profundus. In the hand it supplies the hypothenar muscles (abductor digiti minimi, opponens digiti minimi and flexor digiti minimi), adductor pollicis, all the interossei and the ulnar two lumbricals. The median nerve supplies all of flexor digitorum superficialis.

122. a.   The musculocutaneous nerve (C5–C7) is a branch of the lateral cord of the brachial plexus. The function of the musculocutaneous nerve is to provide muscular innervation to biceps brachii, brachialis and coracobrachialis. It also provides cutaneous innervation to the lateral surface of the forearm via its continuation called the lateral cutaneous nerve of the forearm. Injuries to the musculocutaneous nerve can arise from direct trauma, for example a stab injury, or from violent separation of the neck and shoulder in a fall from a motorcycle or horse. Brachioradialis is supplied by the radial nerve and pronator teres is supplied by the median nerve.

123. b.   The axillary artery is split into three parts. The first part runs from the lateral border of the first rib to the medial border of pectoralis minor. The second part is deep to pectoralis minor. The third part is from the lateral border of pectoralis minor to the inferior border of teres major. The first part has one branch – superior thoracic. The second part has two branches – thoracoacromial and lateral thoracic. The third part has three branches – subscapular, anterior and posterior circumflex humeral. A mnemonic for remembering the order of the arteries from proximal to distal is 'send the Lord to say a prayer' (superior thoracic, thoracoacromial, lateral thoracic, subscapular, anterior circumflex humeral, posterior circumflex humeral).

124. e.   The four muscles of the rotator cuff are supraspinatus, infraspinatus, teres minor and subscapularis. The supraspinatus initiates abduction of the arm. Infraspinatus and teres minor laterally rotate the arm. Subscapularis medially rotates and adducts the arm. Teres major medially rotates and adducts the arm but is not part of the rotator cuff. The tendons of the four muscles blend with the joint capsule of the shoulder and therefore act as a musculotendinous support. The name *rotator cuff* stems from the fact that the muscles rotate the humerus and they all act as a cuff around the head of the humerus. A mnemonic for remembering the four muscles is SITS (supraspinatus, infraspinatus, teres minor and subscapularis).

125. a.   The rhomboid major and minor muscles originate from the spinous processes of the vertebrae and insert on to the medial border of the scapula. Both muscles slope superior to inferior with the rhomboid minor superior to its larger relative. The action of these muscles is to retract the scapula as well as rotate the scapula inferiorly and hold it to the chest wall. Abduction of the humerus is performed by supraspinatus and then deltoid. Adduction of the humerus is performed by pectoralis major, latissimus dorsi, teres major and subscapularis. Elevation of the scapula is carried out by levator scapulae and the superior fibres of trapezius. Medial rotation of the humerus is performed by subscapularis, pectoralis major, latissimus dorsi and the anterior fibres of the deltoid.

126. c.   The acromion forms the edge at the lateral extremity of the scapular spine. The deltoid covers the greater tuberosity of the humerus. The coracoid process, which is easily identified, lies immediately below the clavicle at the junction of the middle and outer thirds and is covered by the anterior fibres of the deltoid muscle. The medial border of the clavicle can be seen and the supraclavicular nerve may be able to be rolled against the clavicle during palpation of slim patients.

127. e.   An above-elbow back slab is the preferred method of holding a fracture until definitive management (i.e. operation). The anterior humeral line is important in radiologically assessing elbow fractures. Posterior fat pads, if visible, usually imply that a fracture has occurred. A hanging cast is employed in proximal humerus fractures and is not the first line in management of elbow fractures.

128. e.   A Bennett fracture is a fracture of the base of the first metacarpal, which may be associated with subluxation or dislocation of the first metacarpal phalangeal joint. The proximal pole of scaphoid may undergo avascular necrosis. Fractures of this bone may take a week to 10 days to be visible on X-ray. A mallet finger injury, whether bony or tendinous, is usually treated with a splint to hold the finger in extension.

129. e.   Neurapraxia is the mildest form of nerve injury. It does not involve loss of continuity and causes transient functional loss. Axonotmesis involves complete interruption of the nerve axon and surrounding myelin with preservation of the surrounding mesenchymal structures. The distal part of the nerve undergoes Wallerian degeneration, but the prognosis is often good as the uninjured mesenchymal latticework provides a path for axonal regeneration. Neurotmesis involves complete disconnection of a nerve; functional loss is complete.

Froment's sign is flexion of the interphalangeal joint of the thumb in order to resist removal of the piece of paper. This is caused by adductor pollicis weakness as a result of ulnar nerve damage and overcompensation by flexor pollicis longus supplied by the median nerve. Ulnar nerve entrapment can occur in Guyon's canal: the pisohamate tunnel at the wrist.

130. a.   The axillary artery starts at the border of the first rib as a continuation of the subclavian artery and continues as the brachial artery at the tip of teres minor. The axillary artery is split into three parts each giving off its own branches, which are:

First part – this extends from the lateral border of the first rub to the superior border of the pectoralis minor muscle, giving off the superior thoracic artery.

Second part – this is deep to pectoralis minor, giving off the thoracoacromial artery and the lateral thoracic artery.

Third part – this extends from the inferior border of pectoralis minor to the inferior border of teres major, giving off the subscapular, anterior and posterior circumflex humeral arteries.

131. c. The history gives a classical presentation of a Colles fracture. This is traditionally described as a transverse fracture of the radius within 1 in. (2.5 cm) from the radiocarpal joint, with a dorsally displaced and dorsally angulated distal fragment. Radial shortening may be present and the fracture may be comminuted. There may, or may not, be involvement of the ulna. An undisplaced fracture can be treated with a cast applied to the forearm in palmer flexion and ulnar deviation. With Colles fractures there is an associated ulna styloid fracture in 60% of cases. A scaphoid fracture is the most common associated carpal bone fracture and typically occurs when a patient has fallen on an outstretched hand or after a crush injury. There is focal tenderness in the anatomical snuffbox. Non-displaced scaphoid fractures can be treated in a thumb spica splint, whereas fractures greater than 1 mm displacement are at risk of non-union and avascular necrosis and would require internal fixation.

132. e. The axillary nerve is a branch of the posterior division of the brachial plexus and comes off at the level of the axilla. It carries fibres from C5 and C6 and supplies the deltoid and teres minor muscles. It can be damaged during dislocation of the shoulder – most commonly anterior dislocation or during manipulation to reduce the dislocation. Fractures of the surgical neck of humerus, which commonly occur in elderly osteoporotic women after a fall, leave the axillary nerve at risk of damage due to its proximity to the humerus at this level. The axillary nerve and posterior circumflex humeral artery both pass through the quadrangular space together. This is a theoretical space bordered superiorly by teres minor, inferiorly by teres major, medially by the long head of the triceps and laterally by the medial border of the humerus. Both these anatomical structures are in close proximity to the surgical neck of humerus and can be damaged in a fracture of the proximal humerus.

133. c. The long thoracic nerve of Bell (C5, C6, C7) supplies the serratus anterior muscle and is responsible for lateral rotation and protraction of the scapula. Owing to its long, relatively superficial course, it is susceptible to damage and can be damaged during breast surgery. Injuries can also result from direct trauma or stretch during sports. The winged scapula is most prominent when the patient pushes the outstretched arm against a wall. The thoracodorsal nerve, which innervates the latissimus dorsi muscle, is also vulnerable to injury during lymph node dissection. The serratus anterior originates from the external surface of ribs 1–8 laterally and inserts into the anteromedial border of the scapula. Pectoralis minor inserts into the coracoid process of the scapula, subclavius muscle inserts into the inferior surface of the clavicle at its middle third, and pectoralis major and teres major insert into the lateral lip and medial lip of the intertubercular groove of humerus, respectively.

134. d. The axilla is the space between the upper arm and thorax. It contains the axillary artery, axillary vein, brachial plexus, axillary lymph nodes, long thoracic nerve of Bell and thoracodorsal neurovascular bundle. The boundaries of the axilla include:

- Anteriorly: Pectoralis major and minor, subclavius
- Posteriorly: Subscapularis, teres major, latissimus dorsi
- Medially: Upper part of serratus anterior, ribs 1–4 with intercostal muscles
- Laterally: Bicipital groove
- Apex: Clavicle, 1st rib and upper border of scapula
- Floor: Axillary fascia from serratus anterior to deep fascia of the arm

135. e. Supraspinatus tendonitis is often associated with shoulder impingement syndrome. The condition is often seen in patients with glenohumeral instability caused by acromioclavicular joint disease or injury. Examination findings may include stiffness on internal and external rotation and a painful arc. The mainstay of treatment is physical therapy, and some patients gain relief with local injections of corticosteroids.

136. c. The breast overlies the second to the sixth ribs resting on both the pectoralis major and the serratus anterior. The arterial supply to the breast is from the lateral and acromiothoracic branches of the axillary artery, the perforating branches of the internal mammary artery and the lateral perforating branches of the intercostal arteries. Venous drainage is to the corresponding veins. Approximately 75% of the lymphatic drainage is to the axillary nodes, which are arranged into five groups: anterior, posterior, lateral, central and apical.

137. a. The anatomical snuffbox is a triangular deepening on the radial aspect of the hand at the level of the carpal bones. The anatomical relationships of the snuffbox include the abductor pollicis longus and extensor pollicis brevis radially, the extensor pollicis longus ulnarly and the radial artery along its floor. The cephalic vein also crosses the snuffbox arising from the dorsal venous complex. Subcutaneously terminal branches of the superficial branch of the radial nerve run across the roof.

A scaphoid fracture is characterized by tenderness when palpating in the anatomical snuffbox.

138. e. The ulnar artery is larger than the radial artery, both of which are branches of the brachial artery. The ulnar nerve lies ulnar to the artery at the flexor retinaculum. The artery is crossed by the median nerve superficially in the proximal forearm; the deep head of the pronator teres separates the two structures. The ulnar artery forms the superficial palmar arch at the wrist through an anastomosis with the radial artery. The ulnar artery becomes superficial in the distal forearm, lying between the muscle tendons of flexor digitorum superficialis and flexor carpi ulnaris.

139. d. The axillary lymph nodes drain the lymphatics of the breast, pectoral region, upper limb and upper abdominal wall. They are arranged into five groups: (1) anterior, (2) posterior, (3) lateral, (4) central and (5) apical. Metastatic axillary node spread is often defined in three levels:

1. Level I – nodes inferior to pectoralis minor
2. Level II – nodes behind pectoralis minor
3. Level III – nodes above pectoralis minor

140. d.   The suprascapular nerve arises from the upper trunk of the brachial plexus supplying both the supraspinatus and infraspinatus muscles. The plexus is formed from the anterior rami of spinal nerves forming five roots (C5–8, T1). Trunks are formed by the merging of the roots – upper (C5, 6), middle (C7), lower (C8, T1). The trunks then split into anterior and posterior divisions which then merge to form cords. The medial cord is formed by the anterior division of the lower trunk, the lateral cord by the anterior divisions of the upper and middle trunks and the posterior cord is formed from the posterior divisions of all three trunks.

141. e.   The coracohumeral ligament runs from the coracoid process to the front of the greater tubercle of the humerus. Providing support to the head of the humerus the coracoacromial ligament runs from the medial border of the acromion to the lateral border of the coracoid process. The suprascapular ligament bridges across the suprascapular notch and converts it into a foramen, which transmits the suprascapular nerve. The suprascapular vessels lie above the ligament. The spinoglenoid ligament bridges the spinoglenoid notch. The suprascapular vessels and nerve pass deep to it. The costoclavicular ligament joins the clavicle to the first costal cartilage and adjacent rib.

142. d.   The triangular space is an axillary space bounded by:

- Teres major inferiorly
- Long head of triceps laterally
- Teres minor superiorly

The triangular space contains the scapular circumflex vessels.

The quadrangular space is a clinically important space as space occupying lesions or trauma in this area may compress the axillary nerve or posterior circumflex artery. The quadrangular space is bounded by:

- Teres minor superiorly
- Teres major inferiorly
- Long head of triceps medially
- Surgical neck of the humerus laterally

143. a.   The thenar eminence is comprised of three muscles – abductor pollicis brevis, flexor pollicis brevis and opponens pollicis. All muscles are supplied by the recurrent branch of the median nerve. The hypothenar eminence is comprised of the abductor digiti minimi, flexor digiti minimi (brevis) and opponens digiti. All muscles are supplied by the deep branch of the ulnar nerve. The two ulnar lumbricals are innervated by the ulnar nerve and the two radial lumbricals by the median nerve. All interossei (palmar and dorsal) are supplied by the deep branch of the ulnar nerve.

144. e.   The carpal tunnel is formed anteriorly at the wrist by a deep arch formed by the carpal bones and the flexor retinaculum. The four tendons of the flexor digitorum profundus, the four tendons of the flexor digitorum superficialis and the tendon of the flexor pollicis longus pass through the carpal tunnel with the median nerve. The palmaris longus lies superficial and partially inserts in to the flexor retinaculum.

145. d. The scapular anastomosis maintains circulation to the upper limb in this clinical situation, which does not involve the superior thoracic artery. An occlusion of the subclavian artery distally, at the outer border of the first rib (e.g. cervical rib) or axillary artery proximally (e.g. axillary metastasis of carcinoma of breast), compromises blood supply to the upper limb. Collateral circulation (scapular) opens up to maintain the circulation to the upper limb. Scapular anastomosis involves branches of proximal subclavian and distal axillary arteries:

- *Subclavian artery* – thyrocervical trunk branches: suprascapular and deep branch of transverse cervical
- *Axillary artery* – subscapular, posterior circumflex humeral and thoracoacromial arteries

146. a. The fascia around the brachial plexus is called the axillary sheath and is a derivative of the prevertebral fascia (PVF). This covers the anterior vertebral muscles and lies on the anterior aspect of the scalenus anterior and medius, thus forming the floor of the posterior triangle of the neck. The brachial plexus and subclavian artery emerge between the scalenus anterior and medius in the neck and pass behind the clavicle to reach the axilla. In the process they carry an extension of PVF over them as a cover (the axillary sheath) toward the axilla. Most of the nerves in the neck are behind the PVF, but the spinal accessory nerve lies superficial to it and may quite often be damaged.

147. d. The triceps attaches to the olecranon and is responsible for extension of the elbow. If olecranon fractures are treated conservatively, an excellent range of movement can be achieved; however, functional outcome is impaired because of a lack of power of extension. This would be most apparent pushing up against gravity, as one has to do when pushing out of a chair. Brushing hair, reaching into cupboards and pouring kettles are functions mainly achieved by movements of the shoulder, while fastening buttons requires dexterity and may be adversely affected by injuries to the wrist or hand.

148. c. There are six extensor compartments in the extensor retinaculum on the dorsum of the wrist. They contain, in order:

1st – extensor pollicis brevis and abductor pollicis longus muscle
2nd – extensor carpi radialis longus and extensor carpi radialis brevis muscle
3rd – extensor pollicis longus muscle
4th – extensor digitorum and extensor indicis muscle
5th – extensor digiti minimi muscle
6th – extensor carpi ulnaris muscle

The second and third compartments are separated by Lister's tubercle.

149. b. This describes the course of the radial artery which starts at the level of the neck of the radius lying on the tendon of the biceps. It passes under the brachioradialis, reaching the wrist where its pulsations are felt against the radius. After that it winds radially and enters the palm between the heads of the first dorsal interosseous muscle; it ends as the deep palmar arch supplying the hand. The ulnar artery passes inferiorly and medially in the anterior compartment of the forearm. It runs radial to the ulnar nerve and flexor carpi ulnaris and ends in the hand, forming the superficial palmar arch. The superficial branch of the radial nerve also passes down the forearm under brachioradialis. The nerve lies just radial to the artery and, in comparison to the artery, pierces the deep fascia approximately 7 cm proximal to the wrist.

150. b. One of the most common lesions at this site is carpal tunnel syndrome, in which the median nerve is compressed as it passes deep to the flexor retinaculum. The usual presentation is with acroparesthesia. This consists of numbness, tingling and burning sensations felt in the hand and fingers; the pain sometimes radiates up the forearm as far as the elbow. Weakness of the thenar muscles develops, particularly with abduction of the thumb, and is associated with atrophy of the thenar eminence. Sensory loss may appear over the tips of the median innervated fingers.

151. c. The axillary nerve (C5, C6) arises from the posterior cord of the brachial plexus and winds around the surgical neck of the humerus. It supplies the deltoid and teres minor muscles and gives off cutaneous branches supplying sensation to skin overlying the deltoid muscle (regimental badge patch). It may be damaged in an anterior dislocation of the shoulder joint as well as fracture of the surgical neck of the humerus. Deltoid muscle is paralyzed; therefore shoulder abduction is affected in these injuries. It is important to assess sensation over the 'regimental badge patch' area, as assessing motor function will be limited by pain. This is especially important before shoulder joint reduction is attempted as the axillary nerve may also be damaged by reduction of the dislocated joint.

152. b. The radial nerve is closely related to the humerus in the middle third of the shaft. It travels within the radial groove of the humerus and is prone to damage with mid-shaft humeral fractures. The axillary nerve may be affected in fractures of the surgical neck of humerus. Distal humerus fractures can damage the median nerve; medial epicondyle fractures of the humerus can damage the ulnar nerve.

153. a. Medial rotation of the humerus is carried out by the subscapularis muscle. The other rotator cuff muscles are responsible for external rotation (infraspinatus and teres minor) and initiation of shoulder abduction (supraspinatus). Other muscles that internally rotate the humerus are the teres major and pectoralis major muscles.

154. b. The superficial flexor muscles of the forearm arise from a common flexor tendon from the medial epicondyle of the humerus. These muscles are attached by this common flexor attachment. In addition to the four muscles mentioned above, the flexor carpi radialis also arises from this attachment. Muscles attached to the common extensor tendon at the lateral epicondyle of the humerus are the extensor carpi radialis brevis, the extensor carpi ulnaris, the extensor digitorum and the extensor digiti minimi. Flexor digitorum profundus originates from the proximal ulnar and interosseous membrane.

LOWER LIMB

155. e. The deep peroneal nerve supplies the first web space of the foot. The superficial peroneal nerve supplies the anterolateral aspect of the calf and most of the dorsum of the foot (excluding the first web space). The lateral and medial sole are supplied by the lateral and medial plantar nerves, respectively. The sural nerve supplies the posterolateral aspect of the calf and foot. The medial aspect of the calf is supplied by the saphenous nerve.

156. d. The Trendelenburg gait results from weakness of the hip abductors and the Trendelenburg test assesses the strength of these muscles. The muscles that cause hip abduction are the gluteus medius and minimus. If the right abductors are weak, a Trendelenburg gait will show the left hip dipping instead of rising when the left foot is lifted off the floor. The trunk also lurches to the right side to move the centre of gravity over the right hip and maintain balance. The iliopsoas muscle flexes the hip; the quadriceps muscles are primarily knee extensors but also slightly flex the hip through the rectus femoris. The gluteus maximus extends the hip and the short external rotators (piriformis, gemelli, obturator internus and quadratus femoris) externally rotate the hip.

157. b. The femoral ring is the superior opening of the femoral canal. The borders of the femoral ring are medially, the lacunar ligament; posteriorly, the pectineal ligament (the fascia covering the pectineus muscle, which overlies the superior ramus); laterally, the femoral vein; and anteriorly, the medial part of the inguinal ligament. The order of the femoral structures (from lateral to medial) is femoral nerve, artery, vein and lymph nodes (acronym NAVY).

158. d. Hunter's canal, also known as the adductor canal or the subsartorial canal, is a narrow, fascial canal approximately 15 cm long that lies in the distal medial thigh. The canal, surrounded by fascia and muscle, provides a channel for the femoral vessels to pass into the popliteal region. The canal is bordered anteriorly by the distal third of the sartorius muscle. It has a roof made up of the sartorius and subsartorial fascia. The vastus medialis lies laterally and the adductor longus and magnus lie posteromedially. The contents of the canal are the femoral vessels, which exit via the adductor hiatus, and the saphenous nerve. This nerve gives off branches to supply the vastus medialis muscle and the knee and then continues down the leg to pierce the deep fascia to join the superficial great saphenous nerve and supply the skin on the medial side of the lower leg. The vastus intermedius lies deep to the vastus medialis.

159. a. Compartment syndrome is a condition whereby the tissue pressure within a fascial compartment exceeds capillary pressure, compromising venous drainage and arterial flow to that compartment. The anterior compartment is supplied by the deep peroneal nerve, the lateral compartment by the superficial peroneal nerve and the deep posterior compartments by the tibial nerve. There is no medial compartment. The first dorsal web space between the second toe and the hallux is an autonomous area of innervation for the deep peroneal nerve.

160. c. The sciatic nerve is formed from the ventral rami of the fourth lumber to third sacral spinal nerves and is a continuation of the upper band of the sacral plexus; it leaves the pelvis through the greater sciatic foramen. The sciatic nerve is the largest nerve in the body and divides at the apex of the popliteal fossa into the tibial nerve and the common peroneal nerve. It supplies articular branches to the hip joint. In general, the sciatic nerve supplies the posterior compartment of the thigh. The biceps femoris, semitendinosus and semimembranosus and the ischial head of the adductor magnus muscles are supplied by the sciatic nerve muscular branches. The medial compartment is supplied by the obturator nerve, and the femoral nerve supplies the anterior compartment.

161. a. At the point where the external iliac artery passes deep to the inguinal ligament it becomes the femoral artery. The vessel courses from behind the inguinal ligament at the point halfway between the anterior superior iliac spine (ASIS) and pubic tubercle downward along the anterior medial aspect of the thigh until it reaches the adductor hiatus, at which point it continues as the popliteal artery. The femoral artery enters the femoral triangle enclosed only by the femoral sheath for the first few centimetres. The vein is only covered by skin and fascia as it courses through the femoral triangle lying superficially. The femoral sheath is a fascial tube that surrounds the femoral artery, vein and the empty space containing lymphatics in the femoral triangle. The sheath is a continuation of the transversalis fascia, an anterior abdominal wall fascia. There are only three compartments of the femoral sheath: lateral, intermediate and medial compartments. The lateral compartment contains the femoral artery, the intermediate the femoral vein and the medial compartment, sometimes referred to as the femoral canal, is an empty space consisting of lymphatics.

162. c. The lesser trochanter is on the medial aspect of the proximal femur and the psoas and iliacus muscles attach to this prominence. These muscles flex the hip. The greater trochanter is on the lateral aspect of the femur and the following muscles attach to this: piriformis, obturator internus and externus, gluteus medius and minimus, and gemelli.

163. c. The adductor canal, which clinically represents the most common site for atherosclerosis in the lower limb and is used to expose and ligate the popliteal artery during surgery, is bounded by the adductor longus and magnus posteriorly, the vastus medialis anterolaterally and a fibrous membrane overlapped by the sartorius anteromedially. It contains the femoral artery and vein as well as the saphenous nerve, the nerve to the vastus medialis and two divisions of the obturator nerve.

164. c. Limb shortening is a common feature of neck of femur (NOF) fracture and is pathognomonic. The blood supply to the femoral head is of note as fractures of the femoral neck are likely to disrupt the blood supply and lead to avascular necrosis. The medial and lateral circumflex arteries supply the extracapsular arterial ring, with the medial artery being the most important. From the arterial ring, delicate retinacular vessels pass underneath the capsular and up the femoral neck into the head.

165. e. Slipped upper femoral epiphysis (SUFE) most commonly affects overweight boys around the age of puberty (10–15 years). Perthes disease more commonly affects boys but presents earlier (4–10 years). Septic arthritis and neck of femur fractures are incredibly rare in this age of patient and the patient is unlikely to be able to bear weight. Congenital hip dysplasia is a disease that presents in the newborn or is diagnosed in the first few years of life (0–5 years).

166. c. If you suspect a patient with compartment syndrome in the lower leg, it is important to be able to clinically isolate all four compartments. Pain on a passive stretch of a muscle is a key diagnostic sign in compartment syndrome. The following are the isolated passive movements for each compartment:

- Anterior – foot plantarflexion
- Lateral – foot inversion
- Superficial posterior – foot dorsiflexion
- Deep posterior – great toe extension

Compartment syndrome develops when oedema creates venous occlusion leading to tissue injury and further oedema. Subsequently, pressure within the compartment builds until the arterial supply is compromised, resulting in tissue death. The patient complains of increasing pain, which is exacerbated on passive stretching. Treatment involves elevation, releasing any constricting bandages or casts and ultimately fasciotomy.

167. e. The hamstring muscles all arise from the ischial tuberosity and insert into the tibia or fibula. They are semimembranosus, semitendinosus and biceps femoris. Semimembranosus extends from the ischial tuberosity to the medial condyle of the tibia. Semitendinosus originates from the medial aspect of the ischial tuberosity and inserts deep to the gracilis on the upper part of the tibia. The long head of the biceps femoris also originates from the ischial tuberosity and the short head originates from the linea aspera. Both heads form one single tendon inserting into the head of the fibula. The hamstring compartment receives its blood supply from the profunda femoris artery.

168. c. The arterial supply from the ligamentum teres contributes more significantly in childhood. The obturator artery gives off a branch via the ligamentum teres, which provides a negligible blood supply to the femoral head in adults. Lateral and medial circumflex femoral arteries supply the femoral head via retinacula, which reflect back in longitudinal bands under the hip capsule. Vessels from the diaphysis of cancellous bone provide a small arterial blood supply in adulthood. Fractures that are *intracapsular* have a high risk of resultant avascular necrosis of the femoral head, as the retinacula vessels are likely to be disrupted. Pertrochanteric fractures leave these vessels undisturbed and thus avascular necrosis is less likely.

169. c. The popliteal fossa is a space located at the back of the knee joint. The boundaries are:

- Superior and medial – semitendinosus
- Superior and lateral – biceps femoris
- Inferior and medial – medial head of gastrocnemius
- Inferior and lateral – lateral head of gastrocnemius

- Roof – deep fascia
- Floor – popliteal surface of the femur, capsule of knee joint and oblique popliteal ligament

The contents include popliteal artery, popliteal vein, tibial nerve, common peroneal nerve and popliteal lymph nodes.

170. b. The anterior compartment contains the tibialis anterior, extensor hallucis longus, extensor digitorum longus and peroneus tertius muscles along with the deep peroneal nerve and anterior tibial vessels. The lateral compartment contains peroneus longus and brevis muscles along with the superficial peroneal nerve and perforations from the peroneal artery. The deep posterior compartment contains tibialis posterior, flexor hallucis longus, flexor digitorum longus, posterior tibial and peroneal arteries and the tibial nerve. The superficial posterior compartment contains soleus, gastrocnemius and plantaris muscles and the medial cutaneous sural nerve.

171. d. The long saphenous vein drains the medial end of the dorsal venous arch of the foot. It passes anterior to the medial malleolus ascending the medial side of the leg with the saphenous nerve. It crosses the knee a palm's breadth medial to the patella and passes along the medial aspect of the thigh through the lower part of the saphenous opening in the cribriform fascia to join the femoral vein 2 cm below and lateral to the pubic tubercle. There are usually four veins that join the long saphenous vein in the region of the saphenous opening: the superficial epigastric vein, superficial external pudendal vein, deep external pudendal vein and superficial circumflex iliac vein. These veins usually correspond to the cutaneous branches of the femoral artery.

172. a. The tibial nerve originates from the roots L4, 5, S1, 2, 3. It traverses the popliteal fossa and descends in the calf deep to the soleus. It is accompanied by the posterior tibial vessels, passes behind the medial malleolus and ends by dividing into the medial and lateral plantar nerves in the foot. In the popliteal fossa muscular branches are given to gastrocnemius, popliteus and soleus with a cutaneous branch of the sural nerve. In the leg and foot, muscular branches are given to the flexor hallucis longus, flexor digitorum longus, tibialis posterior and intrinsic muscles of the foot. Cutaneous supply is via the medial and lateral plantar nerves.

173. b. The muscles of the sole of the foot can be arranged in four layers, consisting of the following pattern at the four layers: three muscles, two muscles and two tendons, three muscles, and two muscles and two tendons.

Layer 1: Flexor digitorum brevis (medial plantar nerve), abductor hallucis (medial plantar nerve) and abductor digiti minimi (lateral plantar nerve)
Layer 2: Quadratus plantae (lateral plantar nerve), lumbricals (shared between medial and lateral plantar nerves like the hand), and the tendons of hallucis longus and flexor digitorum longus
Layer 3: Flexor hallucis brevis (medial plantar nerve), adductor hallucis (lateral plantar nerve) and flexor digiti minimi brevis (lateral plantar nerve)
Layer 4: Dorsal and plantar interossei muscles (lateral planter nerve) and the tendons of tibialis posterior and peroneus longus

174. c.   The posterior cruciate ligament is attached to the lateral surface of the medial femoral condyle and extends down to the posterolateral aspect of the tibia. The ligament is made up of two separate bundles which, in turn, resist hyperextension and hyperflexion. The ligament's main role is to restict posterior displacement of the tibia relative to the femur. The ligament is extrasynovial but intracapsular.

175. a.   The psoas major muscle joins the iliacus muscle, which originates broadly over the inner aspect of the iliac wing of the pelvis. This becomes the iliopsoas tendon and inserts on the lesser trochanter of the femur and thus flexes the thigh at the hip joint.

176. c.   The common peroneal nerve can be compressed by a below-knee cast at the level of the neck of the fibula. It supplies the muscles of the anterior and lateral compartments of the leg, producing dorsiflexion of the foot, ankle and toes, as well as eversion of the foot. The superficial peroneal nerve gives sensory supply to most of the dorsum of the foot. The deep peroneal nerve supplies the first web space.

177. c.   From lateral to medial, the femoral triangle contains the femoral nerve and its branches, the femoral artery and its branches, including the profunda femoris, and the femoral vein with its main tributary, the long saphenous vein.

178. e.   The muscles of the anterior compartment of the leg are tibialis anterior, extensor hallucis longus, extensor digitorum longus and peroneus tertius. They are all supplied by the deep peroneal nerve and receive their blood supply from the anterior tibial artery. Peroneus brevis is found in the lateral compartment of the leg, along with peroneus longus.

179. a.   The sural nerve arises from the tibial nerve. It is purely sensory and supplies the lateral border of the leg and the lateral border of the foot. It lies approximately 1 cm posterior to the distal fibula and may be damaged during operations on the distal fibula. The saphenous nerve supplies the medial aspect of the leg up to the medial malleolus. The deep peroneal nerve supplies the first web space while the superficial peroneal nerve usually supplies the rest of the dorsum of the foot. The tibial nerve supplies the heel and branches into the medial and lateral plantar nerves to innervate the sole of the foot.

180. a.   The popliteal fossa contains the short saphenous vein, which drains into the popliteal vein. The popliteal vein ends at the adductor hiatus where it becomes the femoral vein. The popliteal artery is the deepest structure within the fossa, initially lying medial to the tibial nerve and moving more lateral to it as it travels distally. The popliteal artery is a branch of the superficial femoral artery. Also within the fossa are the common peroneal and posterior cutaneous nerves of the thigh, with popliteal lymph nodes.

181. c.   The adductor canal (subsartorial/Hunter's canal) is a narrow passageway approximately 15 cm in the middle third of the thigh, deep to the sartorius muscle. It begins at the apex of the femoral triangle and ends at the adductor hiatus. Contents of the canal are the femoral artery and vein, saphenous nerve and nerve to the vastus medialis muscle. The femoral artery and vein pass from the canal through the adductor hiatus to enter the popliteal fossa, becoming the popliteal artery and vein, respectively. The adductor longus is innervated by the obturator nerve, which does not travel within the adductor canal.

182. a. The femoral sheath is a fascial tube extending approximately 4 cm below the inguinal ligament that encloses proximal parts of the femoral vessels and femoral canal. It does not contain the femoral nerve, which can be found lateral to the sheath. The femoral sheath allows the femoral vessels to glide deep to the inguinal ligament during hip movements. The femoral canal is the medial part of the sheath and contains Cloquet's node.

183. c. The muscles that are attached to the greater trochanter are the gluteus medius and minimus, piriformis, superior and inferior gemelli and obturator internus and externus. The quadratus femoris is a part of the above short external rotators of the hip but inserts more inferiorly than the other muscles. Gluteus medius and minimus are hip abductors.

184. e. Foot inversion occurs when the foot turns medially at the subtalar joint. The muscles responsible for this movement are tibialis anterior and posterior. When acting independently, the tibialis anterior dorsiflexes the foot and the tibialis posterior plantarflexes the foot. The tibialis anterior is innervated by the deep peroneal nerve, whereas the tibialis posterior is innervated by the tibial nerve.

185. a. The popliteal fossa is formed by the biceps femoris (superolaterally), semimembranosus and semitendinosus (superomedially), and lateral and medial head of the gastrocnemius (inferolaterally and inferomedially, respectively). The main contents of the popliteal fossa are (from superficial to deep) the tibial nerve, popliteal vein and popliteal artery. Other structures within the fossa include the common peroneal nerve, the posterior cutaneous nerve of the thigh, genicular branches of the knee joint, popliteal lymph nodes and lymphatic vessels, and the small saphenous vein (which pierces the fascia of the popliteal fossa to drain into the popliteal vein). The saphenous nerve follows the course of the large saphenous vein, medial to the popliteal fossa.

186. b. The posterior compartment of the leg can be divided into superficial and deep compartments. Muscles in the superficial compartment are the gastrocnemius, soleus and plantaris. Muscles in the deep compartment are the tibialis posterior, flexor hallucis longus, flexor digitorum longus and popliteus. All these muscles are innervated by the tibial nerve and get their blood supply from the posterior tibial artery. The peroneus tertius is found on the anterior compartment of the leg.

187. e. Six main structures pass deep to the flexor retinaculum in the foot. They are, from anterior to posterior, the tendon sheath of the tibialis posterior, flexor digitorum longus and flexor hallucis longus, as well as the posterior tibial artery, vein and tibial nerve. A useful mnemonic is 'Tom, **D**ick and **a v**ery **n**ervous **H**arry':

- T – **t**ibialis posterior
- D – flexor **d**igitorum longus
- A – posterior tibial **a**rtery
- V – posterior tibial **v**ein
- N – tibial **n**erve
- H – flexor **h**allucis longus

188. d. The iliopsoas muscle is formed by the merging of iliacus and psoas major. It is the main flexor of the thigh at the hip joint. The muscle passes deep to the inguinal ligament and attaches to the lesser trochanter of the femur. The psoas major is innervated by the anterior rami of lumbar nerves L1, L2 and L3. Iliacus is innervated by the femoral nerve (L2 and L3). The iliopsoas tendon can be affected by intra-abdominal inflammation (e.g. appendicitis). Movement or contraction of the muscle in such conditions may result in pain.

189. b. The sartorius is a thin, long muscle located superficially on the anterior part of the thigh. It passes obliquely from lateral to medial, attached proximally at the anterior superior iliac spine and distally at the superior part of the medial aspect of the tibia. It acts on both the hip and knee joints. It also abducts and laterally rotates the thigh at the hip joint. Biceps femoris and semimembranosus are posterior muscles, which extend the hip. Rectus femoris crosses both the hip and the knee but extends the knee. Adductor brevis does not cross the knee.

HEAD, NECK AND SPINE

190. e.   The skin consists of five layers, which cover the skull. They are:

- *Skin* – this is relatively thin in most people but has a rich blood and lymphatic supply. Scalp lacerations are common and can bleed profusely.
- *Connective tissue* – this thick layer of subcutaneous tissue has a rich arterial and nerve supply.
- *Aponeurosis* – this is a strong collagenous sheet of tissue and is the tendinous fascia of the epicranial muscles (frontalis and occipitalis).
- *Loose areolar tissue* – this layer has many potential spaces that are able to be filled with pus or blood. Infection is then able to tract intracranially because of the presence of emissary veins, which run from this layer through the cranial vault into the meninges.
- *Pericranium* – this is a dense layer of specialized connective tissue that is held firmly to the skull through 'Sharpey's fibres', which run from the pericranium and attach within the bones themselves.

The layers of the scalp can be remembered with the acronym SCALP. The investing fascia is a deep fascia that surrounds the whole of the neck.

191. e.   The external carotid artery originates from the bifurcation of the common carotid artery. The external carotid artery has eight major primary branches: the superior thyroid artery, the ascending pharyngeal artery, the lingual artery, the facial artery, the occipital artery, the posterior auricular artery, the superficial temporal artery and the maxillary artery. These branches can be remembered by the mnemonic 'some anatomists like fish, others prefer sausages and mash'. The inferior thyroid artery is a branch of the thyrocervical trunk, itself a branch of the subclavian artery.

192. a.   The seventh cranial (facial) nerve emerges from the inferior border of the pons. It then enters the skull via the internal acoustic meatus, which leads to the petrous part of the temporal bone. The nerve then continues in the facial canal to exit the skull via the stylomastoid foramen. Cranial nerve (CN) VIII enters the skull via the internal acoustic meatus to reach the vestibulocochlear complex. CN IX, X and XI exit the skull via the jugular foramen, accompanying the internal jugular vein, inferior petrosal and sigmoid sinuses and meningeal branches of the ascending pharyngeal and occipital arteries.

193. d.   The maxillary nerve, the second part of the trigeminal nerve, exits the skull via the foramen rotundum. The nasal emissary vein passes through the foramen caecum. The middle meningeal artery and vein and the meningeal branch of the mandibular nerve pass through the foramen spinosum. The mandibular nerve, accompanied by the accessory meningeal artery, passes through the foramen ovale. The internal carotid artery and its accompanying sympathetic and venous plexuses pass through the foramen lacerum.

194. e.   The foramen magnum has three particular characteristics: the junction between the medulla and the spinal cord occurs within it; it is the largest foramen; and it is in the midline and so it is unpaired. It lies within the posterior cranial fossa and is oval in shape with its long axis in the anteroposterior plane. The structures that pass through it are the medulla and associated meninges, the anterior and posterior spinal arteries, the dural veins, the spinal roots of the CN XI and the vertebral arteries.

195. d. The neck is divided into two main triangles on each side of the neck, anterior and posterior. The anterior and posterior triangles share a common boundary, the sternocleidomastoid muscle. The anterior triangle has the anterior border of the sternocleidomastoid laterally, the inferior border of the mandible superiorly and the anterior midline medially. The posterior triangle has the posterior border of the sternocleidomastoid anteriorly, the anterior border of the trapezius posteriorly and the clavicle inferiorly. These two triangles are then further subdivided so that in the posterior triangle the occipital and supraclavicular triangles are found. In the anterior triangle one finds the submandibular, submental, carotid and muscular triangles. The muscular triangle is bounded by the midline, the superior belly of the omohyoid and the anterior border of the sternocleidomastoid. Within this triangle lies the infrahyoid muscles and the thyroid and parathyroid glands.

196. d. A transverse cut through the neck will show that there are four deep fascial layers. The investing fascia is the most superficial of these fascias and surrounds the whole of the structures within the neck. The pretracheal fascia surrounds the trachea, thyroid gland, parathyroid glands, oesophagus and their associated vessels and nerves, such as the recurrent laryngeal nerves. The prevertebral fascia surrounds the cervical vertebrae and the posterior neck muscles. The carotid sheath surrounds the carotid arteries, the internal jugular veins and the vagus nerves. These fascias are important as they provide anatomical dissection planes and limit the spread of infection.

197. d. The anterior and posterior triangles of the neck can be further divided into smaller triangles. The anterior triangle is subdivided into the submandibular, submental, carotid and muscular triangles. The posterior triangle is subdivided by the inferior belly of the omohyoid into the occipital triangle superiorly and the supraclavicular triangle inferiorly. Within the occipital triangle you would find the accessory nerve. During neck dissections the accessory nerve is preserved when possible and can be used to divide the occipital triangle in two. Superior to the nerve lie few important structures. However, inferiorly one finds many important structures such as the phrenic nerve, brachial plexus and transverse cervical artery.

198. a. The pterion is the area where the frontal, sphenoid, parietal and temporal bones meet. This junction forms an inconsistently shaped H. This area is 3.5 cm posterior to the frontozygomatic suture and 4 cm superior to the zygomatic arch. It is clinically important as it marks the position of the anterior middle meningeal artery, which is found intracranially. A head injury to this area may fracture the bones and tear the artery, leading to an extradural haematoma.

199. d. A lumbar puncture is performed to enter the subarachnoid space in order to obtain a sample of cerebrospinal fluid or inject medications. Aiming between L3/L4 or L4/L5, the needle pierces the skin and subcutaneous fascia in the midline.

The needle is then advanced through the supraspinous ligament, the interspinous ligament and then the ligamentum flavum. Usually, the operator will feel a 'give' as the needle tip exits the ligamentum flavum and enters the extradural space. To enter the subarachnoid space the needle is then carefully advanced through the dura mater and finally the arachnoid mater. The posterior longitudinal ligament lies immediately posterior to the vertebra (i.e. anterior to the dural sac and spinal nerves).

200. e.   The cavernous sinuses are approximately 2 cm long and 1 cm wide and are situated on either side of the sella turcica and lateral to the sphenoid air sinuses. These sinuses are important clinically because they drain a wide area of the head and have many important structures related to them. The following veins drain into the cavernous sinuses: the superior and inferior ophthalmic veins, the superficial middle cerebral vein and the sphenoparietal sinuses. The sinuses also communicate with each other. Running in the lateral aspect of the sinuses are the internal carotid artery and associated sympathetic plexus, CN III, CN IV, CN V^1, CN V^2 and CN VI. Infections or tumours of the face are able to reach these sinuses through the valveless veins mentioned above and cause thrombosis. The patient would have a painful, oedematous and venous congested ipsilateral eye. Internal and external ophthalmoplegia with papilloedema and palsies of the nerves mentioned above may also present. In addition, if not treated with antibiotics and anticoagulants, the thrombosis can quickly spread to the contralateral side.

201. a.   The right subclavian arises from the brachiocephalic artery directly behind the sternoclavicular joint, where it courses laterally arching over the lung apex behind the scalenus anterior; at the outer border of the first rib it becomes the axillary artery. The left subclavian artery arises directly from the arch of the aorta travelling superiorly along the mediastinum passing over the apex of the lung behind the scalenus anterior entering the arm. The relationship of the scalenus anterior to the subclavian artery is used to descriptively divide the subclavian artery into three parts: medial to the scalenus anterior, behind the scalenus anterior and lateral to the scalenus anterior. The first part of the subclavian artery gives off the following branches: vertebral, internal thoracic and thyrocervical arteries. The second part gives off the costocervical trunk and the third part the dorsal scapular artery.

202. d.   The zygomatic arch is made up of the zygomatic processes of the temporal, malar and maxilla bones. It is important to remember that fractures of the zygomatic branch can damage the zygomatic branch of the facial nerve, which runs along the mid-portion of the arch.

203. b.   The pterion is the meeting of four bones, the fourth of which is the parietal bone. It is situated about 3 cm superoposteriorly to the level of the zygomatic process of the frontal bone. It is the weakest part of the skull. The pterion is clinically relevant because the anterior division of the middle meningeal artery runs beneath it, which may be injured during a traumatic blow creating an extradural haematoma.

204. e.   Temporal bone trauma varies from causing minor concussion to more severe deficits involving the facial and vestibulocochlear nerves and other intracranial contents. Longitudinal fractures comprise 80% of all temporal bone fractures caused by lateral force over the mastoid or temporal bones. The fracture line runs parallel to the long axis of the petrous bone. All of the options except for the cranial nerve IX palsy are signs of longitudinal temporal bone fracture. Other signs include bleeding from the ear. Facial nerve paralysis can be caused by fractures of the temporal bone.

205. e. Temporal bone trauma varies from causing minor concussion to more severe deficits involving the facial and vestibulocochlear nerves and other intracranial contents. All of the above are signs of transverse fractures except abducens nerve injury. Transverse fractures of the temporal bone are less common than a longitudinal fracture (20% vs. 80%). They are usually caused by frontal or parietal trauma. The fracture line runs at a right angle to the petrous bone, commencing in the middle cranial fossa and ending in the foramen magnum. Cochlear and vestibular structures are often damaged leading to vertigo and sensorineural hearing loss.

206. e. Cystic hygromas are classically located in the left posterior triangle of the neck. They are congenital lymphatic lesions and usually benign. Sebaceous cysts are not usually found on the neck but rather on the scalp, ears, back, face and upper arm. This lump is non-fluctuant and therefore would unlikely be a cyst. It is unlikely to be a branchial cyst, which are usually moveable cystic masses. The diagnosis is most likely a lymph node in this patient.

207. b. This vein drains most of the scalp and side of the face. It starts near the angle of the mandible and is formed from the union of the retromandibular and postauricular veins receiving branches from the posterior external and transverse cervical veins. The external jugular has no valves, lies anterior to the scalenus anterior and does pierce the deep fascia.

208. c. A hangman's fracture is a fracture of both pedicles of C2 caused by hyperextension. A clay shoveler's fracture involves the spinous process of C6/7. It is a stable fracture caused by shearing forces with the arms extended. Doctors should always be present for flexion and extension views. The most common site of fracture is C7/T1.

209. b. Cauda equina is a serious neurological (lower motor neuron) emergency leading to loss of function of the nerve roots. Symptoms include back pain, saddle anaesthesia, bladder and bowel dysfunction and absent anal/bulbocavernosus reflexes. Below L1 (transpyloric plane) the anterior and posterior nerve roots pass almost vertically down through the subarachnoid space and form the cauda equina. This consists of only anterior and posterior nerve roots; the subcostal plane begins at L3. A positive Babinski sign indicates an upper motor neuron defect.

210. d. The middle meningeal artery is the third branch of the first part of the maxillary artery. It runs beneath the pterion where it is most vulnerable to injury. Usually occurring as a result of a significant high force, impact bleeding from the middle meningeal causes an extradural haematoma. This is commonly a result of a tear in the anterior branch. A corresponding linear skull fracture may be a common finding. Ipsilateral pupil dilation is usual.

211. e. Relations of the parotid gland include:

- Superior: External acoustic meatus and temporomandibular joint
- Inferior: Digastric muscle (posterior belly)
- Medial: Styloid process
- Anterior: Masseter muscle

Structures traversing the gland include:

- Facial nerve
- Retromandibular vein
- External carotid artery

The gland is enclosed in the deep investing layer of cervical fascia. The parotid duct arises anteriorly and pierces the buccinator opposite the second upper molar tooth.

212. b. The relations of the sublingual glands include:

- Anterior: Submandibular duct, floor of mouth
- Posterior: Deep lobe of the submandibular gland
- Lateral: Mandible
- Medial: Genioglossus, lingual nerve
- Inferior: Mylohyoid

213. e. The thyroid is enclosed in the pretracheal fascia; layers divided from superficial to deep include:

- Skin
- Superficial fascia
- Platysma
- Deep investing layer cervical fascia
- Strap muscles
- Pretracheal fascia
- Thyroid

The thyroid is supplied by the superior thyroid artery (branch of external carotid) and the inferior thyroid artery (branch of thyrocervical trunk, which itself is a branch of the subclavian artery). The internal carotid artery gives off no branches in the neck. The ascending pharyngeal artery is a terminal branch of the external carotid artery.

214. c. Posterior triangle of the neck

- Boundaries – posterior border of sternocleidomastoid, anterior border of trapezius and middle third of the clavicle
- Roof – investing fascia, platysma
- Floor – prevertebral fascia, subclavian artery, trunks of brachial plexus and cervical plexus

Submental triangle

- Boundaries – anterior belly of digastric muscle, midline of the neck, body of hyoid

Muscular triangle

- Boundaries – midline, body of hyoid bone, superior belly of omohyoid and sternocleidomastoid

215. c. Boundaries of the infratemporal fossa include:

- Medial: Lateral pterygoid plate
- Lateral: Ramus of mandible
- Superior: Greater wing of sphenoid
- Anterior: Maxilla
- Inferior: Free
- Posterior: Carotid sheath

216. b. The pretracheal fascia lies deep to the strap muscles; it extends from the hyoid down to the arch of the aorta, splitting to enclose the thyroid, oesophagus and trachea. The investing layer of cervical fascia lies superficial to the pretracheal, but deep to the superficial layer of cervical fascia; superiorly it attaches from the mastoid process, superior nuchal line, zygomatic process and mandible to the manubrium, clavicles, scapulae spines and acromion. The deep investing layer of cervical fascia has anterior and posterior attachments to the manubrium inferiorly, forming the suprasternal space. The deep investing layer of cervical fascia envelops sternocleidomastoid, trapezius and parotid gland bilaterally. Prevertebral fascia forms the floor of the posterior triangle, overlying levator scapulae and the scalenus muscles (i.e. the prevertebral muscles) – it extends from the skull base to the body of T3; laterally, the fascia encloses the subclavian artery and becomes the axillary sheath inferior to the clavicle. The carotid sheath encloses the carotid arteries, the vagus nerve and the internal jugular vein – it extends from the skull base to the root of the neck.

217. d. Branching arteries of the external carotid artery include:

- Ascending pharyngeal
- Superior thyroid
- Lingual
- Facial
- Occipital
- Posterior auricular
- Maxillary (terminal branch)
- Superficial temporal (terminal branch)

218. c. The internal carotid artery is dilated into the carotid sinus at its point of origin, which receives a rich nerve supply from the glossopharyngeal nerve (IX) and acts as a baroreceptor. It enters the base of the skull via the carotid canal in the petrous temporal bone. Its terminal branches include anterior and middle cerebral arteries (**Note:** It also gives off the ophthalmic artery, which provides supraorbital and supratrochlear arteries, but most importantly the central retinal artery, which is the sole source of blood supply to the retina). It passes deep to the posterior belly of the digastric and parotid gland; on entering the base of the skull, it is separated from the external carotid artery by the styloid process. The internal carotid artery gives off no branches before entering the skull base.

219. b. The thyroid isthmus overlies the 2nd and 3rd tracheal rings. The lateral lobes extend from the thyroid cartilage to the 6th tracheal ring. The pyramidal lobe of the thyroid gland (which represents an embryological remnant during descent of the gland in the neck) most often projects from the thyroid isthmus, and usually on the left. The isthmus lies deep to the anterior jugular veins, which course over it, and usually must be ligated when performing a tracheostomy. The external branch of the superior laryngeal nerve (which supplies the cricothyroid muscle) lies deep to the upper pole of the gland and is at risk of damage during thyroid surgery.

220. e. The tip drains to submental nodes. The anterior two-thirds drains to submental and submandibular nodes. The posterior third has a rich lymphatic midline anastomosis, resulting in increased likelihood of contralateral metastasis; conversely, the anterior two-thirds has a poor crossover lymphatic drainage, making contralateral node involvement unlikely until late in the disease. The posterior third drains to the deep cervical chain of nodes.

221. c. The sensory supply to the ear can be summarized as follows:

- Upper lateral half of pinna: Auriculotemporal nerve (branch of VIII)
- Upper medial half of pinna: Lesser occipital (C2)
- External auditory meatus (EAM): Auriculotemporal nerve, facial nerve, vagus nerve (Arnold's nerve)
- Lateral tympanic membrane: As EAM
- Medial tympanic membrane: Facial nerve, glossopharyngeal nerve (Jacobson's nerve)

222. e. The laryngopharynx extends from the tip of the epiglottis to the termination of the pharynx at the vertebral level of C6. The piriform fossa form deep recesses anteriorly. The cricopharyngeus is tonically contracted at rest. Killian's dehiscence refers to an anatomical area of weakness between the two components of the inferior constrictor (thyropharyngeus and cricopharyngeus) and is implicated in the formation of a pharyngeal pouch. The anteriorly located laryngeal inlet is comprised of the arytenoids, aryepiglottic folds and epiglottis.

223. a. The superficial veins of the head and neck may be summarized as follows:

- Superficial temporal + maxillary → retromandibular (anterior and posterior branches: RMa, RMp)
- RMp + posterior auricular → external jugular
- RMa + facial → common facial

The external jugular vein lies within the superficial fascia, superficial to sternocleidomastoid – it crosses the roof of the posterior triangle in the neck and enters deep cervical fascia 1 in. superior to the clavicle to join the subclavian vein. The anterior jugular veins lie either side of the midline of the neck, communicating with each other accordingly, and also passing laterally to join the ipsilateral external jugular vein, deep to the sternocleidomastoid.

224. c. The drainage of the paranasal sinuses may be summarized as follows:

- Sphenoid sinus: Sphenoethmoidal recess
- Frontal sinus: Middle meatus anteriorly (infundibulum of hiatus semilunaris)
- Maxillary sinus: Middle meatus posteriorly
- Ethmoid sinus: Superior and middle meatus
- Nasolacrimal duct: Inferior meatus

225. b. The movements of the lower jaw may be summarized as follows:

- Elevation: Masseter, temporalis, medial pterygoid
- Depression: Mylohyoid, geniohyoid, digastric, lateral pterygoid
- Protraction: Lateral and medial pterygoid together and bilaterally
- Side to side: Lateral and medial pterygoid together, but alternately on each side
- Retraction: Temporalis

The articular surface of the joint is composed of fibrocartilage.
Sensory innervation of the temporomandibular joint is derived from
the auriculotemporal and masseteric branches of the mandibular nerve
(i.e. VIII of the trigeminal nerve).

226. e. There are 33 vertebra in total:

- Cervical: 7
- Thoracic: 12
- Lumbar: 5
- Sacral: 5
- Coccygeal: 4

The atlas (C1) has no body and articulates superiorly with the occipital condyles.
C7 is the vertebrae prominens, due to its long, non-bifid spine, which is relatively
easy to palpate *in vivo*. The axis (C2) bears the dens, which is also referred to as the
odontoid process – this acts as a pivot, allowing rotation at the atlantoaxial joint.
The vertebral arteries course superiorly via the transverse processes of the cervical
vertebrae (**Note:** The transverse process is commonly absent in C7).

227. b. Ninety percent of parathyroid glands are closely related to the thyroid, the
majority lying anteriorly; approximately 10% are aberrant and are invariably the
lower/inferior glands. Aberrant glands may be found in the mediastinum, behind
the oesophagus and anterior to the trachea; in rare situations, parathyroid glands
may be found within the thyroid proper. Superior parathyroid glands are 4th arch
derivatives, whereas inferior glands are 3rd arch derivatives, developing along
with the thymus – in this manner, when the thymus descends in the neck from its
embryological origin, it drags the inferior parathyroid glands inferiorly with it.

228. d. Structures that pass through the superior orbital fissure (from superiorly
to inferiorly) include:

- Lacrimal nerve
- Frontal nerve
- Trochlear nerve
- Superior branch of oculomotor nerve

- Nasociliary nerve
- Inferior branch of oculomotor nerve
- Abducens nerve

The supraorbital nerve is a terminal branch of the frontal nerve and emerges from the supraorbital foramen.

229. c.   The ophthalmic artery enters the orbit below the optic nerve. The ophthalmic artery spirals around the optic nerve to lie laterally to it, supplying muscles, eyelids and conjunctiva. Anterior and posterior ethmoidal arteries accompany branches of the nasociliary nerve and exit via the medial wall of the orbital cavity. Orbital veins do not contain valves, which accounts for a significant spread of infection from the forehead and orbit to the cavernous sinus. Occlusion of the central retinal artery results in unilateral blindness, as it is the sole supply of blood to the retina.

230. a.   Tensor tympani arises from the anterior wall and inserts onto the handle of the malleus by passing around processus trochleariformis (a small bony pulley). The mucous membrane of the Eustachian tube is supplied by the glossopharyngeal nerve. The aditus lies between the mastoid antrum and the epitympanic recess (or attic). The roof is formed by part of the petrous temporal bone, known as the tegmen tympani. The internal jugular vein is related to the floor of the cavity.

231. e.   The ossicles are united by synovial joints. The handle of the malleus is adherent to the tympanic membrane. The stapes footplate lies adherent to the oval window. The long process of the incus runs parallel to the handle of the malleus, lying in the tympanic cavity. The head of the malleus lies in the epitympanic recess.

232. b.   The antrum lies within the petrous part of the temporal bone. The antrum is well developed at birth; however, the mastoid process does not begin to develop until 24 months of life. The medial wall of the antrum is related to the posterior semicircular canal. The mucosa of the mastoid air cells is supplied in part by the mandibular division of the trigeminal nerve (via nervus spinosus, which arises from foramen spinosum), but also from branches of the glossopharyngeal nerve.

233. c.   The strap muscles lie deep to the investing layer of the deep cervical fascia, on either side of the midline below the hyoid and anterior to the laryngeal cartilages. The nerve supply is derived from the upper cervical ventral rami, notably C1 fibres that 'hitch-hike' along the hypoglossal nerve arising from the superior root of the ansa cervicalis. Mylohyoid forms a sling across the floor of the mouth, arising from both sides of the mandible and inserting onto the body of hyoid. Its action is to elevate the hyoid and raise the floor of the mouth.

234. a.   To help recall the different structures it is useful to remember that the thyroid gland is enclosed in pretracheal fascia, which will therefore be encountered at the time of division of the thyroid isthmus.

235. a.   The cartilaginous parts of the larynx and their corresponding vertebral levels include:

- Hyoid C3
- Thyroid cartilage (upper limit) C4

- Cricoid cartilage C6
- Epiglottis C3
- Arytenoid cartilages C5

236. c. The boundaries of the posterior triangle of the neck are the trapezius muscle, the sternocleidomastoid muscle and the clavicle. The contents include the occipital, transverse cervical, subclavian and suprascapular arteries, the accessory nerve, cervical plexus branches and brachial plexus trunks and the suprascapular and external jugular veins.

237. c. The ophthalmic nerve has five cutaneous branches: the lacrimal, supraorbital, supratrochlear, infratrochlear and external nasal nerves. The infraorbital nerve is a cutaneous branch of the maxillary division of the trigeminal nerve, together with the zygomaticofacial and zygomaticotemporal nerves.

238. e. The maxillary artery is a terminal branch of the external carotid artery. It is described in three parts in relation to the lateral pterygoid muscle. The first part gives off the following branches: inferior alveolar, middle meningeal, accessory meningeal and two branches to the ear. The middle meningeal artery passes upward through the foramen spinosum helping to supply the meninges. It may be torn in a skull fracture leading to the formation of an extradural haematoma. The second part of the maxillary artery supplies the pterygoid and masseter muscle. Branches from the third part include the infraorbital, sphenopalatine, posterior superior alveolar and greater palatine arteries which accompany nerves.

239. b. The junction between the oblique fibres of thyropharyngeus and the horizontal fibres of cricopharyngeus near the midline is a potential weak area at the back of the pharyngeal wall through which a pouch of mucosa may protrude.

240. a. The external carotid artery is formed at the level of C4. The artery ends within the parotid gland at the level of the neck of the mandible by dividing into the superficial temporal and internal maxillary arteries. The branches of the external carotid artery are the superior thyroid artery, lingual artery, facial artery, occipital artery, posterior auricular artery and ascending pharyngeal artery. The inferior thyroid artery is a branch of the thyrocervical trunk from the subclavian artery.

241. e. The cavernous sinuses lie on either side of the body of the sphenoid against the fibrous wall of the pituitary fossa. They communicate with each other via the intercavernous sinuses. Traversing the cavernous sinus are the carotid artery and the following cranial nerves: oculomotor, trochlear, ophthalmic, maxillary and abducens. Lying above the sinus are the optic tract, the uncus and the internal carotid artery. The cavernous sinus is prone to sepsis and thrombosis due to spread via the anterior facial and ophthalmic veins.

242. c. Each arch has its own nerve supply, cartilage, muscle and artery, although considerable absorption and migration of these derivatives occur in development. The fifth arch disappears completely. The third arch derives the common and internal carotid arteries, with the fourth arches deriving the subclavian artery on the right side and the aortic arch on the left. The pulmonary arteries and ductus arteriosus arise from the sixth arches.

243. c. Tracheostomies can be performed for a number of reasons including airway obstruction (congenital, trauma, infection or head and neck tumours), respiratory insufficiency (long-term ventilation, chest injuries) or protection of the tracheobronchial tree following trauma or reduced consciousness (head injury, overdose). The structures encountered from superficial to deep include the skin, superficial fascia, platysma, investing layer of the cervical fascia, pretracheal fascia, thyroid isthmus and trachea.

244. d. The parotid is the largest of the salivary glands wedged between the mandible and sternocleidomastoid. The relations are as follows:

- Superiorly – external auditory meatus and temporomandibular joint
- Inferiorly – it overflows the posterior belly of digastric muscle
- Anteriorly – it overflows the mandible with the overlying masseter
- Medially – the styloid process
- Laterally – skin and superficial fascia

245. b. The anterior wall of the posterior cranial fossa is formed by the petrous temporal bone laterally with the body of the sphenoid bone medially. The occipital bone forms most of the floor and lateral walls of the fossa. In the midline on the posterior wall is the internal occipital protuberance. Contents of the posterior cranial fossa include the foramen magnum, jugular foramen, hypoglossal canal and internal acoustic meatus. Fractures of the middle cranial fossa can lead to injuries to cranial nerves VII and VIII as they run in the petrous temporal bone.

246. a. The seven cervical vertebrae are characterized by their small size and by the presence of a foramen in each transverse process. This foramen transverserium is trough shaped. The five lumbar vertebrae are distinguished from vertebrae in other regions by their large size. They also lack facets for articulation with ribs.

247. e. The abducens nerve innervates the lateral rectus muscle of the eye exclusively; the sole effect of damage to this nerve is that the patient is unable to abduct (laterally deviate) the eye. Ptosis results from lesion of the occulomotor nerve. The pupillary light reflex tests function of the optic and occulomotor nerves.

248. e. The pituitary gland occupies the sella turcica, which is a cup-shaped depression in the basisphenoid bone. The roof of the sella is formed by the diaphragma sella, a fold of dura, which is perforated to allow passage of the pituitary stalk. Above the diaphragma lie the suprasellar cistern, the optic chiasma and the anterior cerebral arteries. The lateral walls of the pituitary fossa are formed by the cavernous sinuses, which contain the internal carotid arteries and cranial nerves III, IV, the first and second divisions of V, and VI. Behind the sella is the pontine cistern containing the basilar artery. The cavernous sinus, pituitary gland, and stalk and median eminence all show significant enhancement after the administration of intravenous contrast medium.

249. c. The history suggests a prolapsed intervertebral disc. The quadriceps is supplied by the femoral nerve, whose root is L2–L4. The skin over the patella is usually part of the L3 dermatome, and the root of the knee jerk is L3/L4.

The sciatic nerve innervates the muscles of the posterior compartment of the thigh and the muscles of the leg. It provides sensory innervation for the posterior thigh, the leg and the foot. The ilioinguinal nerve supplies a small area of skin on the medial aspect of the upper thigh as well as the scrotum and penis. Femoral nerve compression at the level of the inguinal ligament is unlikely given the history of injury and back pain.

250. e.   The superior orbital fissure is a foramen in the middle cranial fossa. The structures passing through the foramen are the oculomotor nerve (III), the trochlear nerve (IV), the ophthalmic division of the trigeminal nerve (V_1), the abducens nerve (VI) and the ophthalmic veins. The lesser petrosal nerve passes through a separate hiatus.

251. e.   The posterior cranial fossa has several internal foramina: foramen magnum, condylar canal, internal acoustic meatus and hypoglossal canal. The foramen spinosum is present in the middle cranial fossa and transmits the middle meningeal artery. The foramen magnum transmits the spinal cord and the hypoglossal canal transmits the hypoglossal nerve.

252. b.   The two internal carotid arteries arise as one of the two terminal branches of the common carotid arteries. They proceed superiorly to the base of the skull where they enter the carotid canal. Entering the cranial cavity, each internal carotid artery gives off the ophthalmic artery, the posterior communicating artery, the middle cerebral artery and the anterior cerebral artery. The posterior communicating artery connects the internal carotid artery with the posterior cerebral artery (arterial circle of Willis).

253. c.   The posterior triangle of the neck is on the lateral aspect of the neck in direct continuity with the upper limb. It is bordered anteriorly by the posterior edge of the sternocleidomastoid muscle and posteriorly by the anterior edge of the trapezius muscle. Its base is the middle one-third of the clavicle and its apex is the occipital bone just posterior to the mastoid process where the attachments of the trapezius and sternocleidomastoid come together.

254. c.   Layers that are dissected when approaching the thyroid are skin, platysma, superficial investing layer of the deep cervical fascia, strap muscles, pretracheal fascia and thyroid gland. The prevertebral fascia lies posterior to the thyroid gland, separated by the trachea, oesophagus, alar fascia and retropharyngeal space when moving anteriorly to posteriorly.

255. e.   The borders of the posterior triangle of the neck are the posterior border of sternocleidomastoid, the anterior border of trapezius and the middle one-third of the clavicle. The accessory nerve enters the posterior triangle at the junction of the superior and middle thirds of the sternocleidomastoid. The remaining four structures are found within the anterior triangle of the neck. The borders of the anterior triangle are midline of the neck, anterior border of the sternocleidomastoid muscle and inferior border of the mandible. The submandibular gland lies between the inferior border of the mandible and the anterior and posterior bellies of the digastric muscle. The hypoglossal nerve (CN XII) enters the anterior triangle deep to the posterior belly of the digastric muscle to innervate the tongue. The thyroid and parathyroid glands are contained within the anterior triangle. The vagus nerve leaves the skull through the jugular foramen entering the carotid sheath and continuing to the root of the neck.

256. b. The borders of the posterior triangle are as follows: posterior border of the sternocleidomastoid, medial third of the clavicle and anterior border of the trapezius muscle. Contents of the posterior triangle of the neck include a selection of arteries, veins, nerves and lymphatics. Below is a list of structures found in the posterior triangle using these four headings:

- Artery: Third part of subclavian artery, suprascapular artery, transverse cervical artery, occipital artery
- Vein: Part of external jugular vein, part of subclavian vein
- Lymph nodes: Cervical, supraclavicular nodes
- Nerves: Trunks of brachial plexus, accessory nerve

257. c. The first part of the subclavian artery is from the point of origin (either from the brachiocephalic artery or directly from the aortic arch) to the medial border of the scalenus anterior. The second part lies behind the scalenus anterior, with the third part from the lateral border of the muscle to the outer border of the first rib. The costocervical trunk lies behind the scalenus anterior, with the dorsal scapula artery in the third part. The vertebral artery, internal thoracic artery and thyrocervical trunk originate from the first part.

258. b. The arteries supplying the thyroid artery include the superior and inferior thyroid arteries and the thyroid ima artery, present in 10% of people. The superior thyroid artery is usually the first branch of the external carotid artery, with the inferior thyroid artery originating from the thyrocervical trunk, a branch of the subclavian artery. The thyroid ima originates from the brachiocephalic trunk. There is no middle thyroid artery. The veins draining the gland are the superior, middle and inferior thyroid veins. The superior and middle veins drain into the internal jugular vein, with the inferior thyroid artery draining into the brachiocephalic vein.

259. d. The arteries supplying the thyroid artery include the superior and inferior thyroid arteries and the thyroid ima artery, present in 10% of people. The superior thyroid artery is usually the first branch of the external carotid artery, with the inferior thyroid artery originating from the thyrocervical trunk, a branch of the subclavian artery. The thyroid ima originates from the brachiocephalic trunk. The veins draining the gland are the superior, middle and inferior thyroid veins. The superior and middle veins drain into the internal jugular vein, with the inferior thyroid vein draining into the brachiocephalic vein.

260. c. When ligating the inferior thyroid artery, there is risk of damage to the recurrent laryngeal nerve. To reduce risk of damage to this structure, the artery is ligated some distance lateral to the gland. The superior thyroid artery is ligated more proximal to the gland. There is risk of damage to the external laryngeal nerve in this area. The thyroid lies deep to the pretracheal fascia and overlies the 2nd and 4th tracheal rings.

261. e. The facial vein descends along the lateral border of the nose and then travels obliquely across the face to cross the inferior border of the mandible. The facial nerve and the external carotid artery pass through the gland. The retromandibular vein is formed by the unification of the superficial temporal and maxillary veins. It also passes through the parotid gland lying deep to the facial nerve and superficial to the external carotid artery. The parotid lymph node is contained within the parotid gland.

262. d. The parotid capsule is supplied by the greater auricular nerve (C2). The capsule itself is derived from the investing layer of deep cervical fascia. Any inflammation within the gland causes exquisite pain in front of the temporomandibular joint due to the unyielding nature of this fascia. Frey syndrome is a complication of parotidectomy and is characterized by gustatory sweating (sweating on the cheek during a meal). This is caused by inappropriate cross-regeneration of the sympathetic and parasympathetic nerve fibres. The parotid duct runs over the lateral surface of the masseter muscle, piercing the buccinator muscle and opening into the mouth opposite the second upper molar. The facial nerve arises from the stylomastoid foramen before passing through the parotid gland.

263. a. Such an injury can cause damage to the pterion, which is the junction of the greater wing of sphenoid, squamous temporal, frontal and parietal bones. The pterion overlies the anterior division of the middle meningeal artery, which, when disrupted, can lead to an extradural haematoma. Typically, the history consists of a period of unconsciousness, followed by a lucid interval, leading to a progressive hemiparesis, stupor and ipsilateral dilated pupil. The autonomic fibres of the oculomotor nerve are superficial and so are affected first when the nerve is compressed. Compression of CN III (oculomotor nerve) against the crest of the petrous part of the temporal bone is a consequence of middle meningeal artery damage.

264. b. The middle meningeal artery and vein pass through the foramen spinosum. This can be remembered by the mnemonic 'may marry a spinster' (middle meningeal artery: foramen spinosum). The internal carotid artery passes across the foramen lacerum. The facial nerve and stylomastoid artery pass through the stylomastoid foramen. The maxillary nerve exits the skull through the foramen rotundum. The mandibular nerve passes through the foramen ovale.

The hypoglossal nerve exits through the hypoglossal canal. Other foramina of the skull include the jugular foramen where the sigmoid sinus and CNs IX, X and XI exit the skull.

265. b. The recurrent laryngeal nerve is in close relation to the inferior thyroid artery, so it is good practice to tie this artery lateral to the inferior pole. It supplies all muscles of the larynx except the cricothyroid muscle, which is supplied by the external branch of the superior laryngeal nerve. Fine nasoendoscopy is usually performed before thyroidectomy to detect any pre-existing loss of vocal cord function. As the left recurrent laryngeal nerve lies inferior to the arch of the aorta, it is at risk of damage during cardiac surgery.

266. c. Damage to the superior laryngeal nerve, especially during thyroidectomy, causes anaesthesia of the laryngeal mucosa superior to the vocal cords. This increases aspiration risk owing to loss of ability to sense, and therefore clear, any foreign material. The posterior cricoarytenoid muscle abducts the vocal cord, whereas the lateral cricoarytenoid muscle adducts the vocal cord. The cricothyroid muscle stretches and tenses the vocal cord and is the only laryngeal muscle supplied by the external branch of the superior laryngeal nerve as opposed to the recurrent laryngeal nerve. The thyroarytenoid muscle relaxes the vocal cord.

267. d. The pharynx extends from the base of the skull to the inferior border of the cricoid cartilage, at the level of C6, and can be divided into the nasopharynx, oropharynx and laryngopharynx. The posterior wall of the pharynx lies against the prevertebral layer of deep cervical fascia. A pharyngeal pouch is a pulsion diverticulum through Killian's dehiscence. This is an area that lies between the cricopharyngeus and thyropharyngeus, which form the inferior constrictors of the pharynx. A patient with a pharyngeal pouch therefore has an increased risk of aspiration pneumonia owing to retained food products within the pouch being regurgitated at a later time and aspirated. The presence of the pouch leads to an increased risk of fistula formation. Of note, stylopharyngeus acts to elevate the pharynx and larynx and arises from the styloid process passing between the middle and superior constrictors.

268. d. There is increased risk of damage to the teeth when performing a tonsillectomy because of the use of a metal mouth gag. The palatine tonsils are derived from the second pharyngeal pouch. The adenoids lie in the mucous membrane of the roof and posterior wall of the nasopharynx. The tonsils lie between the palatoglossal and palatopharyngeal arches in adults. During a tonsillectomy, the paratonsillar vein is at risk of damage and is therefore a common cause of post-tonsillectomy bleeding. The tonsils are supplied by the tonsillar branch of the facial artery.

269. d. The pterion is formed by the frontal, parietal, temporal and greater wing of sphenoid bones, united by an H-shape formation of sutures. It is an important clinical landmark because it is a weak part of the skull that is easily fractured by a blow to the side of the head. Also, the anterior branch of the middle meningeal artery runs beneath the pterion, and a rupture of this vessel causes an extradural haemorrhage, which is a compressive injury exerting pressure on the cerebral cortex. An emergency burr hole may be required to decompress the brain.

270. b. The common carotid artery bifurcates into the internal carotid and the external carotid artery. The branches of the external carotid artery are the superior thyroid, ascending pharyngeal, lingual, facial, occipital, posterior auricular, superficial temporal and maxillary arteries. The superficial temporal and the maxillary arteries are the terminal branches of the external carotid artery. The internal carotid does not give off any branches until it enters into the cranium. This is a useful method of differentiating between the internal and external carotid during neck dissection. The inferior thyroid artery is a branch of the thyrocervical trunk, which arises from the first part of the subclavian artery.

271. b. The common carotid artery bifurcates into the internal and external carotid arteries. The internal carotid artery does not give off any branches in the neck and face and enters the cranium to supply the brain (forms part of the circle of Willis). The external carotid artery gives off eight branches: ascending pharyngeal, superior thyroid, lingual, facial, occipital, posterior auricular and two terminal branches, superficial temporal and maxillary artery. The middle meningeal artery is a branch of the maxillary artery, running beneath the pterion where it is vulnerable to injury.

272. b. Structures within the parotid gland, from superficial to deep, are the facial nerve (and its branches), retromandibular vein and external carotid artery. It is important to avoid damage to these structures during surgery to the parotid gland. Lymph nodes are found on the parotid sheath as well as within the gland itself. Malignant parotid tumours can present with facial nerve palsy.

273. c. All the intrinsic laryngeal muscles are supplied by the recurrent laryngeal nerve except the cricothyroid muscle, which is supplied by the external laryngeal nerve, a branch of the superior laryngeal nerve. Both the recurrent and superior laryngeal nerves are branches of the vagus nerve. These nerves are susceptible to damage during surgical procedures in the neck (e.g. thyroidectomy).

274. b. The thyroid gland consists of two lateral lobes joined in the middle by the thyroid isthmus. The lobes extend inferiorly up to the 6th tracheal rings, whereas the isthmus is usually between the 2nd and 3rd tracheal rings. The arterial supply is from the superior thyroid artery from the external carotid artery (closely related to the external branch of the superior laryngeal nerve) and the inferior thyroid artery from the first part of the subclavian artery (closely related to the recurrent laryngeal nerve). The thyroid gland also occasionally receives additional supply from the thyroidea ima branches from the aortic arch. There are four main types of thyroid malignancy, the most common being papillary carcinoma, followed by follicular, medullary and anaplastic (rare). Thyroid malignancy is very rarely associated with Hashimoto thyroiditis.

275. a. The right subclavian arises from the brachiocephalic artery directly behind the sternoclavicular joint, where it courses laterally arching over the lung apex behind the scalenus anterior; at the outer border of the first rib it becomes the axillary artery. The left subclavian artery arises directly from the arch of the aorta travelling superiorly along the mediastinum passing over the apex of the lung behind the scalenus anterior entering the arm. The relationship of the scalenus anterior to the subclavian artery is used to descriptively divide the subclavian artery into three parts: medial to scalenus anterior, behind the scalenus anterior and lateral to the scalenus anterior. The first part of the subclavian artery gives off the following branches: vertebral, internal thoracic and thyrocervical arteries. The second part gives off the costocervical trunk and the third part the dorsal scapular artery.

CENTRAL, PERIPHERAL AND AUTONOMIC NERVOUS SYSTEMS

276. b. The brachial plexus is a cluster of interconnecting nerves within the supraclavicular and axillary areas of the upper limb. It consists of five roots (C5–T1), three trunks (superior, middle and inferior), six divisions (anterior and posterior for each trunk), three cords (lateral, posterior and medial – named by their respective anatomical position relative to the axillary artery), five terminal branches (musculocutaneous, median, ulnar, radial and axillary) and multiple side branches from the superior trunk and all three cords. The mnemonic for remembering the order of the structures from proximal to distal is 'Robert Taylor drinks cold beer' (roots, trunks, divisions, cords, branches).

277. a. The thoracodorsal nerve (C6–8) supplies the latissimus dorsi muscle and is a branch from the posterior cord of the brachial plexus. It arises from between the upper and lower subscapular nerves and then runs inferolaterally, deep to the subscapularis and teres major. The teres major is supplied by the lower subscapular nerve. The supraspinatus is supplied by the suprascapular nerve. The deltoid is supplied by the axillary nerve, and the rhomboid major is supplied by the dorsal scapular nerve.

278. d. A high stepping gait is characteristic of a patient not being able to dorsiflex his foot (foot drop). The main muscles that dorsiflex the foot are found in the anterior compartment of the lower leg and are supplied by the deep fibular nerve (L4–S1). The muscles involved are the tibialis anterior, the extensor hallucis longus, the extensor digitorum longus and the fibularis tertius. The muscles of the lateral compartment, the peroneus longus and brevis, are mainly evertors of the foot but do play a minor role in plantarflexion. These muscles are supplied by the superficial peroneal nerve (L5–S2). The superficial and deep peroneal nerves are formed from the common peroneal nerve, which itself is part of the sciatic nerve.

279. d. The nerves of the lumbar plexus are classified based on their anatomical position as they exit the psoas major muscle. These are:

- Anterior – genitofemoral nerve (L1, L2)
- Medial – obturator nerve (L2–L4)
- Lateral – subcostal nerve (T12) (contributes in over 50% of people), iliohypogastric (L1), ilioinguinal (L1), lateral cutaneous nerve of the thigh (L2, L3), femoral nerve (L2–L4)

The posterior femoral cutaneous nerve (S1–S3) arises from the sacral plexus.

280. e. The deep peroneal nerve supplies the first web space of the foot. The superficial peroneal nerve supplies the anterolateral aspect of the calf and most of the dorsum of the foot (excluding the first web space). The lateral and medial sole are supplied by the lateral and medial plantar nerves, respectively. The sural nerve supplies the posterolateral aspect of the calf and foot. The medial aspect of the calf is supplied by the saphenous nerve.

281. a.   The saphenous nerve (L3, L4) supplies the medial aspect of the calf and is a cutaneous branch of the femoral nerve. The saphenous nerve accompanies the femoral artery as it runs down the anterior aspect of the thigh and into the adductor canal (or subsartorial canal). The saphenous nerve does not run through the adductor hiatus like the femoral vessels but crosses the femoral artery to lie medially and then passes between the sartorius and the gracilis. The nerve then pierces the deep fascia on the medial aspect of the leg to then run inferiorly with the great saphenous vein.

282. a.   The seventh cranial (facial) nerve emerges from the inferior border of the pons. It then enters the skull via the internal acoustic meatus, which leads to the petrous part of the temporal bone. The nerve then continues in the facial canal to exit the skull via the stylomastoid foramen. CN VIII enters the skull via the internal acoustic meatus to reach the vestibulocochlear complex. CN IX, X and XI exit the skull via the jugular foramen, accompanying the internal jugular vein, inferior petrosal and sigmoid sinuses and meningeal branches of the ascending pharyngeal and occipital arteries.

283. d.   The maxillary nerve, the second part of the trigeminal nerve, exits the skull via the foramen rotundum. The nasal emissary vein passes through the foramen caecum. The middle meningeal artery and vein and the meningeal branch of the mandibular nerve pass through the foramen spinosum. The mandibular nerve, accompanied by the accessory meningeal artery, passes through the foramen ovale. The internal carotid artery and its accompanying sympathetic and venous plexuses pass through the foramen lacerum.

284. e.   Once the facial nerve has exited the skull via the stylomastoid foramen the nerve gives off the posterior auricular nerve, a branch to the stylohyoid and a branch to the posterior belly of digastric. The nerve then enters the parotid gland and divides into five branches: temporal, zygomatic, buccal, mandibular and cervical. These branches supply the muscles of facial expression. The supraorbital nerve ultimately originates from the trigeminal nerve.

285. e.   The auricle is mainly supplied by the great auricular nerve (C2). This nerve supplies the skin of the lateral and superior aspects. The auriculotemporal nerve (mandibular nerve, CN V^3) only provides sensation superior to the external acoustic meatus. The external acoustic meatus is innervated by three cranial nerves: the auriculotemporal nerve (CN V^3), branches from the tympanic plexus of the facial nerve (CN VII) and the auricular branch of the vagus nerve (CN X). C1 does not contribute.

286. c.   The sacrotuberous and sacropinous ligaments divide the pelvis into two important foramina, the greater and lesser sciatic foramen. The pudendal nerve and internal pudendal artery and vein pass through both the lesser and greater sciatic foramen. However, the sciatic nerve, superior and inferior gluteal nerves and posterior femoral cutaneous nerve pass through the greater sciatic foramen. The pudendal nerve (S2, 3, 4) provides sensory innervation to the external genitalia and perianal region. Its motor supply is to the external anal sphincter and muscles associated with ejaculation in the male and the muscles of the urogenital diaphragm. The nerve is commonly injured in prolonged cycling or difficult childbirth.

287. b.   The common peroneal nerve originates from the upper part of the popliteal fossa. It travels inferolaterally medial to the head of the biceps femoris; once arriving at the posterior aspect of the fibular head, it wraps around the lateral aspect of the fibular neck when it enters the peroneus longus muscle. This superficial location leaves it vulnerable to injury from compression from a tight plaster of Paris (POP) or from direct injury during surgery or trauma. Here it divides into its two terminal branches: the superficial peroneal nerve and the deep peroneal nerve. A foot drop occurs due to paralysis of the dorsiflexor and evertor muscles supplied by the common peroneal nerve.

288. b.   The ilioinguinal nerve innervates the muscles of the lower abdomen, specifically the skin overlying the inguinal region, upper part of the thigh and anterior third of the scrotum or labia in women. This nerve is at risk in the muscle-splitting incision made for appendicectomy. Damage during appendicectomy would lead to the inability to pull the falx inguinalis over the thin area of weak fascia on the posterior wall of the inguinal canal, thereby predisposing the patient to develop an inguinal hernia.

289. e.   The thigh is surrounded by a thick facial sheath. The deep fascia divides the thigh into three compartments, each having its own muscles, nerves and blood supply. The anterior compartment is supplied by the femoral artery and its nervous supply from the femoral nerve. The medial compartment is supplied by the profunda femoris and obturator and has its nerve supply derived from the obturator nerve. The posterior compartment derives its nerve supply from the sciatic nerve and blood supply from the profunda femoris.

290. b.   The brachial plexus has three trunks – upper, midline and lower – with each trunk dividing into an anterior and posterior division. These divisions unite to form cords. These cords are named according to their position with respect to the axillary artery: posterior, medial and lateral. The lateral cord contains nerve fibres from C5 to C7. The lateral cord gives rise to the musculocutaneous nerve (C5, C6 and C7) and contributes partly to the median nerve. The medial cord contributes to the median nerve via fibres C8 and T1.

291. e.   The medial plantar nerve supplies the first lumbrical, flexor digitorum brevis, flexor hallucis brevis and abductor hallucis. All other muscles in the sole of the foot are supplied by the lateral plantar nerve. The sural nerve innervates the skin overlying the posterior surface of the lower leg and lateral side of the foot. The saphenous nerve provides cutaneous innervation to the overlying skin of the medial aspect of the leg and foot.

292. c.   The musculocutaneous nerve arises from the lateral cord of the brachial plexus, supplying coracobrachialis, biceps and brachialis muscles. It also gives rise to the lateral cutaneous nerve of the forearm, which supplies the sensory innervation to the lateral aspect of the forearm. The axillary nerve supplies the lateral upper arm and the musculocutaneous nerve supplies the lateral aspect of the forearm. The median nerve supplies the palmar aspect of the index finger. The dorsal web space is supplied by the radial nerve, with the ulnar nerve supplying the little finger.

293. b. The median nerve arises from the lateral and medial cords of the brachial plexus and supplies the flexor compartment of the forearm. Axillary nerve supplies the lateral upper arm and the musculocutaneous nerve supplies the lateral aspect of the forearm. The median nerve supplies the palmar aspect of the index finger. The dorsal web space is supplied by the radial nerve, with the ulnar nerve supplying the little finger.

294. e. The ulnar nerve arises from the medial cord of the brachial plexus and supplies the two ulnar-sided lumbricals, while the median nerve supplies the two radial-sided lumbricals. The axillary nerve supplies the lateral upper arm and the musculocutaneous nerve supplies the lateral aspect of the forearm. The median nerve supplies the palmar aspect of the index finger. The dorsal web space is supplied by the radial nerve, with the ulnar nerve supplying the little finger.

295. c. A very useful guide for nerve root examination is the American Spinal Injury Association (ASIA) score sheet. The nerve roots are assigned to the following actions - C5 - elbow flexion, C6 - wrist extension, C7 - elbow extension, C8 - flexion of middle finger distal phalanx, T1 - little finger abduction.

296. b. A very useful guide for nerve root examination is the American Spinal Injury Association (ASIA) score sheet. The nerve roots are assigned to the following actions - C5 - elbow flexion, C6 - wrist extension, C7 - elbow extension, C8 - flexion of middle finger distal phalanx, T1 - little finger abduction.

297. d. A very useful guide for nerve root examination is the American Spinal Injury Association (ASIA) score sheet. The nerve roots are assigned to the following actions - C5 - elbow flexion, C6 - wrist extension, C7 - elbow extension, C8 - flexion of middle finger distal phalanx, T1 - little finger abduction.

298. b. Deficits caused by a facial nerve lesion proximal to the internal acoustic meatus will lead to decreased salivation due to loss of innervation to the submandibular and sublingual glands. Unilateral facial paralysis is due to loss of facial muscle innervation. Loss of the chorda tympani taste fibres leads to loss of taste in the anterior two-thirds of the tongue and hyperacusis due to loss of innervation to the stapedius muscle of the inner ear which normally dampens sound.

299. a. The sciatic nerve is the largest nerve in the body including the roots from L4, 5, S1–3. It emerges from the greater sciatic foramen passing (in most people) under piriformis and crossing over the obturator internus and quadratus femoris to descend on the adductor magnus. The nerve terminates by dividing into the tibial and common peroneal nerves (commonly at mid-thigh level). Injuries to the sciatic nerve can occur via penetrating trauma or posterior dislocation of the hip leading to paralysis of hamstring muscles and all muscles of the leg and foot, causing a foot drop deformity. There is almost complete sensory loss below the knee.

300. b. The spinal root L4 contributes to segmental innervation of vastus medialis and lateralis responsible for knee extension. Spinal root L1 innervates the cutaneous dermatome of the hip girdle and groin area. L2 and L3 roots innervate the anterior aspects of the thigh (think 3 to the knee) and L4 and L5 innervate the medial and lateral lower leg dermatomes (think 4 to the floor). Injury to L4 will therefore lead to reduced sensation over the shin area and reduced extension of the knee.

301. a.　Radial nerve injuries are associated with humeral shaft fractures, in particular of the mid-humerus. The most commonly reported symptom, wrist drop, occurs as a result of the muscles on the posterior compartment of the forearm being paralyzed. There is also associated sensory loss which will manifest as paraesthesia or numbness on the dorsum of the hand and forearm in the distribution of the radial nerve. The affected individual will also report an inability to extend the metacarpophalangeal joints. In general, if the lesion occurs above the elbow, numbness of the forearm may occur. Forearm lesions typically preserve sensation in spite of wrist drop. Lesions at the wrist may lead to isolated sensory changes and paraesthesia over the back of the hand without motor weakness. Axillary lesions will lead to involvement of all the radial innervated muscles, with decreased reflexes of the triceps and brachioradialis, decreased sensation over triceps, posterior forearm and dorsum of the hand. Compression at the spiral groove is common leading to weakness in all radial-innervated muscles distal to the triceps; the triceps reflex is preserved, but brachioradialis is decreased. There is sensory loss over the radial dorsal part of the hand and the posterior part of the forearm. In distal radial lesions at the wrist, no motor weakness occurs, although numbness of the dorsal hand is noted, sparing the ulnar one third.

302. d.　The vagus exits the cranium via the jugular foramen. It descends in the neck posterior to the oesophagus between the internal jugular vein and common carotid artery in the carotid sheath. It gives off a superior laryngeal branch, which supplies the inferior constrictor muscles, cricothyroid and sensation to the interior of the larynx above the vocal cords. On the right side, it gives off the recurrent laryngeal branch as it crosses the subclavian artery; it then descends in the superior mediastinum, closely related to the great veins. On the left side, it gives off the recurrent laryngeal branch as it crosses the aortic arch: this subsequently passes below the ligamentum arteriosum.

303. a.　The radial nerve arises from C5–T1, which gives rise to the posterior cord of the brachial plexus. It passes between the medial and long heads of the triceps. In the axilla, the radial nerve gives off the posterior cutaneous nerve of the forearm. The spiral groove lies on the posterior aspect of the humerus – fracture of the humerus in this location puts the radial nerve at risk of damage.

304. d.　The ulnar nerve arises from nerve roots C8 and T1; it is formed from the medial cord of the brachial plexus; it travels down from the axilla between the axillary vein and artery to lie on coracobrachialis, medial to the brachial artery; in the forearm it passes between the two heads of the flexor carpi ulnaris and then lies between this muscle and flexor digitorum profundus. Note that as it enters the wrist, it lies superficial to the carpal tunnel and does not travel through it.

305. b.　The median nerve arises from spinal roots C5, C6, C7, C8 and T1. After crossing from the lateral to medial aspect of the brachial artery at the midpoint of the humerus, it then enters the forearm, separated from the ulnar artery by the deep head of pronator teres. The anterior interosseous branch is given off in the forearm, supplying the pronator quadratus, flexor pollicis longus and flexor digitorum profundus. The median nerve becomes superficial on the ulnar side of, but deep to, the flexor carpi radialis at the wrist.

306. b.　The superior cervical ganglion lies at vertebral levels C2 and C3. The middle cervical ganglion lies at vertebral level C6. The inferior cervical ganglion lies at vertebral level C7, often fusing with the first thoracic ganglion at the level of the first rib to become the 'stellate ganglion'. Grey rami pass from the superior ganglion to cranial nerves VII, IX, XI and XII.

307. b.　The phrenic nerve arises from the anterior cervical rami of C3, 4 and 5, passing between scalenus medius and scalenus anterior, the latter of which it courses on in the neck. The right and left phrenic nerves travel anterior to the vagus nerve bilaterally. The right phrenic nerve courses inferiorly, lateral to the superior vena cava, and onto the fibrous pericardium overlying the right atrium; it travels anterior to the root of the lung, then pierces the central tendon of the diaphragm. The left phrenic nerve crosses anterior to the aortic arch (in contrast to the left vagus nerve, which crosses posteriorly) and courses inferiorly, anterior to the left pulmonary artery and fibrous pericardium of the left ventricle; after crossing the root of the left lung anteriorly, it passes through the caval orifice of the diaphragm at T8.

308. b.　The trochlear nerve arises from the back of the midbrain and runs under the free edge of the tentorium; it enters the dura of the lateral wall of the cavernous sinus (inferior and lateral to the oculomotor nerve); it then passes through the superior orbital fissure (outside the tendinous ring) and medially to supply the superior oblique muscle. Its action can be tested by asking the patient to look toward the nose, then downward.

309. a.　The ciliary ganglion lies in the apex of the orbit lateral to the optic nerve. It receives sensory roots from the nasociliary nerve, sympathetic (postganglionic) roots from the plexus on the internal carotid artery and preganglionic parasympathetic fibres from the Edinger–Westphal nucleus. The postganglionic efferent fibres from the ganglion pass via the ciliary nerves to the muscles of the iris and ciliary muscle. Stimulation results in papillary constriction and accommodation of the lens.

310. d.　The fibres of the vagus nerve originate in the medulla. The nerve exits the cranium through the jugular foramen, passing down the neck in the carotid sheath. The superior, internal and external laryngeal branches are given off in the neck. The right recurrent laryngeal nerve is given off in the root of the neck and hooks behind the subclavian artery, whereas the left recurrent laryngeal nerve is given off at the level of the arch of the aorta and hooks behind it at the level of the ligamentum arteriosum. Both vagi enter the abdomen through the oesophageal opening in the diaphragm – the left vagus travels anterior and the right vagus posterior to the oesophagus.

311. d. The stellate ganglion is located at the level of C7, lying anterior to the C7 transverse process and below the subclavian artery. The ganglion itself is formed by the unification of the inferior cervical ganglion with the first thoracic ganglion and predominantly causes vasoconstriction within the upper limb. Damage to the stellate ganglion can lead to Horner's syndrome. Blockade of the T2–3 ganglia by performing a thoracic sympathectomy may be used to treat Raynaud's and hyperhydrosis.

312. b. The cremasteric muscle is dependent on nerve roots L1 and L2. It is innervated by the genital branch of the genitofemoral nerve. The reflex is elicited by stroking the superior and medial aspect of the thigh causing the cremaster to retract the testes. The cremaster covers the spermatic cord and testes and is derived from the internal oblique muscle.

313. b. Meralgia paraesthetica is a painful mononeuropathy of the lateral femoral cutaneous nerve, commonly caused by focal entrapment of this nerve as it passes just under or through the inguinal ligament. Treatment is based on symptoms. Weight reduction, less compressive clothing, non-steroidal anti-inflammatory drugs (NSAIDs), local anaesthetic infiltration and surgical release have been described as treatment modalities.

314. d. The femoral nerve is the largest branch of the lumbar plexus (L2–4). It forms in the abdomen within the substance of the psoas major muscle and descends posterolaterally through the pelvis to the midpoint of the inguinal ligament. It supplies the anterior thigh muscles (the quadriceps group extends the leg at the knee); it also supplies other anterior thigh muscles (iliacus and sartorius) which allow flexion of the thigh at the hip joint. The femoral nerve also gives several branches to the skin on the anteromedial side of the lower limb.

315. a. The lateral cutaneous nerve of the thigh supplies the anterolateral aspect of the thigh. It has no motor branches. Meralgia paraesthetica is a condition where there is irritation of the nerve causing sensory changes in the distribution of the lateral cutaneous nerve of the thigh without any motor changes. L2 and L3 supply part of the dermatome described but both have motor branches. The femoral nerve supplies the quadriceps muscle, and the saphenous nerve runs with the saphenous vein to supply an area of skin below the knee on the medial aspect of the leg.

316. d. The history described is typical of carpal tunnel syndrome. Entrapment of the median nerve at the carpal tunnel affects the muscles of the thenar eminence. These are the abductor pollicis brevis, flexor pollicis brevis and opponens pollicis. The nerve supply to the thenar eminence muscles can be variable apart from abductor pollicis brevis, which is always supplied by the median nerve and makes it the muscle to test. In addition, the motor branch of the median nerve after the level of the carpal tunnel also innervates the radial two lumbricals.

317. b. A C5/C6 lesion, Erb palsy, produces sensory loss over the lateral aspect of the upper arm (deltoid paralysis), with loss of shoulder abduction, and paralysis of the biceps, brachialis and coracobrachialis. In addition to loss of elbow flexion, the biceps is also a powerful supinator of the forearm, so the forearm assumes a pronated position. A T1 lesion produces a claw hand (Klumpke palsy). Sympathetic chain injury results in Horner syndrome, with ptosis of the upper eyelid and constriction of the pupil (meiosis) on the affected side.

318. a. The inferior alveolar nerve, a branch of the mandibular division of the trigeminal nerve (V), traverses the inferior alveolar, or dental canal of the mandible, to supply all the teeth of that hemimandible. The mental branch of the nerve emerges through the mental foramen to supply the lower lip, which becomes numb in a successfully performed block. The muscles of the tongue, of mastication and of facial expression are not affected.

319. c. An injury to the ilioinguinal nerve within the inguinal canal may result in paraesthesia over the pubis and anterior scrotum. The ilioinguinal nerve (L1) passes through the internal oblique muscle to enter the inguinal canal laterally. It passes anterior to the cord and exits the superficial ring to provide sensation to the root of the penis, mons pubis and anterior scrotum in the male and labia majora in the female.

320. b. The femoral nerve may be damaged from fractures of the pelvis or femur, or dislocations of the hip, and hip or hernia surgery. It can also be involved in psoas abscesses, thigh wounds and frequently in large psoas haematomas in patients with haemophilia and diabetic amyotrophy. Partial lesions are common from thigh wounds with the nerve to the quadriceps most frequently involved and causing great problems in walking, with the knee often giving way, especially when descending stairs. It leads to a loss of power in the knee extension. In addition, there are quadriceps wasting, loss of knee jerk and impaired sensation over the front of the thigh.

321. c. Morton's neuroma is an enlarged common plantar nerve, usually in the third interspace between the third and fourth toes. Patients present with pain in the third interspace, which may be sharp or dull and is usually worsened by wearing shoes and walking. Treatment may include injection of anti-inflammatory drugs or surgical excision.

322. d. The brachial plexus forms from the anterior rami of cervical nerves C5 to C8 and thoracic nerve T1. The contributions of each of these nerves, which are between the anterior and middle scalene muscles, are the roots of the brachial plexus. As the roots emerge from between these muscles they form the next component of the brachial plexus (the trunks) as follows:

- The anterior rami of C5 and C6 form the upper trunk.
- The anterior ramus of C7 forms the middle trunk.
- The anterior rami of C8 and T1 form the lower trunk.

323. a. The vagus nerve (CN X) arises bilaterally from the medulla. It exits the cranium via the jugular foramen and enters the carotid sheath, together with the internal carotid artery and the internal jugular vein. It then enters the superior thoracic aperture. The right vagus nerve branches around the right subclavian artery to form the right recurrent laryngeal nerve. The left vagus nerve branches around the arch of aorta forming the left recurrent laryngeal nerve. These nerves provide sensorimotor supply to the larynx together with the superior laryngeal nerve, another branch of the vagus nerve. The vagus nerve passes through the diaphragm at the level of T10 with the oesophagus. It provides parasympathetic supply to organs of the thorax and abdomen right up to the left colic flexure.

324. b.   The median nerve supplies five hand muscles. They are the lateral two lumbricals, opponens pollicis, abductor pollicis brevis and flexor pollicis brevis (they can be remembered using the mnemonic LOAF). All other hand muscles are supplied by the ulnar nerve. The radial nerve does not supply any muscles in the hand.

325. c.   The nucleus of cranial nerve (CN) VI is located in the pons, along with nuclei of CNs VII and VIII. The motor nucleus and a portion of the sensory nucleus of CN V is also located in the pons. Cranial nerve nuclei III and IV and a portion of the sensory nucleus of CN V are found in the midbrain. The nuclei of the remaining cranial nerves, IX, X, XI and XII, are in the medulla.

326. b.   Cranial nerve (CN) III supplies the sphincter pupillae and ciliary muscles. CN VII supplies glands in the face, mainly lacrimal, submandibular, sublingual and nasal cavity glands, as well as mucosa of the palate. CN IX supplies the parotid gland. CN X supplies thoracic and abdominal viscera up to the left colic flexure.

327. c.   Parasympathetic supply is limited to viscera and glands of the body, sparing skin and skeletal muscles. The majority of the supply arises from the cranial nerves. Cranial nerve (CN) III supplies the sphincter pupillae and ciliary muscles of the eye. CN VII supplies the lacrimal, submandibular and sublingual glands, mucosa of the palate, as well as glands in the nose. CN IX supplies the parotid gland. CN X supplies the thoracic and abdominal viscera up to the left colic flexure.

328. d.   The common peroneal nerve (L4, L5, S1, S2) is a branch of the sciatic nerve, along with the tibial nerve. It begins at the superior angle of the popliteal fossa, travelling superolaterally in the fossa and then superficial to the lateral head of the gastrocnemius. It winds around the neck of the fibula and is vulnerable to injury at this point. It then gives off deep and superficial branches. The deep branch supplies muscles in the anterior compartment of the leg, whereas the superficial branch supplies muscles in the lateral compartment of the leg. These branches also give sensory supply to the anterior surface of the leg and dorsum of the foot. Injury to the common peroneal nerve commonly presents with a foot drop: patients are unable to dorsiflex their feet owing to weakness of tibialis anterior and peroneus tertius muscles. The tibialis posterior muscle is supplied by the tibial nerve.

329. b.   The radial nerve (C6–C8, T1) runs down the arm between the lateral and medial heads of triceps and around the spiral groove of the humerus where is it vulnerable to injury when there is a mid-shaft fracture of the humerus. Once on the lateral aspect of the arm the radial nerve runs between brachialis and brachioradialis just proximal to the elbow. The posterior interosseous nerve is a continuation of the deep branch of the radial nerve, supplying most of the extensor muscles of the forearm. It starts approximately at the level of the radial head and is therefore suceptible to damage from fractures. Supply to extensor carpi radialis longus is directly from the main radial nerve before it splits; hence wrist extension is still possible if the posterior interosseous nerve is damaged. The brachioradialis muscle is the only upper limb flexor muscle to be innervated by the radial nerve. The median nerve crosses from lateral to medial to the brachial artery at the mid-humeral level.

PART II

PHYSIOLOGY

CHAPTER 3
PHYSIOLOGY

Questions

RESPIRATORY SYSTEM

1. A 42-year-old lifelong smoker is about to have an abdominoperineal resection for rectal carcinoma. He is sent for pulmonary function tests as part of his preoperative assessment. All of the following lung volumes can be measured directly using simple spirometry except:
   a. Functional residual capacity (FRC)
   b. Expiratory reserve volume (ERV)
   c. Tidal volume (TV)
   d. Vital capacity (VC)
   e. Inspiratory reserve volume

2. The anatomical dead space of the lungs is defined as which one of the following?
   a. The volume of air left in the lungs after a tidal breath
   b. The amount of air left in the lungs after a maximal breath
   c. After breathing out normally, the remainder of air that can be expired
   d. The volume of air in the conducting airways
   e. The amount of air breathed in or out during a normal breath cycle

3. Which one of the following statements is false regarding surfactant?
   a. It is produced in the granular mitochondrial bodies of type II alveolar epithelial cells.
   b. It helps reduce alveolar surface tension.
   c. Dipalmitoylphosphatidylcholine (DPPC) is a major constituent of surfactant.
   d. Surfactant deficiency is an important cause of infant respiratory distress syndrome (IRDS).
   e. Cigarette smoking decreases lung surfactant production.

4. Within the alveoli, which of the following produce surfactant?
   a. Type I alveolar cells
   b. Type II alveolar cells
   c. Macrophages

d. Capillary endothelial cells
e. Interstitial connective tissue

5. Which of the following statements concerning breathing and pulmonary compliance is correct?
   a. Surfactant is produced by pulmonary macrophages in response to injury of type II pneumocytes.
   b. Compliance of the lung is greater during expiration.
   c. Surfactant increases alveoli surface tension.
   d. In the context of expiration, compliance is also referred to as elastance.
   e. Decreased lung compliance is seen in chronic obstructive pulmonary disease.

6. Carbon dioxide is primarily transported in the arterial blood as which one of the following?
   a. Dissolved CO_2
   b. Carbonic acid
   c. Carbaminohaemoglobin
   d. Bicarbonate
   e. Calcium carbonate

7. When considering the physiological changes that take place during acclimatization to high altitude, which of the following statements is true?
   a. The partial pressure of oxygen is increased.
   b. The oxyhaemoglobin saturation is increased.
   c. Ventilation is decreased.
   d. 2,3-Diphosphoglycerate (2,3-DPG) concentration increases.
   e. Oxyhaemoglobin affinity is increased.

8. Which one of the following is a feature of the pulmonary circulation?
   a. Vasoconstriction in hypoxia
   b. Increased basal vasoconstrictor tone in response to a rising pH
   c. Decreased blood volume during systole
   d. Vasodilation in hypoxia
   e. Increased blood volume during diastole

9. The following areas of the brain have to play a role in the control of respiration except:
   a. The pons
   b. The cerebral cortex
   c. The midbrain
   d. The medulla oblongata
   e. The limbic system

10. The following statements regarding the chemical regulation of respiration are true except:
    a. Central chemoreceptors are sensitive to changes in arterial PCO_2.
    b. Levels of PO_2 play a significant role in central regulation of respiration.
    c. CO_2 is able to cross the blood–brain barrier.

d. High levels of CO_2 cause an increase in respiratory rate.

e. A drop in pH will stimulate increasing respiration.

11. Which statement concerning the control of respiration is correct?

a. The peripheral chemoreceptors of the carotid body primarily sense changes in pH.

b. Central chemoreceptors lie outside the blood–brain barrier.

c. Central chemoreceptors primarily sense direct changes in PCO_2.

d. The apneustic and pneumotaxic centres can be voluntarily overridden by the cortex.

e. The peripheral chemoreceptors of the aortic arch are largely insensitive to changes in PO_2.

12. Which of the following conditions shift the oxygen dissociation curve to the left?

a. Increased temperature

b. High 2,3-DPG

c. Low pH

d. High carbon dioxide

e. High carbon monoxide

13. All of the following causes the oxygen–haemoglobin dissociation curve to shift to the right except:

a. High PCO_2

b. High 2,3-DPG

c. High temperature

d. Low carbon monoxide (CO)

e. Low $[H^+]$

14. Which of the following features causes the sigmoid shape of the oxygen–haemoglobin dissociation curve?

a. The binding of one oxygen molecule increases the affinity of binding of other oxygen molecules.

b. The binding of one oxygen molecule decreases the affinity of binding of other oxygen molecules.

c. The Bohr effect.

d. Adenosine diphosphate (ADP) in the cells.

e. Surfactant.

15. The following statements regarding pulse oximetry are true except:

a. It does not provide information on the adequacy of ventilation.

b. It has a linear relationship with O_2 arterial carriage.

c. It does not provide a direct indication of arterial PO_2.

d. It may overestimate O_2 saturations in inhalational burn cases.

e. Saturation below 70% is unreliable.

16. Concerning pulse oximetry, which one of the following statements is true?

a. It measures arterial O_2 partial pressure.

b. Readings are inaccurate with the presence of carbon monoxide.

c. It gives a good indication of ventilation.

d. Readings are usually reliable despite poor peripheral perfusion.
e. It usually uses three wavelengths of light.

17. Which statement regarding the haemoglobin molecule is correct?
    a. It is comprised of six subunits to bind oxygen.
    b. Each subunit binds one oxygen molecule.
    c. Adult haemoglobin has a higher affinity for oxygen than carbon monoxide.
    d. Fetal haemoglobin contains δ rather than α subunits.
    e. As haemoglobin binds more oxygen molecules, there is a reduction in affinity for further oxygen.

18. Which one of the following statements concerning haemoglobin is correct?
    a. It consists of eight peptide chains.
    b. It carries eight oxygen atoms.
    c. It is only able to carry oxygen.
    d. It releases oxygen more easily in less acidic conditions.
    e. It contains one haem group.

19. A 35-year-old man is brought into the emergency department following a road traffic collision. The following changes can usually be detected in a patient with tension pneumothorax except:
    a. Reduced venous return
    b. Increased respiratory rate
    c. Reduced heart rate
    d. Reduced PO_2
    e. Increased jugular venous pressure

20. Your Foundation Year 1 doctor bleeps to say that one of your postoperative patients is saturating at 85% on air and the blood gas shows a PO_2 of 7.59 kPa and a PCO_2 of 3.4 kPa. Which of the following are included in your differential diagnosis?
    a. Airway obstruction
    b. Chronic obstructive pulmonary disease
    c. Opiate overdose
    d. Pulmonary oedema
    e. None the above

21. A 23-year-old woman has been stabbed in the chest. Which one of the following is not a sign of a massive haemothorax?
    a. Reduced breath sounds
    b. Hypovolemic shock
    c. Increased jugular venous pressure (JVP)
    d. Evidence of penetrating injury
    e. Dull percussion tone

22. An 89-year-old man is brought in by ambulance as a trauma call. He was found unconscious at the bottom of a flight of stairs. On arrival in the emergency department, the patient is very agitated with a respiratory rate of 35 and a heart rate of 126. On your primary survey, you note the patient's

trachea is deviated to the left, with hyperresonant percussion notes on the right and absent breath sounds. Which is the emergency step for this patient?

a. Request a chest X-ray
b. Insert a chest drain
c. Perform pericardiocentesis
d. Perform immediate needle thoracocentesis
e. Request for the patient to be intubated

CARDIOVASCULAR SYSTEM

23. A pregnant lady requires an appendicectomy. Which of the following cardiovascular physiological changes would not be expected in pregnancy?
    a. Increase in heart rate of around 35%
    b. Increase in stroke volume of around 35%
    c. Venous dilatation of around 150%
    d. Red cell mass increased by 20–30%
    e. Ventricular enlargement with cardiac hypertrophy

24. Which one of the following statements best describes the Frank–Starling law of the heart?
    a. Cardiac output is a factor of stroke volume and heart rate.
    b. Stroke volume is not affected by peripheral vascular resistance.
    c. Stroke volume is directly proportional to end-diastolic volume.
    d. Stroke volume does not change with sympathetic stimulation.
    e. Stroke volume is a function of end-diastolic volume.

25. What is the typical blood pressure of the pulmonary artery?
    a. 10/5 mmHg
    b. 25/15 mmHg
    c. 40/15 mmHg
    d. 80/40 mmHg
    c. 120/80 mmHg

26. Regarding pulmonary artery wedge pressure monitoring, the following statements are true except:
    a. Normal values of the pulmonary artery wedge pressure are between 6 and 12 mmHg.
    b. It is useful in the treatment of septic patients.
    c. 'Wedge' pressure is a good reflection of right atrial pressure.
    d. It can be used to measure cardiac output.
    e. The catheter is often introduced via the internal jugular vein.

27. Which of the following statements regarding the monitoring of circulation is correct?
    a. A normal central venous pressure ranges from 15 to 20 mmHg.
    b. Pulse oximetry pulses light in the red and infrared wavelengths.
    c. Normal pulmonary artery occlusion pressure is between 2 and 5 mmHg.
    d. Central venous pressure can be used to calculate cardiac output.
    e. Pulmonary artery occlusion pressure reflects right atrial pressure.

28. Which of the following statements about the third heart sound is true?
    a. It is caused by closure of the atrioventricular valves.
    b. It indicates ventricular hypertrophy.
    c. It is caused by rapid ventricular filling.
    d. It is heard loudest in the aortic area.
    e. It is caused by closure of the aortoventricular valves.

29. Which of the following correctly describes the Wenckebach phenomenon of heart block?
   a. Fixed prolonged PR interval.
   b. Some P waves are not followed by a QRS complex – consistent 2:1, 3:1.
   c. No recognizable relationship between P waves and QRS complexes.
   d. PR interval becomes progressively more prolonged until a QRS complex is dropped.
   e. Every P wave is always followed by a QRS complex.

30. All of the following conditions cause a high cardiac output owing to reduced peripheral resistance except for which one?
   a. Beriberi
   b. Arteriovenous fistula
   c. Hyperthyroidism
   d. Anaemia
   e. Massive haemorrhage

31. Which of the following factors helps a person recover from moderate degrees of shock?
   a. Baroreceptor reflexes
   b. Reverse stress–relaxation of the circulatory system
   c. Formation of angiotensin by the kidneys
   d. All of the above
   e. a and c only

32. During myocardial contraction, which of the following is the most important factor controlling myocardial contractility?
   a. Intracellular Na^+
   b. Extracellular Na^+
   c. Intracellular K^+
   d. Intracellular Ca^{2+}
   e. Extracellular Ca^{2+}

33. Which statement is correct regarding fluid movement through capillary membrane?
   a. Capillary pressure tends to force fluid out from the capillary.
   b. Interstitial fluid pressure tends to force fluid into the capillary when positive but out from the capillary when negative.
   c. Capillary plasma colloid osmotic pressure tends to cause osmosis of fluid into the capillary.
   d. Interstitial fluid colloid osmotic pressure tends to cause osmosis of fluid out from the capillary.
   e. All the above.

34. Which of the following statements relating to the Starling equilibrium is true?
   a. Filtration is favoured at the arterial end of the capillary.
   b. Retention of plasma proteins within the vasculature maintains the oncotic pressure.
   c. Oncotic pressure is relatively higher at the arterial end.

d. All of the above.

e. a and b only.

35. Concerning the coronary circulation, which of the following statements is correct?

a. The heart receives 10% of the overall cardiac output.

b. The coronary blood flow at rest is 300–400 mL/min per 100 g of cardiac tissue.

c. Myocardial oxygen consumption is approximately 8 mL O_2/min per 100 g of cardiac tissue.

d. Approximately 95% of the oxygen delivered to the myocardium is extracted.

e. Increased myocardial oxygen demand during exercise is predominantly accounted for through an increase in the oxygen extraction ratio.

36. Which of the following statements regarding the oxygen consumption of cardiac muscle is correct?

a. O_2 consumption by the non-beating heart is about 2 mL O_2/100 g per minute.

b. O_2 consumption by the beating heart at rest is about 8 mL O_2/100 g per minute.

c. O_2 consumption by the heart can be estimated in humans by utilizing the Fick principle.

d. All of the above.

e. Only b and c.

37. Concerning the distribution of body water in a healthy 70 kg man, which of the following statements is correct?

a. There is approximately 30 L of water in total.

b. Interstitial fluid would amount to approximately 9 L.

c. Extracellular fluid would amount to approximately 9 L.

d. Intravascular fluid would amount to approximately 2 L.

e. Transcellular fluid would amount to approximately 5 L.

38. The volume of water in the intracellular compartment is what approximate percentage of body weight?

a. 20%

b. 30%

c. 40%

d. 50%

e. 60%

39. Which of the following increases turbulence in blood flow?

a. A Reynolds number less than 2000

b. A decrease in velocity of blood

c. A decreased density of blood

d. An increase in diameter of blood vessel

e. All of the above

40. Which of the following is the main site of red blood cell formation in adults?

a. Long bones

b. Flat bones

c. Liver
d. Spleen
e. Kidneys

41. Which one of the following statements regarding shock is not true?
    a. Shock is defined as inadequate tissue perfusion and oxygen delivery to the tissues.
    b. In cardiogenic shock the systemic vascular resistance decreases.
    c. In cardiogenic shock the cardiac output decreases.
    d. In neurogenic shock there is a decrease in systemic vascular resistance.
    e. In septic shock the systemic vascular resistance decreases.

42. A 25-year-old male has cut his arm with an electric saw while doing some DIY at home. He comes in fully conscious but appears a little restless. His shirt is clearly blood soaked. All of his observations come back as normal apart from a raised blood pressure. Which (if any) class of shock is he in?
    a. Not shocked
    b. Class I
    c. Class II
    d. Class III
    e. Class IV

43. A 50-year-old barely conscious man has been brought in by ambulance with multiple stab wounds. His blood pressure on arrival was 70/50 mmHg, heart rate 145 bpm, respiratory rate 40. He has been catheterized for at least an hour but has passed no urine. Which of the following is his likely percentage loss of blood?
    a. 0–10%
    b. 15–20%
    c. 25–30%
    d. 35–40%
    e. >40%

44. A 43-year-old woman is brought by ambulance to the accident and emergency department having been stabbed in the upper abdomen with a kitchen knife. On examination, there is no evidence of active bleeding; however, she has a heart rate of 132 bpm, blood pressure of 94/68 and is pale. Which one of the following responses of the body to blood loss is correct in this scenario?
    a. There is an increase in heart rate.
    b. There is an increase in cardiac output.
    c. There is an increase in central venous pressure.
    d. Splanchnic vasodilation occurs.
    e. Cerebral blood flow and perfusion will rise.

45. You are called to the accident and emergency department to assess a 25-year-old male patient. On examination, he is pale with evidence of a penetrating right-sided chest wall injury. His heart rate is 145 bpm,

blood pressure 75/50 mmHg and he is combative during your examination. You want to raise his cardiac output and address his state of shock. Which of the following fluids is most suitable in this situation?

a. Dextrose-saline
b. 5% dextrose
c. Blood
d. Colloid
e. Hartmann's solution (Ringer's lactate)

46. A 75-year-old man is 10 days post left hemicolectomy. He has been progressing well but becomes short of breath and complains of central chest pain, which is worse when he takes a deep breath. On examination he is confused, tachycardic and tachypnoeic. You also notice an erythematous, oedematous and tender left calf. You take a set of observations, which reveal a blood pressure of 85/40 mmHg and a pulse of 120 bpm. You diagnose that the man is in shock, but which type of shock is he in?

a. Cardiogenic
b. Hypovolaemic
c. Septic
d. Anaphylactic
e. Obstructive

47. Which one of the following statements regarding septic shock is true?

a. In septic shock there is significant vasoconstriction.
b. In septic shock there is a decrease in cardiac output.
c. In septic shock there is a reduced afterload.
d. In septic shock there is reduced sympathetic drive.
e. Septic shock after biliary surgery is commonly caused by Gram-positive organisms.

48. Which of the following electrocardiogram (ECG) changes is not associated with hyperkalaemia?

a. Tented T waves
b. Small P waves
c. Wide QRS complex
d. Prominent U waves
e. Sine wave formation

49. Concerning the jugular venous waveform, which of the following statements is correct?

a. The C wave is due to atrial contraction.
b. The X descent occurs at the end of atrial systole.
c. The A wave is caused by bulging of the mitral valve into the left atrium.
d. The Y descent occurs following opening of the aortic valve.
e. The V wave occurs due to contraction of the right ventricle.

50. With reference to the jugular venous pressure (JVP), the rise in right atrial pressure before the tricuspid valve opens is known as what?

a. A wave
b. C wave

c. V wave
d. X descent
e. Y descent

51. Which one of the following statements is true regarding the waveform of the jugular venous pressure (JVP)?
    a. The A wave is seen in ventricular systole.
    b. A raised A wave suggests right ventricular hypertrophy.
    c. C waves are produced when the tricuspid valve opens.
    d. Large V waves are seen in mitral stenosis.
    e. None of the above.

52. In the cardiac cycle, which one of the following statements is correct?
    a. The first heart sound is caused by the opening of the mitral valve.
    b. The second heart sound is caused by the closing of the mitral valve.
    c. The P wave on the electrocardiogram (ECG) corresponds to atrial repolarization.
    d. The C wave of the jugular venous pressure (JVP) occurs because of closure of the tricuspid valve during ventricular contraction.
    e. The T wave on the ECG represents ventricular depolarization.

53. Elevation of the jugular venous pressure (JVP) is seen in all of the following conditions except which one?
    a. Poorly controlled heart failure
    b. Cardiac tamponade
    c. Constrictive pericarditis
    d. Overtransfusion of blood and fluids
    e. Haemorrhage

54. All of the following features are noted in cardiac muscle except:
    a. Cardiac muscle cells have multiple nuclei.
    b. The dark areas crossing the cardiac muscle fibres are called intercalated discs.
    c. It is a syncytium of many heart muscle cells.
    d. Cardiac muscle has a branched structure on electron microscopy.
    e. Cardiac muscle is involuntary striated muscle.

55. You are asked to review a 75-year-old man who is complaining of central dull chest pain. You ask for an electrogardiogram (ECG), which shows raised ST segments in leads I, aVL and V4–V6. The location of the myocardial infarction is likely to be in which area of the heart?
    a. Inferior wall
    b. Lateral wall
    c. Anterolateral
    d. Septal
    e. Posterior wall

56. Which one of the following comments is true regarding stroke volume?
    a. Increasing the preload increases the stroke volume.
    b. It is the volume of blood pumped by the heart over 1 min.
    c. Women have higher stroke volumes than men.

d. Increasing the afterload increases the stroke volume.

e. It can be calculated by subtracting the diastolic from the systolic blood pressure.

57. Regarding inotropes, the following statements are true except:
    a. All inotropes increase the rate of contraction of the heart.
    b. Endogenous inotropes are derived from the medulla of the adrenal gland.
    c. Noradrenaline has mild β-stimulating properties.
    d. Adrenaline acts on both α and β receptors.
    e. Noradrenaline causes peripheral vasoconstriction.

58. While reviewing one of your patients in the high-dependency unit, you notice that she has been started on noradrenaline. Which of the following statements is true?
    a. Noradrenaline does not cause limb ischaemia.
    b. Noradrenaline is used to primarily act on α-adrenergic receptors.
    c. Noradrenaline decreases the cardiac strain.
    d. Noradrenaline decreases the end-diastolic volume.
    e. Noradrenaline is mainly used to decrease peripheral vascular resistance.

59. Which of the following organs does not contain β_2 receptors?
    a. Heart
    b. Blood vessels
    c. Lungs
    d. Uterus
    e. Liver

60. The following statements regarding the clotting cascade are true except:
    a. Clotting factor X is not part of the extrinsic pathway.
    b. The extrinsic pathway requires tissue thromboplastin.
    c. Thrombin is formed in the final common pathway.
    d. Prolonged prothrombin time (PT) may be caused by a deficiency in clotting factor V.
    e. Activated partial thromboplastin time (APTT) measures the integrity of the intrinsic system.

61. On standing, the body employs various mechanisms to maintain blood pressure. Which one of the following is true?
    a. Stroke volume rises on standing.
    b. Standing causes a reduction in carotid baroreceptor stimulation.
    c. There is reduced sympathetic stimulation on standing.
    d. To increase arterial pressure, the body attempts to increase cardiac output and reduce systemic vascular resistance.
    e. Vagal cardiac stimulation rises.

62. The following can increase the rate of stimulation of erythrocyte production except:
    a. Respiratory disease
    b. High altitude

c. Vasodilatation
d. Haemorrhage
e. Increased levels of red blood cell degradation products

63. Myoglobin is an oxygen-binding porphyrin. Which one of the following statements regarding myoglobin in skeletal muscle is correct?
a. It binds and stores oxygen for rapid release during falling PO_2.
b. It is found in fast fibres only.
c. It releases O_2 at high PO_2.
d. It exhibits cooperative binding with O_2 (sigmoid dissociation curve).
e. It is devoid of iron.

64. Which one of the following statements regarding pulse pressure is correct?
a. A high pulse pressure suggests significant blood loss or dehydration.
b. A high pulse pressure is seen in aortic stenosis.
c. Pulse pressure can increase with exercise.
d. Angiotensin-converting enzyme inhibitors are ineffective at reducing pulse pressure.
e. A high pulse pressure can be caused by mitral regurgitation.

65. Which haemoglobin type makes up the majority of the haemoglobin (Hb) molecules in the fetus?
a. HbA1
b. HbA2
c. HbS
d. HbF
e. HbE

66. Which of the following is not a recognised function of a central venous catheter (CVC)?
a. Central venous pressure (CVP) monitoring
b. Total parenteral nutrition delivery
c. Drug infusion
d. Rapid intravenous fluid resuscitation in trauma
e. Haemodialysis

67. Which of the following statements is incorrect regarding the sinoatrial (SA) node?
a. It is located near the entrance of the superior vena cava into the heart.
b. Its parasympathetic supply is from the vagus.
c. Its sympathetic supply is from T1–T4.
d. Blood supply is mainly from the left coronary artery.
e. The SA node initiates cardiac contraction in normal individuals.

68. During vigorous exercise, which one of the following occurs?
a. The heart rate remains the same.
b. Cardiac contractility remains unaltered.
c. End-systolic volume increases.
d. Central venous pressure always drops.
e. Stroke volume falls.

69. During a preoperative clinic you look through the echocardiography report of a patient waiting for an elective total hip replacement. The report states that the ejection fraction (EF) is normal. Which of the following is the approximate EF of the normal heart in a resting state?
    a. 15%
    b. 30%
    c. 45%
    d. 60%
    e. 75%

70. The blood pressure is closely monitored on a beat-to-beat basis. All of the following are features of baroreceptors except:
    a. The carotid sinus and aortic arch receptors monitor the arterial circulation.
    b. The baroreceptors are stimulated by distension of the structures in which they are located.
    c. Baroreceptors are more sensitive to pulsatile pressure than to constant pressure.
    d. The afferent nerve fibres from the carotid sinus form a distinct branch of the vagus nerve.
    e. The threshold for eliciting activity in the carotid sinus nerve is about 60 mmHg.

71. Which of the following statements are false regarding control of blood pressure?
    a. Renin is synthesized in the juxtaglomerular apparatus.
    b. Aldosterone is released in response to angiotensin II.
    c. Conn syndrome is a secondary cause of hyperaldosteronism.
    d. The Anrep effect is a response to acute increase in afterload.
    e. The Bowditch effect is a response to change in heart rate.

72. During the preoperative clinic you see a patient who is due an elective right hemicolectomy. The patient has a diagnosis of Addison's disease. Which of the following would you not expect to find in the patient's serum biochemistry?
    a. Raised adrenocorticotropic hormone (ACTH)
    b. Low cortisol
    c. Low sodium
    d. Low potassium
    e. Raised urea

73. The following statements concerning cardiac physiology are true except:
    a. Coronary blood flow is increased during diastole.
    b. Cardiac index is measured as stroke volume per square metre of body surface area.
    c. Coronary blood flow can increase up to 1 L/min during strenuous exercise.
    d. Occlusion of the left coronary artery can lead to death.
    e. Papillary muscles contract prior to ventricular contraction.

74. Concerning the lymphatic circulation, which statement is correct?
    a. Collecting lymphatics lack valves.
    b. Collecting lymphatics are found in skeletal muscle.
    c. Initial lymphatics contract in a peristaltic fashion.
    d. The normal 24 h lymph turnover is 5–6 L.
    e. Initial lymphatics lack smooth muscle.

75. Concerning oedema, which of the following statements is correct?
    a. It is defined as an excess accumulation of fluid in the interstitial space.
    b. An exudate is a consequence of imbalanced hydrostatic forces.
    c. Nephrotic syndrome leads to a transudate.
    d. Increased capillary permeability leads to a transudate.
    e. Transudates are rich in fibrinogen and protein.

76. Concerning capillary pressure, which of the following statements is correct?
    a. The pressure of nail-bed capillaries at the arteriolar end is roughly 20 mmHg.
    b. The pressure of nail-bed capillaries at the venous end is roughly 25 mmHg.
    c. The pulse pressure of nail-bed capillaries at the arteriolar end is roughly 5 mmHg.
    d. The pulse pressure of nail-bed capillaries at the venous end is roughly 5 mmHg.
    e. The pulse pressure of nail-bed capillaries at the arteriolar end is roughly 35 mmHg.

77. Which of the following represent the correct composition of intravenous fluids?
    a. Hartmann's solution – Na 131 mmol/L, K 0 mmol/L, Cl 111 mmol/L, HCO_3 29 mmol/L
    b. Normal saline – Na 145 mmol/L, Cl 155 mmol/L
    c. 5% dextrose – osmolality – 308 mosmol/L
    d. Hartmann's solution – osmolality – 278 mosmol/L
    e. Normal saline – osmolality – 278 mosmol/L

GASTROINTESTINAL SYSTEM

78. The following statements about gallstones are true except:
    a. They can be found in stools.
    b. There is an increased incidence in haemolytic diseases.
    c. They are most commonly mixed types.
    d. They are most commonly formed in the bile duct.
    e. They can cause jaundice.

79. Concerning functions of the liver, which of the following statements is correct?
    a. Bile is secreted by hepatocytes.
    b. Approximately 400 mL of bile is produced by the liver each day.
    c. The liver is responsible for synthesis of all essential amino acids.
    d. Glycogenolysis involves the breakdown of glucose to ketone bodies during periods of starvation.
    e. The cytochrome P450 system of the liver is inhibited by phenytoin.

80. Within the stomach, hydrogen potassium ATPase is unique to which type of cell?
    a. Parietal cells
    b. Chief cells
    c. Endocrine (G-cell)
    d. Mucous cells
    e. Enterochromaffin cells

81. Which of the following statements regarding gastrin is incorrect?
    a. Gastrin stimulates gastric acid secretion from parietal cells.
    b. Gastrin is released by G-cells in the stomach.
    c. Gastrin is released by G-cells in the duodenum.
    d. Gastrin is released by parietal cells.
    e. Gastrin production is stimulated by stomach distension.

82. Gastrin production is inhibited by which one of the following?
    a. Stomach distension
    b. Acid within the duodenum
    c. Vagal stimulation
    d. The presence of partly digested proteins in the duodenum
    e. Intrinsic factor

83. Concerning the stomach secretions, which statement is correct?
    a. G-cells secrete HCl and pepsinogen.
    b. HCl secretion is inhibited by secretin.
    c. Chief cells produce intrinsic factor.
    d. Parietal cells produce gastrin.
    e. Gastric secretion is approximately 2–3 L/day.

84. Which of the following statements regarding oxyntic glands and parietal cells is incorrect?
    a. Oxyntic glands have three types of cells.
    b. The oxyntic glands are located on the inside surfaces of the body and fundus of the stomach.

c. Parietal cells produce pepsinogen.

d. Intrinsic factor produced by the parietal cell helps in absorption of vitamin B_{12}.

e. Parietal cells have canaliculi.

85. You are managing a patient with acute pancreatitis. All of the following changes usually indicate a more severe attack of acute pancreatitis except:
    a. Raised corrected calcium levels
    b. Raised white blood cells
    c. Respiratory failure
    d. Raised glucose levels
    e. Raised urea levels

86. All of the following features are noted with regard to saliva except:
    a. The average daily secretion of saliva is 250 mL.
    b. Saliva has a pH range of 6–7.
    c. Serous secretion of saliva contains ptyalin.
    d. Saliva contains factors that destroy bacteria.
    e. Concentration of bicarbonate ions in saliva is about two to three times that of plasma.

87. When calculating the volume of fluid movement within the gastrointestinal tract (GIT), how many litres of fluid are secreted by the stomach under normal conditions?
    a. 250 mL
    b. 1 L
    c. 2.5 L
    d. 4 L
    e. 8 L

88. Which is the major enzyme found in saliva?
    a. Pepsin
    b. Lipase
    c. Trypsin
    d. Amylase
    e. Elastase

89. The following statements regarding vomiting are true except:
    a. It can be caused by severe pain.
    b. Excessive vomiting can lead to metabolic alkalosis.
    c. Vomiting is commonly preceded by autonomic symptoms.
    d. It may result from a labyrinth dysfunction.
    e. It usually leads to aspiration pneumonia.

90. A 6-week-old baby boy is brought to hospital with projectile vomiting, weight loss and persisting hunger. Examination reveals dehydration and a small olive-sized swelling in the upper abdomen. The diagnosis of pyloric stenosis is made. Which of the following explain the commonly identified biochemical abnormality with pyloric stenosis?
    a. Hypokalaemic hypochloraemic alkalosis
    b. Hyperkaleamic hypochloraemic alkalosis

    c. Hypokalaemic hypochloraemic acidosis

    d. Hypokalaemic hyperchloraemic alkalosis

    e. Hypokalaemic hyperchloraemic acidosis

91. The following statements regarding jaundice are true except:

    a. Pre-hepatic jaundice is caused by raised levels of unconjugated bilirubin.

    b. Conjugated bilirubin is water soluble.

    c. Pruritus is a common feature of pre-hepatic jaundice.

    d. It can be caused by pancreatic cancer.

    e. Pale stool is a sign of cholestatic jaundice.

92. Concerning the physiology of the colon, which of the following statements is correct?

    a. There is a net absorption of potassium.

    b. There is a net absorption of bicarbonate.

    c. There is minimal absorption of water.

    d. It has a direct role in the synthesis of vitamin K and various B vitamins.

    e. Mass action contraction occurs one to three times per day.

93. A patient has recently undergone a pancreatic resection for a tumour. Which of the following changes would you not expect?

    a. Protein malnutrition

    b. Deficiency of vitamin B12

    c. Failure to neutralize gastric chyme

    d. Hypocalcaemia

    e. Anaemia

94. Which of the following statements relating to pancreatic physiology are true?

    a. Acinar cells respond to cholecystokinin.

    b. The ratio of pancreatic enzyme secretion with different diets is always the same.

    c. Chloride is secreted from duct cells.

    d. The enzyme trypsin acts on triglycerides.

    e. Secretin is released from the stomach before acting on the pancreas.

95. An elderly woman is admitted with acute pancreatitis secondary to gallstones. The team uses the Glasgow scoring system to assess her severity. Which of the following is a correct criterion of the Glasgow (Imrie) scoring system?

    a. PO_2 <8 KPa

    b. Neutrophils >12 × 10^9/L

    c. Albumin <36 g/L

    d. Corrected calcium <2.4 mmol/L

    e. Age <55 years

96. Motility within the wall of the intestine propels food through the gastrointestinal tract. Which one of the following statements is correct regarding intestinal activity?

    a. It is decreased by parasympathetic stimulation.

    b. It is inhibited by serotonin.

c. It is greater in movements of segmentation than in peristalsis.
d. It is caused by the rhythmic contraction of paced depolarizations called fast waves.
e. It is greater in the large bowel than it is in the small bowel.

97. Concerning swallowing, which of the following statements is correct?
a. There are two main phases.
b. The pharyngeal phase of swallowing is voluntary.
c. The oesophageal phase of swallowing is the shortest.
d. Contraction of the inferior constrictor muscle prevents food entering the nasopharynx.
e. Normal resting pressure of the lower oesophageal sphincter is 30 mmHg.

98. Which of the following hormones stimulates insulin release?
a. Gastrin
b. Guanylin
c. Cholecystokinin
d. Secretin
e. Gastric inhibitory peptide

99. Which of the following statements about bile physiology is true?
a. Gallbladder contraction is stimulated by the hormone secretin.
b. Urobilinogen colours faeces brown.
c. Bile acids are produced from the breakdown of haemoglobin.
d. Bile is used in the digestion and absorption of proteins.
e. Urobilinogen is only secreted in the faeces.

100. Which of the following enzymes helps protein digestion in the stomach?
a. Trypsin
b. Chymotrypsin
c. Pepsin
d. Carboxypeptidase
e. Proelastase

101. Stimulation of the myenteric plexus leads to which of the following?
a. Increased tonic contraction of the gut wall
b. Increased intensity of the rhythmical contractions
c. Rapid movement of the gut owing to peristaltic waves
d. All of the above
e. a and c only

102. Which cranial nerve (CN) is involved in the autonomic motor control of oesophageal swallowing?
a. X
b. XI
c. XII
d. VII
e. VIII

103. Which neurons function to relax the lower oesophageal sphincter during swallowing?
    a. Inhibitory neurons of the myenteric plexus
    b. Excitatory neurons of the myenteric plexus
    c. Inhibitory neurons of the coeliac plexus
    d. Inhibitory neurons of the mesenteric plexus
    e. Inhibition of the vagus nerve

104. What is the approximate rate of primary peristalsis of food in the oesophagus?
    a. 1 cm/s
    b. 5 cm/s
    c. 10 cm/s
    d. 20 cm/s
    e. 1 m/s

105. You are seeing a patient in the intensive care unit who is on total parenteral nutrition. Which of the following is not a recognized metabolic complication of parenteral nutrition?
    a. Hypoammonaemia
    b. Hyperlipidaemia
    c. Hyperglycaemia
    d. Essential fatty acid deficiency
    e. Hyperchloraemic metabolic acidosis

106. The liver uses vitamin K to synthesize which clotting factor?
    a. Factor VII
    b. Prothrombin
    c. Factor X
    d. Protein C
    e. All of the above

107. Which of the following inhibits gastric acid secretion?
    a. Nausea
    b. Gastrin
    c. Vagal stimulation
    d. Histamine
    e. Pepsinogen

RENAL SYSTEM

108. Which of these statements regarding the physiology of micturition is true?
    a. Intravesical pressure is approximately 10 cmH$_2$O.
    b. The sympathetic nervous system (SNS) decreases contraction of the internal sphincter.
    c. The parasympathetic nervous system (PNS) decreases detrusor contraction.
    d. The sympathetic nerves arise from L4–L5.
    e. The parasympathetic nerves arise from S2–S4.

109. The following can reduce serum potassium levels except:
    a. Insulin
    b. β-Adrenergic stimulation
    c. Aldosterone
    d. Renal failure
    e. Theophylline

110. The following statements on renal physiology are true except:
    a. The proximal convoluted tubule reabsorbs the majority of filtered Na$^+$.
    b. Filtrate at the end of the descending limb will be in a highly dilute state.
    c. The ascending loop is impermeable to water.
    d. Furosemide inhibits Na$^+$ reabsorption at the ascending limb.
    e. Thiazide diuretic inhibits Na$^+$ reabsorption at the distal convoluted tubule.

111. The following statements regarding the loop of Henle are true except:
    a. The descending limb is permeable to urea.
    b. Tubular filtrate is increasingly more concentrated heading down the loop.
    c. Sodium is co-transported out of the ascending limb.
    d. The ascending limb is permeable to water.
    e. The U-shape allows solute to be continuously recycled in order to maintain a high medullary osmolality.

112. The kidney plays an important role in the acid–base balance of the body. Which of the following statements regarding the kidney is true?
    a. The distal convoluted tubule reabsorbs 90% of filtered bicarbonate.
    b. The proximal convoluted tubule has a low concentration of carbonic anhydrase.
    c. Carbonic anhydrase converts carbonic acid into carbon dioxide and water.
    d. Secretion of hydrogen ions in the kidney from the body mainly occurs in the proximal tubule segments.
    e. Hydrogen ions cross passively down their concentration gradient into the tubular lumen in exchange for sodium ions.

113. Concerning sodium and water balance, which statement is correct?
    a. The physiological daily requirement of sodium is 2 mmol/kg.
    b. 30% of the body's sodium is found in the intracellular compartment.
    c. Atrial natriuretic peptide is secreted by the cardiac atria following a drop in circulating volume.

    d. Glucocorticoids increase sodium and water reabsorption.

    e. Arginine vasopressin is produced by the anterior pituitary gland.

114. An 85-year-old man with a past medical history of medically controlled hypothyroidism undergoes a transurethral resection of prostate under general anaesthesia. The procedure takes approximately 2 h. One hour after the operation he is restless and confused. His blood pressure is 134/78 mmHg and heart rate is regular at 80 bpm. Blood tests, including full blood count, urea and electrolytes, and an arterial blood gas are taken from the patient. Which of the following results is most likely to indicate an explanation for his situation?

    a. Sodium 110 mmol/L

    b. Haemoglobin 74 g/L

    c. PO_2 9.8 kPa

    d. Potassium 3.5 mmol/L

    e. PCO_2 5.8 kPa

115. Which of the following ions does not form part of the calculation for the anion gap?

    a. Sodium

    b. Bicarbonate

    c. Potassium

    d. Chloride

    e. Calcium

116. Which one of the following can stimulate the release of renin from the kidneys?

    a. Hyperkalaemia

    b. Hypertension

    c. Beta-blocker

    d. Aldosterone

    e. Salt depletion

117. The following statements regarding atrial natriuretic peptide (ANP) are true except:

    a. It increases glomerular filtration.

    b. It is released in response to a decrease in extracellular fluid (ECF).

    c. It inhibits Na^+ reabsorption.

    d. It is a vasodilator.

    e. It reduces the secretion of renin.

118. Regarding the renin–angiotensin–aldosterone (RAA) system, the following statements are true except:

    a. The juxtaglomerular apparatus monitors changes in the renal circulation.

    b. Angiotensin I is converted into angiotensin II in the liver.

    c. The macula densa detects changes in Na^+ load.

    d. Angiotensin II stimulates release of antidiuretic hormone (ADH).

    e. Aldosterone stimulates reabsorption of Na^+.

119. Which one of the following is the principal site of action for antidiuretic hormone (ADH).

    a. The posterior pituitary gland

    b. The distal convoluted tubule

c. The collecting duct
d. The proximal convoluted tubule
e. The afferent arteriole within Bowman's capsule

120. The adrenal gland is responsible for the production of multiple hormones? Which of the following statements is correct?
a. The zona glomerulosa is responsible for glucocorticoid production.
b. The zona fasciculata is responsible for mineralocorticoid production.
c. The zona reticularis is responsible for androgen production.
d. The zona fasciculata is superficial to the zona glomerulosa and zona reticularis.
e. The zona fasciculata can respond to Adrenocorticotropic hormone (ACTH) released by the anterior pituitary to produce aldosterone.

121. Which of the following play a crucial role in the regulation of H^+ concentration?
a. The respiratory centre
b. The kidneys
c. The chemical acid–base buffer systems
d. b and c only
e. All of the above

122. Which of the following substances is the most suitable for calculating renal clearance?
a. Creatinine
b. Urea
c. Insulin
d. Inulin
e. Glucose

123. An arterial blood gas on an unwell patient has the following values: pH 7.23, PCO_2 7.3 kPa, HCO_3^- 24 mmol/L. Which of the following is the most likely acid–base disturbance?
a. Metabolic acidosis
b. Metabolic alkalosis
c. Respiratory acidosis
d. Respiratory alkalosis
e. Respiratory acidosis with metabolic compensation

124. A 70-year-old insulin-dependent diabetic man returns from theatre having had a laparotomy for a perforated duodenal ulcer. The operation was uncomplicated. On return to the ward, he is noted to have a raised respiratory rate at 24, tachycardia at 132 bpm, but is normotensive at 126/86 mmHg. His oxygen saturations are 100% in room air. His blood gas shows pH 7.52, PCO_2 3.2 kPa, PO_2 18 kPa, oxygen saturation 100%, bicarbonate 24 mmol/L. Which of the following is the most likely diagnosis?
a. Pain
b. Pulmonary embolism
c. Pneumonia

d. Diabetic ketoacidosis

e. Type II respiratory failure

125. Which statement regarding metabolic acidosis is correct?
    a. Metabolic acidosis may result in an increased anion gap.
    b. The PCO_2 levels increase to compensate metabolic acidosis.
    c. Anion gap is calculated using Na, K, HCO_3 and Ca^2 ions.
    d. Diabetic ketoacidosis has a normal anion gap.
    e. A normal anion gap is between 5 and 10 mmol/L.

126. A 50-year-old barely conscious male has been brought in by ambulance with multiple stab wounds. His blood pressure on arrival is 70/50 mmHg, heart rate 160 bpm, respiratory rate 42. He has been catheterized for at least an hour but has passed no urine. Currently, the patient is not on any supplemental oxygen. A helpful medical student presents you with an arterial blood gas (ABG). Which of the following would be the likely result?
    a. pH 7.40, PO_2 11.5, PCO_2 4.4, base excess (BE) 1, lactate 0.5
    b. pH 7.30, PO_2 8, PCO_2 7, BE –5.0, lactate 1.0
    c. pH 7.28, PO_2 11, PCO_2 3.0, BE –10, lactate 6.2
    d. pH 7.49, PO_2 10.7, PCO_2 2.6, BE –3.0, lactate 2.0
    e. pH 6.5, PO_2 5, PCO_2 15, BE –25, lactate 25

127. Concerning acid–base homeostasis, which of the following statements is correct?
    a. An acidosis is an excess of bicarbonate in the blood.
    b. The normal pH of blood ranges from 7.30 to 7.40.
    c. A buffer consists of a weak base and a weak acid.
    d. Haemoglobin and plasma proteins are the most important buffers in the blood
    e. The renal system can act quickly in order to maintain acid–base homeostasis.

128. Regarding urinary and plasma concentrations of substances in a normal physiological state, all of the following features are true except:
    a. Urine has no glucose.
    b. The sodium concentration is the same in plasma and urine.
    c. Urine has a higher concentration of urea.
    d. Plasma has lower concentrations of creatinine.
    e. Chloride concentration is higher in plasma.

129. When considering the regulation of the glomerular filtration rate (GFR), which of the following statements is true?
    a. Increased sympathetic nerve activity dilates afferent arterioles.
    b. Under autoregulation a decrease in blood pressure leads to a decrease in GFR.
    c. Under autoregulation a decrease in blood pressure leads to a constriction of afferent arterioles.
    d. Increased sympathetic nerve activity increases GFR.
    e. Under autoregulation, increased blood pressure leads to a constriction of afferent arterioles.

130. All of the following are features of normal renal physiology except:
    a. The distal convoluted tubule always receives a hypo-osmotic solution.
    b. The afferent artery supplies the glomerulus.
    c. Glomerular filtration rate (GFR), is controlled by the afferent and efferent arterioles.
    d. About 5% cardiac output is received by the kidney.
    e. Each human kidney has approximately 1.3 million nephrons.

131. When deciding on a solute, in order to accurately measure the Glomerular filtration rate (GFR), which of the following solute characteristics is not required?
    a. Produced endogenously
    b. Detectable in the urine
    c. Freely filtered by the kidney
    d. No absorption
    e. No alteration in renal blood flow

ENDOCRINE SYSTEM (INCLUDING GLUCOSE HOMEOSTASIS)

132. The following statements concerning growth hormone are true except:
    a. Secretion is stimulated by high glucose levels.
    b. Secretion is inhibited by somatostatin.
    c. Secretion follows a circadian pattern.
    d. It is secreted in response to trauma.
    e. It stimulates mitosis in epiphyseal plates.

133. The following statements regarding cortisol are true except:
    a. It stimulates gluconeogenesis.
    b. It stimulates lipolysis.
    c. The highest levels are present around midnight.
    d. It is increased in an acute infection.
    e. It inhibits complement.

134. Concerning the physiological effects of aldosterone, which of the following statements is correct?
    a. It stimulates sodium reabsorption at the proximal convoluted tubule.
    b. It acts to decrease water retention.
    c. It may lead to a metabolic acidosis.
    d. Its release is stimulated by hypokalaemia.
    e. Its release is reduced by increased circulating Atrial natriuretic peptide (ANP).

135. A 70-year-old woman presents with a prolonged history of fatigue and generalized headache. She is found to have uncontrolled high blood pressure at the general practitioner surgery. She has a history of congestive cardiac failure. Blood tests show that she is hypernatraemic and hypokalaemic. Plasma renin levels are raised. Which one of the following is the most likely diagnosis?
    a. Conn syndrome
    b. Primary hyperaldosteronism
    c. Secondary hyperaldosteronism
    d. Cushing syndrome
    e. Essential hypertension

136. Which one of the following hormones is produced by the posterior pituitary gland?
    a. Growth hormone
    b. Thyrotropin-releasing hormone
    c. Prolactin
    d. Adrenocorticotropic hormone
    e. Vasopressin

137. Concerning endocrine functions of the kidney, which statement is correct?
    a. Atrial natriuretic peptide (ADH) causes epithelial cells of the distal convoluted tubule to increase the synthesis of water channels.
    b. The ADH system will predominate over the renin–angiotensin system if there are conflicting interests in blood tonicity and volume.

    c. Aldosterone causes increased absorption of sodium in the collecting duct of the nephron.

    d. Erythropoietin is secreted in response to acute hypoxia.

    e. The kidney is involved in the hydroxylation of 25-hydroxycholecalciferol.

138. Concerning insulin, which one of the following statements is true?

    a. It has a long half-life in the circulation.

    b. Sympathetic stimulation increases insulin secretion.

    c. It promotes uptake of glucose by brain cells.

    d. It promotes protein degradation.

    e. It inhibits lipolysis.

139. Concerning potassium balance, which of the following statements is correct?

    a. Ninety percent of the body's potassium is intracellular.

    b. Aldosterone promotes the excretion of potassium in the distal convoluted tubule.

    c. Insulin promotes hyperkalaemia.

    d. Addison's disease is associated with hypokalaemia.

    e. Conn syndrome promotes hyperkalaemia.

140. Which one of the following statements is incorrect regarding the synthesis and function of vitamin D?

    a. Ultraviolet light is involved in the synthesis of cholecalciferol.

    b. Cholecalciferol is converted to 25-hydroxy-cholecalciferol in the liver.

    c. 25-Hydroxy-cholecalciferol is converted to 1,25-dihydroxy-cholecalciferol in the liver by 1-α-hydroxylase.

    d. 1-α-Hydroxylase is regulated by parathyroid hormone.

    e. 1,25-Dihydroxy-cholecalciferol increases gut calcium absorption.

141. Concerning antidiuretic hormone (ADH), which of the following statements is correct?

    a. It is released by anterior pituitary gland.

    b. It acts mainly on the proximal convoluted tubule.

    c. It is stimulated by alcohol.

    d. Lack of production causes cranial diabetes insipidus.

    e. It causes the production of a high volume of urine.

142. The following hormones and physiological effects are correctly paired except:

    a. Growth hormone: Secretion of Insulin-like growth factor 1

    b. Prolactin: Milk secretion

    c. Oxytocin: Uterine contraction

    d. Vasopressin: Water retention

    e. Adrenocorticotropic hormone: Cortisol secretion

143. A 42-year-old man is referred to the endocrine surgical unit with a history of bitemporal hemianopia, weight gain and skin hyperpigmentation. Dexamethasone suppression test shows a high Adrenocorticotropic hormone, with a cortisol level that suppresses with high-dose steroid. Which of the following comments regarding his condition is correct?

    a. He has a diagnosis of Cushing syndrome.

    b. ACTH is released from the anterior pituitary decreasing cortisol production.

    c. Pro-opio-melanocortin (POMC) is cleaved from ACTH.

    d. Melanocyte-stimulating hormone (MSH) is cleaved from ACTH.

    e. ACTH levels in Cushing disease are typically high.

144. A 75-year-old man attends your preoperative assessment clinic for elective open inguinal hernia repair under general anaesthetic. In his history you note that he is a long-standing heavy smoker with a productive cough and recurrent chest infections. He has a cut on his forearm that has taken several weeks to heal, with multiple bruises and striae across his abdomen. A chest X-ray shows a small lesion in the left mid-zone with some patchy consolidation in the left base. As his appearance is Cushingoid, you suspect he has a lung malignancy with ectopic Adrenocorticotropic hormone (ACTH) production. Which of the following findings on blood test would confirm this?

    a. Low ACTH, low cortisol

    b. Low ACTH, high cortisol

    c. High ACTH, low cortisol

    d. High ACTH, high cortisol

    e. Normal ACTH, high cortisol

145. A young woman is admitted following a fire in her home. She has sustained severe burns to most of her body. Following initial resuscitation she is transferred to a specialist burns unit. Which of the following is not a recognized systemic complication of severe burns?

    a. Hypokalaemia

    b. Hypothermia

    c. Gastric ulceration

    d. Sepsis

    e. Coagulopathy

146. Which one of the following statements regarding hypermagnesaemia is true?

    a. High magnesium is often associated with a low potassium.

    b. High magnesium seen in chronic renal failure is caused by impaired renal excretion.

    c. High magnesium may be caused by loop diuretics.

    d. Treatment commonly requires artificial ventilation due to respiratory depression.

    e. Intravenous calcium gluconate can be used to promote magnesium excretion.

147. Which one of the following statements regarding hypomagnesaemia is true?

    a. Hypomagnesaemia can be caused by acute pancreatitis.

    b. Hypomagnesaemia can result in respiratory depression.

    c. Hypomagnesaemia is typically associated with hyperkalaemia.

    d. Hypomagnesaemia is seen commonly in chronic renal failure.

    e. An electrocardiogram may show a shortened QT interval.

148. Which statement regarding magnesium balance is correct?

    a. A normal serum level of magnesium is 0.2–0.4 mmol/L.

    b. Total body magnesium is approximately 10 g.

c. Hypermagnesaemia can lead to bradycardia.

d. Electrocardiogram changes with hypomagnesaemia include a shortened PR interval.

e. Diuretics are a common cause of hypermagnesaemia.

149. Which of the following electrocardiogram changes are found with hypokalaemia?
   a. ST segment elevation
   b. U waves
   c. Tall T waves
   d. Shortened PR interval
   e. Wide QRS complex

150. Which of the following statements is false regarding the basal metabolic rate (BMR)?
   a. Skeletal muscle accounts for 20–30% of the BMR.
   b. Thyroid hormone increases the BMR.
   c. Malnutrition decreases the BMR.
   d. BMR is low during sleep.
   e. The average BMR for a 70 kg individual is 100 kcal/h.

151. Adrenaline is an endogenous catecholamine. Its effects include which one of the following?
   a. Decreased glucagon secretion by pancreatic alpha cells
   b. Decreased insulin secretion by pancreatic beta cells
   c. Increased glycogen synthesis in liver
   d. Increased glycogen synthesis in muscles
   e. Increased lipolysis

152. The adrenal gland is responsible for the production of multiple hormones? Which one of the following statements is incorrect?
   a. The cortex produces cortisol.
   b. The cortex produces aldosterone.
   c. The medulla produces adrenaline and noradrenaline.
   d. The medulla is responsible for androgen production.
   e. The cortex can be divided into the zona glomerulosa, zona fasciculata and zona reticularis.

153. Which of the following is not a correct paired hormone and response of the body in response to surgery/trauma?
   a. Glucagon – glycogenolysis, gluconeogenesis
   b. Insulin – low in ebb phase, with increased levels in flow phase
   c. Serotonin – vasodilatation, bronchodilatation
   d. Aldosterone – reabsorption of Na and secretion of K
   e. Growth hormone – lipolysis and protein synthesis

154. Which of the following statements regarding the actions of cortisol is incorrect?
   a. Metabolic effects of cortisol include lipolysis.
   b. Cortisol acts with vasopressors to increase vascular tone.
   c. Immunosuppressive effects include an increase in T-cell number.

d. Cortisol increases the effect of triiodothyronine (T$_3$) in maintaining body temperature.
e. Cortisol produces euphoria.

155. Which of the following statements relating to glucocorticoids is true?
    a. Hydrocortisone is secreted from the adrenal medulla.
    b. Glucocorticoids enhance insulin uptake by lymphatic tissue.
    c. Cortisol decreases nitrogen excretion.
    d. Cortisol increases insulin secretion.
    e. Glucocorticoid secretion is increased during prolonged exercise.

156. Which of the following statements is true regarding histamine?
    a. It is released by mast cells and basophils by immunoglobulin G (IgG).
    b. It causes relaxation of intestinal smooth muscle.
    c. It causes bronchiole dilatation.
    d. It decreases vascular permeability.
    e. It is released by enterochromaffin-like cells in the stomach.

157. Concerning the adrenal cortex, which of the following statements is correct?
    a. The zona glomerulosa is the superficial layer.
    b. The zone fasciculata is the superficial layer.
    c. The two most superficial layers are for production of glucocorticoids, oestrogens and androgens.
    d. Progestogens are only produced during pregnancy.
    e. Mineralocorticoid production occurs in the zona reticularis.

158. Which of the following combinations of body site and normal temperature is correct?
    a. Tympanic – 36°C
    b. Tympanic – 37°C
    c. Oral – 37°C
    d. Oesophageal – 37.5°C
    e. Axillary – 35°C

159. You are looking after a patient who has undergone an abdominoperineal resection. The patient has entered a catabolic state in the postoperative period. Which of the following physiological changes is not normally associated with a catabolic state?
    a. Insulin resistance
    b. Increased fatty acid oxidation
    c. Increased liver glycogen levels
    d. Increased urinary nitrogen excretion
    e. Increased plasma cortisol levels

160. Concerning the physiological properties of calcium, which of the following statements is correct?
    a. 5% of total body calcium is free.
    b. 60% of free calcium is bound to albumin.
    c. Acidosis increases the amount of ionized calcium in the blood.

d. It is stored in bone as calcium carbonate.

e. The normal serum calcium level is 2.6–2.8 mmol/L.

161. All of the following are effects of angiotensin II except:
    a. Stimulates release of antidiuretic hormone
    b. Increases thirst
    c. Vasodilatation
    d. Stimulates aldosterone release
    e. Facilitates release of norepinephrine

162. Concerning the pituitary gland and its hormones, which statement is correct?
    a. Vasopressin is produced by the neurohypophysis.
    b. Adrenocorticotropic hormone acts on the zona reticularis.
    c. Growth hormone is produced by the neurohypophysis.
    d. Prolactin stimulates dopamine production from the hypothalamus.
    e. Oxytocin initiates parturition.

163. Which of the following statements regarding the renin–angiotensin–aldosterone system physiology is true?
    a. Aldosterone is secreted from the zona fasciculata of the adrenal gland.
    b. Renin converts angiotensin I into angiotensin II.
    c. Aldosterone acts to increase K^+ reabsorption.
    d. The juxtaglomerular complex is in contact with the efferent arteriole.
    e. The macula densa inhibits renin secretion.

164. A 72-year-old man is admitted to hospital and is diagnosed with having hyponatraemia secondary to alcoholic liver disease. Which of the following types of hyponatraemia is the most likely to be associated with liver cirrhosis?
    a. Hypervolaemic hyponatraemia
    b. Euvolaemic hyponatraemia
    c. Hypovolaemic hyponatraemia
    d. Hypertonic hyponatraemia
    e. Hypotonic hyponatremia

NERVOUS SYSTEM

165. A 37-year-old woman is shot on the right paramedian side of the thoracic spine. What would you expect to find on examination in the emergency department?
    a. Ankle joint hyperreflexia on the left leg
    b. Reduced proprioception and vibration sense of the right leg
    c. Reduced pain and temperature sensation on the right side of the body below the level of the lesion
    d. Spastic paralysis of the left side of the body below the level of the lesion
    e. Reduced two-point discrimination on the left side of the body below the level of the lesion

166. A 54-year-old man has recently undergone an open reduction internal fixation of a distal radius fracture. After the procedure he has been placed in a backslab. A few hours after the operation you are called to see the patient on the ward after he develops increasing pain in the forearm with paresthesia in the index and middle fingers. What would the most appropriate first cause of action be?
    a. Book the patient for theatre for a revision procedure as you suspect a damaged nerve.
    b. Return the patient to theatre for an urgent carpal tunnel decompression.
    c. Reassure the patient and observe for an hour.
    d. Increase analgesia and leave the arm in a dependent position.
    e. Split the backslab bandage and elevate the arm.

167. A patient sustained a head injury following a fall from a third-storey flat and has now developed an ulcer in his stomach. What is this type of ulcer known as?
    a. Punched-out ulcer
    b. Curling's ulcer
    c. Marjolin's ulcer
    d. Cushing's ulcer
    e. Neuropathic ulcer

168. During a carotid endarterectomy, your patient suffers a stroke. You identify that the patient's speech has become affected and need to test the gag reflex. Which one of the following nerves supplies the afferent limb of the gag reflex?
    a. Glossopharyngeal nerve
    b. Maxillary division of the trigeminal nerve
    c. Vagus nerve
    d. Ophthalmic division of the trigeminal nerve
    e. Mandibular division of the trigeminal nerve

169. A 27-year-old man has been brought into the emergency department after being involved in a road traffic collision. While assessing him, you observe the signs of the fight or flight response. Which of the following clinical signs would you not expect to find?
    a. Decreased lacrimation
    b. Tachycardia

c. Sweating
d. Miosis
e. An increase in peripheral vascular resistance

170. A 23-year-old female is knocked from her horse sustaining a major head injury. She is brought into the emergency department and following a rapid primary survey undergoes a full trauma series computed tomography (CT) scan. Her initial Glasgow Coma Scale (GCS) is 12, but this rapidly deteriorates to 6. Her CT scan reveals a large frontal contusion with midline shift. Management of a serious head injury involves which of the following parameters?
    a. Hypotension to minimize bleeding
    b. Prevention of hypoxia, hypotension and hypercapnia
    c. Hypercapnia
    d. Mannitol alone
    e. Anticonvulsants alone

171. Regarding the nervous supply of the cardiovascular system, which one of the following is true?
    a. β_2 receptors predominate in the heart.
    b. β_1 receptors predominate in the vascular smooth muscle.
    c. M_2 muscarinic receptors are found in the sinoatrial node.
    d. β adrenergic stimulation enhances sodium influx into cells.
    e. Under basal conditions, the sympathetic nervous system predominantly affects the heart functions.

172. You are looking after a patient in the neurosurgical Intensive Therapy Unit (ITU). The patient does not have an intracranial bolt *in situ* but you are concerned of increasing intracranial pressure (ICP). The following changes may be expected in a patient with raised ICP except:
    a. Raised heart rate
    b. Reduced respiratory rate
    c. Raised blood pressure
    d. Increased pulse pressure
    e. Pupillary constriction

173. A 25-year-old woman was involved in a road traffic accident and suffered a significant head injury. She is being monitored in the neurosurgical intensive care unit. Her blood pressure is 100/70 mmHg and she has a heart rate of 80 bpm. Her current ICP is 10 mmHg. Which of the following is her cerebral perfusion pressure?
    a. 70 mmHg
    b. 170 mmHg
    c. 90 mmHg
    d. 180 mmHg
    e. 40 mmHg

174. Concerning cerebral blood flow, which statement is correct?
    a. It accounts for 5% of the cardiac output.
    b. The rate of flow is directly proportional to the arterial pressure.

c. Hypoxia produces cerebral vasoconstriction.
d. Cerebral perfusion pressure is the difference between mean arterial pressure and intracranial pressure.
e. Hypercarbia produces cerebral vasoconstriction.

175. Concerning cerebral spinal fluid (CSF), which statement is correct?
    a. The volume of CSF is 400 mL.
    b. It is produced at a rate of 150 mL/day.
    c. It is produced by the choroid plexus and blood vessels lining ventricular walls.
    d. From the lateral ventricles it flows into the 3rd ventricle via the aqueduct of Sylvius.
    e. From the lateral ventricles it flows into the 4th ventricle via the foramen of Magendie.

176. Action potentials cause changes in membrane potential by which one of the following mechanisms?
    a. Chloride ions outward
    b. Potassium ions inward
    c. Potassium ions outward
    d. Sodium ions inward
    e. Sodium ions outward

177. Which of the following statements regarding action potentials is correct?
    a. The resting potential in a nerve is −49 mV.
    b. Depolarization of the membrane is caused by an influx of potassium ions.
    c. Myelinated fibres have a conduction velocity of 5–10 m/s.
    d. Depolarization brings the membrane potential to +20 mV.
    e. α motor fibres have a diameter of 15–20 μm.

178. Action potentials involve the transport of ions across a membrane. Approximately how many millivolts are reached during a typical stimulation?
    a. −70 mV
    b. −10 mV
    c. +10 mV
    d. +40 mV
    e. +70 mV

179. While on the neurosurgical ITU, your consultant considers a patient brain-dead. Which of the following is not a criterion for brainstem death?
    a. Fixed pupils
    b. Absent corneal reflex
    c. Absent vestibulo-ocular reflex
    d. No muscle relaxants
    e. Mild hypothermia

180. Regarding cerebral blood flow, which statement is incorrect?
    a. The brain receives approximately 10–15% of the cardiac output.
    b. Increases in PCO_2 levels are associated with a decrease in cerebral blood flow.

c. The range of autoregulation is at a cerebral perfusion pressure of 60–160 mmHg.

d. Hypoxia impairs myogenic autoregulation of cerebral blood flow.

e. Cerebral circulation receives some sympathetic vasoconstrictor fibres.

181. A patient is brought into the emergency department with a stab to the neck in the midline. Which of the following statements is correct regarding spinal shock?

a. At the onset of spinal shock, the arterial blood pressure falls instantly.

b. Blood pressure returns to normal within a few days.

c. Reflexes may be hyperexcitable in the initial stages.

d. All of the above.

e. Only a and b are correct.

182. Which of the following describe the role of blood–brain barrier?

a. Protection of the brain from endogenous and exogenous toxins in the blood

b. Prevention of the escape of neurotransmitters into the general circulation

c. Maintaining the constancy of the environment of the neurons in the central nervous system

d. All of the above

e. a and c only

183. Which of these statements about cerebrospinal fluid is correct?

a. Cerebrospinal fluid lies in the epidural space.

b. The total volume is 250 mL.

c. Daily production is approximately 250 mL.

d. Cerebrospinal fluid flows from the third ventricle via the foramen of Luschka.

e. Normal cerebrospinal fluid pressure is 0.5–1.0 kPa.

184. All of the following features are noted in glial cells except:

a. There are two major types of glial cells.

b. Oligodendrocytes, Schwann cells and astrocytes are types of macroglia.

c. Astrocytes help regulate the blood–brain barrier.

d. Astrocytes are involved in myelin formation.

e. Microglia are able to perform phagocytosis.

185. Concerning the autonomic nervous system, which of these statements is correct?

a. Pre-ganglionic fibres are myelinated.

b. The neurotransmitter in pre-ganglionic cells is noradrenaline.

c. Post-ganglionic cells are located at the lateral horns of the spinal grey matter.

d. Nicotinic receptors are post-ganglionic.

e. The adrenal medulla receives parasympathetic innervation from pre-ganglionic parasympathetic fibres.

186. Considering muscle physiology, which one of the following statements is correct?
    a. A motor unit is defined as all the muscles producing one type of movement at a joint.
    b. Motor units are all the same size.
    c. A lower innervation ratio gives a finer degree of muscle control.
    d. Contractile force is increased by increasing the strength of the nerve stimulus.
    e. When a muscle contracts, all of its motor units are involved.

187. Which of the following component layers of peripheral nerves protects from stretching forces?
    a. Endoneurium
    b. Perineurium
    c. Epineurium
    d. Panneurium
    e. Transneurium

188. A patient comes into hospital following a car accident where her head hit the dashboard. On examination the patient only opens her eyes to pain and withdraws her limbs; she only communicates by making noises to pain. Which of the following is her GCS?
    a. 5
    b. 6
    c. 7
    d. 8
    e. 9

189. A young man is admitted with a head injury following a fall. Which of the following criteria of the GCS is correct?
    a. Eyes opening to speech – 4
    b. Abnormal flexion to pain – 3
    c. Confused conversation – 3
    d. Incomprehensible sounds – 1
    e. Localizes pain – 6

190. Which of the following statements is false regarding nerve fibres?
    a. The fibres are divided into types A and C.
    b. Type A fibres are the typical large and medium-sized myelinated fibres of spinal nerves.
    c. Type C fibres are further subdivided into α, β, γ and δ fibres.
    d. Type C fibres constitute more than one-half of the sensory fibres in most peripheral nerves.
    e. All of the above.

THYROID AND PARATHYROID

191. Which one of the following statements regarding the physiology of the thyroid gland is correct?
    a. About 50% of T_3 and thyroxine (T_4) is bound to proteins.
    b. Free T_4 is in lower concentration than free T_3.
    c. Iodide crosses from the plasma down its concentration gradient.
    d. Iodide is converted to iodine by thyroid peroxidase.
    e. Thyroid-stimulating hormone (TSH) inhibits T_3 and T_4 release.

192. All of the following are physiological effects of thyroid hormones except:
    a. Inotropic effect on cardiac muscle
    b. Decreased protein breakdown of muscle
    c. Normal growth and skeletal development
    d. Increased rate of carbohydrate absorption
    e. Lipolysis

193. Concerning the thyroid gland, which of the following is correct?
    a. Triiodothyronine is the principal hormone of the gland.
    b. Calcitonin is produced by follicular cells.
    c. Organification involves the binding of tetraiodothyronine to amino acids.
    d. Tyrosyl units bind with T_4 to form thyroglobulin.
    e. Thyroglobulin is stored in the colloid of follicles.

194. Concerning the action and regulation of parathyroid hormone (PTH), which of the following statements is correct?
    a. Hyperparathyroidism results in increased renal calcium excretion.
    b. PTH acts directly on bone to cause calcium reabsorption.
    c. PTH directly increases phosphate reabsorption at the proximal tubules of the kidney.
    d. PTH directly increases calcium reabsorption at the proximal tubules of the kidney.
    e. PTH directly increases calcium absorption from the intestine.

195. Concerning the physiological effects of thyroid hormones, which of the following statements is correct?
    a. Large doses of thyroid hormones result in increased peripheral resistance.
    b. Hypothyroid patients are found to have decreased cerebral oxygen consumption.
    c. Hyperthyroid patients are found to have increased cerebral blood flow.
    d. Thyroid hormones result in increased formation of hepatic low-density lipoprotein (LDL) receptors.
    e. Hypothyroid patients are found to have decreased cerebral glucose concentrations.

196. Concerning the mechanism of action of thyroid hormones, which of the following statements is correct?
    a. Thyroid receptors are extracellular.
    b. Thyroid receptor α_2 is found solely in the brain.

c. Thyroid receptor α_2 binds T_3.

d. T_4 has a more rapid mode of action than T_3.

e. T_3 is more potent than T_4.

197. Osteoclasts are inhibited by which of the following hormones/factors?

a. Parathyroid hormone

b. Calcitonin

c. 1,25-Dihydroxycholecalciferol

d. Tumour necrosis factor

e. None of the above

198. Which one of the following statements regarding the action of parathyroid hormone (PTH) is correct?

a. PTH decreases cyclic Adenosine monophosphate (AMP) production.

b. PTH is produced in response to high calcium.

c. PTH increases osteoclastic resorption of bone.

d. PTH decreases intestinal absorption of calcium.

e. PTH decreases renal tubular reabsorption of calcium.

199. Which of the following results does not fit with a diagnosis of primary hyperparathyroidism?

a. Raised serum calcium

b. Raised serum phosphate

c. Normal serum alkaline phosphatase

d. Raised 24 h calcium in urine

e. Normal vitamin D levels

200. A 58-year-old man with renal failure is diagnosed with secondary hyperparathyroidism. Which of the following is a characteristic of this pathology?

a. High serum calcium

b. Low parathyroid hormone levels

c. Low phosphate

d. Low vitamin D levels

e. Low serum alkaline phosphatase

201. A 65-year-old woman has had a renal transplant and is diagnosed as having tertiary hyperparathyroidism. Which one of the following is not characteristic of tertiary hyperparathyroidism?

a. Low serum calcium

b. Raised serum phosphate

c. Raised serum alkaline phosphatase

d. Raised parathyroid hormone

e. Developing after long-standing secondary hyperparathyroidism

202. Which one of the following statements regarding calcitonin is true?

a. Calcitonin is produced by parafollicular C-cells of the thyroid.

b. Levels rise in response to low calcium.

   c. It stimulates osteoclastic bone resorption.

   d. It decreases renal excretion of calcium.

   e. It decreases renal excretion of phosphate.

203. Concerning calcitonin, which of the following statements is correct?

   a. Oestrogen decreases secretion.

   b. β-Adrenergic agonists increase the rate of secretion.

   c. Glucagon decreases the rate of secretion.

   d. The plasma level is decreased in Zollinger–Ellison syndrome.

   e. It has a half-life of 12 h.

204. Thyroid stimulating hormone has all of the following effects on thyroid gland except for which one?

   a. Increased proteolysis of thyroglobulin

   b. Decreased activity of the iodide pump

   c. Increased number of thyroid cells

   d. Increased size and increased secretory activity of the thyroid cells

   e. Fibrosis of the glandular tissue

205. During a total thyroidectomy, there is a risk of damage to or removal of the parathyroid glands causing hypocalcaemia. Which of the following statements is true?

   a. There is a low risk of tetany with hypocalcaemia.

   b. Trousseau's sign is abnormal wrist extension with the fingers drawn together in extension after a blood pressure cuff is inflated on the arm for 3 min.

   c. Chvostek's sign is generally present in hypercalcaemia only.

   d. Circumoral numbness is a sign of hypocalcaemia.

   e. Shortened QT interval on an electrocardiogram may be seen in hypocalcaemia.

206. The following are clinical features of hypercalcaemia except:

   a. Abdominal pain

   b. Renal stones

   c. Depression

   d. Tetany

   e. Confusion

207. In a normal individual, a decrease in serum calcium leads to which one of the following?

   a. A reduction in parathyroid hormone (PTH)

   b. A decrease in osteoclastic activity

   c. An increase in calcium reabsorption from the distal convoluted tubules of the kidney

   d. PTH downregulation of the 1-hydroxylation of 25-hydroxy vitamin D

   e. An overall rise in phosphate levels

208. An elderly man presents to accident and emergency with abdominal pain, bone changes and renal colic. Baseline investigations confirm a raised serum calcium level. Which of the following conditions is unlikely to cause a raised serum calcium?
    a. Pancreatitis
    b. Primary hyperthyroidism
    c. Sarcoidosis
    d. Milk alkali syndrome
    e. Thiazide diuretics

209. Following either a traumatic insult to the body or surgery, how are circulating levels of T_3 and T_4 affected?
    a. No change
    b. Increase for 2 h
    c. Increase for a few days
    d. Decrease for 2 h
    e. Decrease for a few days

210. A 47-year-old male is admitted to the intensive care unit following an emergency laparotomy after a road traffic collision. His morning blood tests reveal low serum levels of T_3, with a normal T_4 and thyroid stimulating hormone level. Which of the following diagnosis is correct?
    a. Hashimoto's thyroiditis
    b. Sick euthyroid syndrome
    c. De Quervain's thyroiditis
    d. Iodine deficiency
    e. Hyperthyroidism

211. Which of the following medications has an effect on levothyroxine absorption?
    a. Iron supplements
    b. Histamine receptor antagonists
    c. Glucocorticoids
    d. Proton pump inhibitors
    e. a and d only

212. Which of the following cells are responsible for calcitonin production?
    a. Follicular cells of the thyroid gland
    b. Oxyphil cells of the parathyroid gland
    c. Chief cells of the parathyroid gland
    d. Parafollicular C-cells of the thyroid gland
    e. c and d only

CHAPTER 4
PHYSIOLOGY

Answers

RESPIRATORY SYSTEM

1. a.   Most lung volumes and capacities can be measured but residual volume and any lung capacity containing residual volume cannot be measured using simple spirometry. Functional residual capacity (FRC) is the volume of gas in the lungs at the end of a passive expiration and is calculated by adding the expiratory reserve volume (ERV) and residual volume. ERV is the additional volume that can be expired after a normal expiration. Tidal volume (TV) is the amount of air that enters or leaves the lung in a single respiratory cycle. Vital capacity (VC) is the maximal volume that can be expired after a maximal inspiration.

2. d.   The volume of air in the conducting airways is known as the anatomical dead space. Tidal volume is the amount of air that is inspired or expired during a normal breath cycle. After breathing out normally, the remainder of air that can be expired is defined as the expiratory reserve volume. The residual volume is, therefore, the remaining volume of air after a maximal breath.

3. a.   Surfactant is a lipid surface tension–lowering agent produced in the lamellar bodies of type II alveolar epithelial cells. Dipalmitoylphosphatidylcholine (DPPC) constitutes almost 60% of surfactant, with phospholipids and proteins making up the remainder. Surfactant deficiency at birth leads to high surface tension in the lungs and collapse of alveoli (atelectasis). Cigarette smoking decreases surfactant production. Other causes include invasive cardiac surgery, occlusion of the main bronchus and long-term inhalation of 100% oxygen.

4. b.   Alveoli are polyhedral structures clustered into honeycomb-like units, found at the end of respiratory bronchioles. The walls of alveoli are made up of type I and type II alveolar cells. Surfactant (a contraction of the term *surface active agent*) is produced by type II alveolar cells and acts to lower the surface tension of water. The surfactant molecules diffuse through the water and reduce the attractive forces within it, thereby preventing the alveoli from collapsing. As part of the pathogenesis of acute respiratory distress syndrome (ARDS), inflammation causes increased capillary and alveolar permeability that leads to an accumulation of protein-rich fluid in the lungs. The resultant decrease in lung compliance is accompanied by reduced surfactant, which further lowers compliance. The condition results in potentially fatal levels of hypoxaemia.

5. b.   Surfactant is produced by type II alveolar cells (pneumocytes). Surfactant decreases alveoli surface tension and reduces the work of breathing. Elastance has a reciprocal relationship to compliance, that is elastance = 1/compliance. Chronic obstructive pulmonary disease (COPD) is characterized by increased compliance; pulmonary fibrosis results in decreased compliance.

6. d.   The solubility of CO_2 in blood is about 20 times that of O_2; therefore, considerably more CO_2 than O_2 is present in simple solution at equal partial pressures. The CO_2 that diffuses into red blood cells is rapidly hydrated to H_2CO_3 because of the presence of carbonic anhydrase. The H_2CO_3 dissociates to H^+ and HCO_3^-, and the H^+ is buffered, primarily by haemoglobin, while the HCO_3^- enters the plasma. There is 49 mL of CO_2 in each decilitre of arterial blood (2.6 mL is dissolved, 2.6 mL as carbamino compound and 43.8 mL as HCO_3^-). So CO_2 is primarily transported in the arterial blood as bicarbonate.

7. d.   When a person moves to a significantly higher altitude, several adjustments need to be made to counter the decrease in PO_2 at the higher altitude. At altitudes as low as 1500 m the hypoxic ventilatory response produces tachypnoea in response to the decreased PO_2 and low oxyhaemoglobin saturation, and leads to a lower PCO_2 and a respiratory alkalosis. The alkalosis controls the tachypnoea and, after 2–3 days, the total minute volume stabilizes 2.5 L/min higher than at sea level. The total haemoglobin increases owing to stimulation of the kidneys to secrete erythropoietin, but the oxyhaemoglobin affinity decreases because of increased concentrations of 2,3-diphosphoglycerate (2,3-DPG) within circulating erythrocytes. The rise in 2,3-DPG helps unloading of oxygen at the peripheral capillaries.

8. a.   Systemic hypoxia causes the pulmonary arterioles to constrict with a resultant increase in pulmonary arterial pressure. The O_2 deficiency acts directly on vascular smooth muscle in the area to produce constriction shunting blood away from the hypoxic area. Accumulation of CO_2 leads to a drop in pH in the area, and the decline in pH also produces vasoconstriction in the pulmonary circulation as opposed to the vasodilation it produces in other tissues. The pulmonary circulation increases during systole not diastole.

9. c.   Respiratory control is aimed primarily to maintain levels of PO_2 and PCO_2 within a normal range. This is done via chemical and neurological control mechanisms. Several areas of the brain exert varying degrees of control on respiration. Within the medulla oblongata, there are inspiratory and expiratory neurons that produce alternating rhythms of action potentials with intervening periods of inactivity. The neurons stimulate different muscle groups involved in breathing. Two areas in the pons, the apneustic and pneumotaxic centres, influence the pattern of breathing by prolonging or shortening inspiration, respectively. The cerebral cortex controls voluntary breath holding or hyperventilation. The limbic system play a role in the respiratory system in extreme states of emotion, for example fear or anger.

10. b. The level of PCO_2 is the most important stimulus to respiration. A change in the level of PCO_2 will be detected by chemoreceptors, found centrally and peripherally. Central chemoreceptors are found close to the medulla oblongata and are very sensitive to changes in arterial PCO_2. CO_2 readily crosses the blood–brain barrier and reacts with water to produce H^+, causing the pH to fall. This central acidosis triggers the chemoreceptors to stimulate an increase in respiratory rate in order to remove CO_2 rapidly. Peripheral chemoreceptors are located in the carotid body and respond to PO_2 only when the levels are abnormally low (i.e. <8 kPa). Peripheral regulation of respiration plays a more important role in patients with chronic lung disease that retains CO_2 and depends on hypoxic drive to maintain respiration. Peripheral chemoreceptors also respond to changes in pH.

11. d. The peripheral chemoreceptors are largely sensitive to changes in PO_2 and to a lesser extent changes in pH. Central chemoreceptors (situated on the ventrolateral surface of the medulla) lie within the blood–brain barrier. They are sensitive to changes in pH; however, H^+ is not able to permeate the barrier. Thus, changes in pH are brought about indirectly through diffusion of CO_2 across the barrier, which subsequently dissociates into hydrogen ions: $H_2O + CO_2 \leftrightarrow H_2CO_3 \rightarrow \leftarrow H^+ + HCO_3^-$. The apneustic and pneumotaxic centres produce an involuntary respiratory cycle but can be voluntarily overridden by the cortex.

12. e. The oxygen dissociation curve is shifted to the left in conditions increasing its affinity for oxygen. The changes are listed in the table below.

Factor	Left shift	Right shift
Temperature	Low	High
2,3-DPG	Low	High
$P(CO_2)$	Low	High
$P(CO)$	High	Low
pH (Bohr effect)	High (alkalosis)	Low (acidosis)

13. e. A right shift of the oxygen–haemoglobin dissociation curve represents a decrease in affinity for haemoglobin and oxygen; hence the haemoglobin will offload the oxygen easier. Conditions where this would be useful would be in a respiring cell requiring oxygen. In a respiring cell, PCO_2, 2,3-DPG and temperature would be high, whereas pH would be low. The causes of shift to the right can be remembered using the mnemonic 'Cadet, face right!' for high CO_2, high acid, high 2,3-DPG, exercise and high temperature.

14. a. The oxygen–haemoglobin dissociation curve relates the percentage saturation of the oxygen (SO_2) carrying power of haemoglobin (Hb) to the saturation of oxygen (PO_2). This curve has a characteristic sigmoid shape. Combination of the first haem protein in the Hb molecule with O_2 increases the affinity of the second haem protein for O_2, and oxygenation of the second increases the affinity of the third, and so on, so that the affinity of Hb for the fourth O_2 molecule is many times that for the first. The decrease in O_2 affinity of Hb when the pH of blood falls is called the Bohr effect.

15. b.   Pulse oximetry measures the O_2 saturation of haemoglobin. It uses red and infrared light to measure the ratio of the differences in absorption of oxyhaemoglobin and deoxyhaemoglobin; however, it does not measure the partial pressure of O_2 in arterial blood. Pulse oximetry readings can be understood using the O_2–haemoglobin dissociation curve, which is a sigmoid curve. As a molecule of oxygen binds to haemoglobin, the structure of haemoglobin changes, making it easier for the next molecule of oxygen to bind. However, pulse oximetry does not provide a direct indication of ventilation, which is best provided by the PCO_2 levels. In carbon monoxide (CO) poisoning (e.g. burn cases), CO preferentially binds to haemoglobin compared with O_2. Pulse oximetry is unable to discern between oxyhaemoglobin and carboxyhaemoglobin (both bright red molecules) and hence may give a falsely high reading despite a low PO_2.

16. b.   Pulse oximetry measures arterial oxygen saturation (not partial pressure). It uses two wavelengths of light (red and infrared) and calculates the difference in absorption of light by oxyhaemoglobin and deoxyhaemoglobin. Oxygen saturation is then calculated from this data. Only the pulsation component of arterial blood is measured and the constant background (skin, fat and venous blood) is subtracted. However, it has several drawbacks. It does not give a good indication of ventilation (better reflected by the partial pressure of CO_2). In the presence of carbon monoxide, pulse oximetry readings are unreliable. Carbon monoxide competes with oxygen binding to haemoglobin, forming carboxyhaemoglobin, which also appears bright red and gives a falsely high saturation reading. Patients with poorly perfused peripheries owing to hypotension or hypothermia may also not give reliable saturation readings.

17. b.   Haemoglobin is comprised of two α and two β subunits. A subunit is comprised of a globin molecule (i.e. polypeptide chain) and a haem molecule – each subunit may bind one oxygen molecule. Adult haemoglobin has a higher affinity for carbon monoxide than oxygen, which is the basis of carbon monoxide poisoning. Fetal haemoglobin contains δ rather than β subunits, resulting in increased affinity for oxygen than adult haemoglobin. Affinity for oxygen is further increased with subsequent binding of oxygen molecules.

18. b.   Haemoglobin is an iron-containing protein found in red blood cells. The basic structure of adult human haemoglobin consists of four peptide chains (two α and two β) with each peptide chain having its own haem group. A haem group is made up of a protoporphyrin ring surrounding an iron molecule. Each haemoglobin molecule can carry four oxygen molecules (hence eight oxygen atoms). Oxygen–haemoglobin dissociation has a sigmoid relationship and haemoglobin dissociates with oxygen more readily in metabolizing tissues (with lower pH, higher temperature and higher PCO_2).

19. c.   In a tension pneumothorax, the pressure within the pleural cavity increases with time. As a result, there is an increase in mediastinal and thoracic pressure. Venous return is diminished, with a backlog of venous blood as evidenced by distended jugular veins. The heart responds by increasing the rate of contraction to maintain cardiac output. Respiratory compromise is evidenced by increased respiratory rate and low PO_2.

20. d. The patient in this question has type I respiratory failure, which is defined as a PO_2 of <8 kPa and a PCO_2 of <6.5 kPa. Type I respiratory failure is known as a hypoxaemic respiratory failure and is caused by ventilation–perfusion mismatching. The PCO_2 is low or normal because tachypnoea is able to clear the CO_2 from the alveoli. Type II respiratory failure is defined as a PO_2 of <8 kPa and a PCO_2 of >6.5 kPa. Type II respiratory failure is known as ventilatory failure because of lack of air movement within the chest. The relative state of hypoventilation causes the PO_2 to fall and the PCO_2 to rise.

21. c. A haemothorax is the accumulation of blood within the pleural cavity. A massive haemothorax can be caused by blunt or penetrating trauma. Signs suggestive of a massive haemothorax are reduced breath sounds, dullness to percussion and mediastinal shift and haemodynamic instability. JVP is not directly associated with a massive haemothorax; however it can be raised if there is a concomitant tension pneumothorax. A haemothorax should be treated with formal pleural drainage and if the initial volume of blood drained exceeds 1500 mL or persists at a rate of >200 mL/h, urgent referral to a thoracic unit is necessary.

22. d. This scenario describes a tension pneumothorax. This is a life-threatening condition caused by the progressive build-up of air in the pleural space. Most often this occurs from a laceration of the lung, which allows air to enter the pleural space but not leave. As the pressure builds up the lung collapses and the trachea and mediastinum are pushed to the opposite side. The clinical picture is of a distressed cyanotic patient with the findings described in the question. Diagnosis is a clinical one and treatment is immediate decompression with a cannula into the second intercostal space mid-clavicular line. This converts the tension pneumothorax into a simple one which can then be managed with a chest drain.

CARDIOVASCULAR SYSTEM

23. a.   Cardiac output is increased mainly through an increase in stroke volume of around 35% with a relatively smaller increase in resting heart rate of 15%. This causes the heart to enlarge during pregnancy. Owing to increased plasma volume and red cell mass, the venous system distends about 150%, reducing blood flow within the capillary system.

24. e.   The Frank–Starling law states that the greater the volume of blood entering the heart during diastole (the end-diastolic volume), the greater the volume of blood ejected during systolic contraction (stroke volume). Therefore, the greater the stretch of the ventricle in diastole, the greater the stroke volume. The stretching of the muscle fibres increases the affinity of Ca^{2+} to troponin C. This leads to a greater number of cross-bridges to form within the muscle fibres, resulting in an increase in the contractile force of the cardiac muscle. The increase in end-diastolic volume and stroke volume is not directly proportional and beyond a critical point further increases in end-diastolic volume, actually lead to a drop in stroke volume. This is because the muscle fibres have been stretched beyond their capacity. With sympathetic stimulation there is a similar relationship but there is a greater stroke volume for the same end-diastolic volume. Similarly, for a failing heart, there is an increase in stroke volume, but the increase is less than in normal states and the volume is less for the same end-diastolic volume.

25. b.   A knowledge of intracardiac and pericardiac blood pressures is important when floating a Swan–Ganz catheter so that an estimation of the position of the catheter tip can be established. The catheter can be used to measure the pulmonary artery wedge pressure, which is an indirect method of monitoring a patient's fluid balance. Below is a list of the normal intracardiac, aortic and pulmonary artery blood pressures:

- *Right atrium:* 0–4 mmHg
- *Right ventricle:* 25/0–4 mmHg
- *Pulmonary artery:* 25/15 mmHg
- *Left atrium:* 5–10 mmHg
- *Left ventricle:* 120/0–10 mmHg
- *Aorta:* 120/80 mmHg

26. c.   Pulmonary artery wedge pressure is measured using a pulmonary artery catheter (Swan–Ganz catheter) and is used to approximate cardiac output. This is done via a thermodilution technique using Fick's law. When the catheter is wedged in a pulmonary artery, there is an uninterrupted continuous column of blood right up to the left atrium; hence the wedge 'pressure' is an indirect measurement of the left atrial pressure. Wedge pressure monitoring also assumes that left ventricular end-diastolic pressure is correlated with left ventricular end-diastolic volume, giving an approximation of left ventricular preload.

27. b.   Central venous pressure gives a good indication of preload. It is a useful guide to fluid replacement. Normal pressures range from 8 to 12 mmHg. A low pressure indicates hypovolaemia and a high pressure fluid overload.

Pulse oximetry measures arterial oxygen saturation. It pulses red and infrared light at wavelengths of 660–940 nm. Pulmonary artery occlusion pressure reflects left atrial pressure. A normal pressure ranges from 6 to 12 mmHg. It has the advantage of being used to measure cardiac output.

28. c. The third heart sound is caused by rapid ventricular filling and is best heard in children. It is heard just after the second heart sound, and to help differentiate it from the fourth heart sound, think of the word *Kentucky*. During auscultation the 1st, 2nd and 3rd heart sounds should fall on the syllable stresses of the word *Ken... TucKy*. The 4th heard sound is a word like *TeNNe...SSee*. The first and second heart sounds are caused by closure of the atrioventricular and aortoventricular valves, respectively. The presence of a 4th heart sound indicates ventricular hypertrophy or heart failure. It results from ventricular distension caused by forceful atrial contraction. The aortic area is the best location for listening for aortic stenosis.

29. d. First-degree heart block – prolonged PR interval, constant in timing. Every P wave is followed by a QRS complex; second degree (Wenckebach) – progressive lengthening of PR interval until a P wave fails to be conducted; second degree (Mobitz II) – PR intervals normal and constant, occasional P wave is not conducted; third degree – P waves bear no relationship to the QRS complexes.

30. e. Beriberi, arteriovenous fistula, hyperthyroidism and anaemia all cause a high cardiac output from chronically reduced total peripheral resistance. None of them result from excessive excitation of the heart itself. In contrast, haemorrhage results in peripheral vasoconstriction and an increase in heart rate to maintain adequate perfusion of vital organs.

31. d. The factors that cause a person to recover from moderate degrees of shock are all the negative feedback control mechanisms of the circulation that attempt to return cardiac output and arterial pressure to normal levels. Baroreceptor reflexes elicit powerful sympathetic stimulation of the circulation. Reverse stress–relaxation of the circulatory system causes the blood vessels to contract around the diminished blood volume, so that the blood volume that is available more adequately fills the circulation. The formation of angiotensin by the kidneys constricts the peripheral arteries and causes decreased output of water and salt by the kidneys, both of which help prevent progression of shock.

32. d. Intracellular Ca^{2+} is the most important factor controlling myocardial contractility, where increased calcium concentration increases contractility and decreased calcium concentration decreases contractility. When the action potential arrives at the myocardium, Ca^{2+} is able to move from the sarcoplasmic reticulum into the cytoplasm. There, the Ca^{2+} binds to troponin C leading to activation of the actin–myosin complex and contraction. The cardiac action potential has a characteristic plateau phase, and this is caused by the influx of further Ca^{2+}, which prolongs and enhances the contraction.

33. e. The four primary forces that determine fluid movement through capillary membrane are called Starling forces, after the physiologist who first demonstrated their importance. The net filtration pressure (NFP) is calculated as NFP = Pc – Pif – Πp + Πif. Pc is capillary pressure, Pif is interstitial fluid pressure,

Πp is plasma colloid osmotic pressure and Πif is interstitial fluid colloid osmotic pressure. If the sum of these forces is positive there will be a net fluid filtration across the capillaries. If the sum of the forces is negative there will be a net fluid absorption from the interstitial spaces into the capillaries.

34. e. The Starling equilibrium explains the relationship between hydrostatic pressure, colloid osmotic pressure and the flow of fluid across the capillary membrane. The hydrostatic pressure is greater at the arterial end than at the venous end. The colloid osmotic pressure (i.e. the ability of proteins to draw water by osmosis) of the plasma and tissue fluid is the same throughout the capillary because large proteins are unable to leave the capillary. At the arterial end there is net filtration because of the higher hydrostatic pressure compared with the colloid osmotic pressure; at the venous end there is net absorption because the hydrostatic pressure is lower than the colloid osmotic pressure. Overall, there is a net excess of fluid left in the extracellular space as not all of the fluid is able to be drawn back into the plasma. This excess is returned to the circulation via the lymphatics.

35. c. The heart receives approximately 5% of the overall cardiac output. The coronary blood flow during exercise is 300–400 mL/min per 100 g of cardiac tissue; at rest it is approximately 70–80 mL/min. Myocardial oxygen consumption is approximately 8 mL O_2/min per 100 g of cardiac tissue, which is some 15–20 times that of skeletal muscle. Approximately 70% of the oxygen delivered to the myocardium is extracted. Increased oxygen demand during exercise is predominantly accounted for by increased blood flow through the myocardium.

36. d. The O_2 consumption by non-beating myocardium is considerably higher than that of resting skeletal muscle at about 2 mL O_2/100 g per minute. The O_2 consumption by the beating heart is about 8 mL O_2/100 g per minute at rest. The Fick principle relates to the relationship between the mL O_2/100 g, coronary blood flow (CBF) and extraction of oxygen from the blood allowing the O_2 consumption by the heart to be estimated.

37. b. In a healthy 70 kg man, the approximate fluid distribution would be summarized as follows:

- Two-thirds of body weight is water = 42 L.

Of that 42 L

- Two-thirds is intracellular = 28 L.
- One-third is extracellular = 14 L, of which:
  - Interstitial = 9 L
  - Intravascular (i.e. plasma) = 4 L
  - Transcellular (i.e. '3rd space') = 1 L

38. c. In a healthy 70 kg man, the approximate fluid distribution would be summarized as follows:

- Approximately 60% of body weight is water.

Of that 60%,

- Two-thirds is intracellular (40% of body weight).

- One-third is extracellular:
  - Interstitial = 13%
  - Intravascular (i.e. plasma) = 6%
  - Transcellular (i.e. 3rd space) = 1%

39. d. The tendency for turbulent flow is determined by the equation $Re = (vd\rho)/\eta$. Re is the Reynolds number and is the measure of the tendency for turbulence to occur, v is the mean velocity of blood flow (in centimetres per second), d is the vessel diameter, ρ is density and η is the viscosity (in poise). The viscosity of blood is normally about 1/30 P, and the density is only slightly greater than 1. When the Reynolds number rises above 2000, turbulent flow will occur in vessels.

40. b. The bone marrow of essentially all bones produces red blood cells until a person is 5 years old. The marrow of the long bones, except for the proximal portions of the humeri and tibiae, becomes quite fatty and produces no more red blood cells after about age 20 years. Beyond this age, most red cells continue to be produced in the marrow of the membranous bones, such as the vertebrae, sternum, ribs and ilia. Even in these bones, the marrow becomes less productive as age increases.

41. b. Shock is defined as inadequate tissue perfusion and oxygen delivery to the tissues. There are several different types of shock: hypovolaemic, septic, cardiogenic, neurogenic and anaphylactic. Cardiogenic shock is characterized by an increase in systemic vascular resistance in response to the heart being unable to maintain an adequate stroke volume resulting in a decrease in cardiac output. In neurogenic shock, loss of autonomic control leads to decreased systemic vascular resistance. In septic shock there is increased vasodilation leading to a reduced cardiac afterload and there is a sympathetic response to increase the cardiac output.

42. b. It is likely this patient is in class I shock as indicated by his altered mental status but stable observations. This indicates he may have lost anywhere up to 750 mL or 15% of his blood volume. Young adults are very good at preserving normal physiological readings despite quite sizeable blood losses because of their physiological reserve. This patient will need volume replacement with crystalloid. The table below describes the classes of shock.

For an average 70 kg man	Class I	Class II	Class III	Class IV
Blood loss (mL)	<750	750–1500	1500–2000	>2000
Blood loss (%)	<15	15–30	30–40	>40
Heart rate	<100	>100	>120	>140
Blood pressure (mmHg)	Normal or increased	Normal	Decreased	Decreased
Respiratory rate	14–20	20–30	30–40	>40
Urine output (mL/h)	>30	20–30	5–15	Negligible
Mental status	Slightly anxious	Mildly anxious	Anxious/ confused	Confused/ lethargic

43. e. If the answer is more than 40%, this indicates a blood loss of more than 2 L. This man therefore has signs of class IV shock. He has signs of tachycardia, tachypnoea, hypotension, anuria and confusion. He will need fluid replacement with crystalloid and blood. The table below describes the classes of shock.

For an average 70 kg man	Class I	Class II	Class III	Class IV
Blood loss (mL)	<750	750–1500	1500–2000	>2000
Blood loss (%)	<15	15–30	30–40	>40
Heart rate	<100	>100	>120	>140
Blood pressure (mmHg)	Normal or increased	Normal	Decreased	Decreased
Respiratory rate	14–20	20–30	30–40	>40
Urine output (mL/h)	>30	20–30	5–15	Negligible
Mental status	Slightly anxious	Mildly anxious	Anxious/ confused	Confused/ lethargic

44. a. During haemorrhagic shock, there is an increase in heart rate with an overall fall in cardiac output and fall in central venous pressure. There is reduced perfusion to the peripheries. In an effort to maintain cerebral blood flow, there is splanchnic vasoconstriction. Despite this, cerebral blood flow will fall.

45. c. The cause of the low cardiac output is true hypovolaemia and the patient is in class IV shock. This level of shock represents a blood loss volume of >40%. Resuscitation with a crystalloid (or colloid) is required, but due to the large volume of blood loss apparent, it is more important to resuscitate the patient with blood. Resuscitating with just a crystalloid would dilute the remaining circulating blood to a fatal level. There is no evidence to show that giving colloid over a crystalloid in the acute setting changes outcome; therefore, crystalloid use prevents the risk of allergic reaction to colloid. Five percent dextrose solution is hypotonic and the dextrose is rapidly metabolized by the liver, resulting in the fluid being distributed around the body equally. For every litre of 5% dextrose administered, only 95 mL will remain in the plasma in a 70 kg patient. (A healthy 70 kg patient will have 42 L of water, of which 4 L are in the plasma. Therefore, for every 1000 mL only a factor of 4/42 will remain in the plasma [95 mL].)

46. e. This scenario describes a pulmonary embolism secondary to a deep venous thrombosis. The embolism is large enough to lodge proximally within the pulmonary circulation and affect the cardiac output. The blockage prevents venous blood reaching the left side of the heart, leading to an obstructive type of shock. Shock is defined as circulatory collapse leading to decreased tissue perfusion and cellular hypoxia. It is important to remember that although blood pressure is a good guide to tissue perfusion, it is not completely reliable. For example, a patient may be maintaining his blood pressure through vasoconstriction. However, if the vasoconstriction is severe enough to cause decreased tissue perfusion, then cellular hypoxia results. Other types of shock include cardiogenic (e.g. myocardial infarction), true hypovolaemia (e.g. blood loss) and apparent hypovolaemia (e.g. anaphylaxis).

47. c. Shock is defined as inadequate tissue perfusion and oxygen delivery to the tissues. There are several different types of shock: hypovolaemic, septic, cardiogenic, neurogenic and anaphylactic. Cardiogenic shock is characterized by an increase in systemic vascular resistance in response to the heart being unable to maintain an adequate stroke volume. In septic shock there is increased vasodilation leading to a reduced cardiac afterload and there is a sympathetic response to increase the cardiac output. Septic shock after biliary surgery is commonly caused by Gram-negative organisms.

48. d. Changes associated with hyperkalaemia include:

- Tented T waves
- Small P waves
- Wide QRS complex
- Shortened PR interval
- Eventual disappearance of P waves, resulting in a sine wave

Changes associated with hypokalaemia include:

- Inverted T waves
- S–T depression
- Prolonged PR interval
- Atrial/ventricular tachyarrhythmias
- Appearance of a U wave

49. b. The jugular venous pressure (JVP) is identified in the neck by observing a double pulsation in the internal jugular vein. The pressure within the internal jugular results from cyclical atrial contraction and dilatation. Below is an explanation of the waveforms:

- *A wave:* Represents atrial systole and is absent in atrial fibrillation and is increased in tricuspid or pulmonary stenosis. During complete heart block atrial contraction may occur at a time when the tricuspid valve is closed causing 'cannon' waves.
- *C wave:* Represents closure of the tricuspid leaflets in the right atrium at the start of ventricular systole.
- *X descent:* The pressure inside the atrium drops as a result of the atrium relaxing and the tricuspid valve moving down during ventricular systole.
- *V wave:* The rise in atrial pressure is caused by rapid blood filling prior to opening of the tricuspid valve.
- *Y descent:* The tricuspid valve opens and blood passively flows into the right ventricle.

50. c. The jugular venous pressure (JVP) is identified in the neck by observing a double pulsation in the internal jugular vein. The pressure within the internal jugular results from cyclical atrial contraction and dilatation. Below is an explanation of the waveforms:

- *A wave:* Represents atrial systole and is absent in atrial fibrillation and is increased in tricuspid or pulmonary stenosis. During complete heart block atrial contraction may occur at a time when the tricuspid valve is closed causing 'cannon' waves.
- *C wave:* Represents closure of the tricuspid leaflets in the right atrium at the start of ventricular systole.
- *X descent:* The pressure inside the atrium drops as a result of the atrium relaxing and the tricuspid valve moving down during ventricular systole.
- *V wave:* The rise in atrial pressure is caused by rapid blood filling prior to opening of the tricuspid valve.
- *Y descent:* The tricuspid valve opens and blood passively flows into the right ventricle.

51. b. The A wave is produced by atrial systole. A raised A wave suggests increased resistance to ventricular filling, such as in right ventricular hypertrophy and tricuspid or pulmonary stenosis. Cannon waves are large A waves that occur when the atrium contracts against a closed tricuspid valve. C waves represent closure of the tricuspid leaflets in the right atrium at the start of ventricular systole. V waves develop as the atrium is filled during ventricular contraction. Large V waves are seen in tricuspid regurgitation.

52. d. The first heart sound is caused by the closure of the atrioventricular valves (mitral and tricuspid) and the second heart sound is caused by the closure of the aortic and pulmonary valves. The jugular venous pressure (JVP) has several waveforms. The C wave results from the closure of the tricuspid valve during ventricular contraction. This bulges the cusps upward causing the C wave. The P wave and the T wave on the electrocardiogram (ECG) correspond to atrial depolarization and ventricular repolarization, respectively.

53. e. All of the above conditions cause a rise in the JVP, except for haemorrhage, which leads to hypovolaemia and therefore a drop in JVP. In constrictive pericarditis and cardiac tamponade, ventricular filling is reduced. Fluid overload with either intravenous fluids or blood leads to a rise in JVP.

54. a. Cardiac muscle cells are uninucleate. The junction of two muscle fibres has an extensive series of folds at Z lines, which appear as dark areas – intercalated discs. Cardiac muscle is a syncytium of many heart muscle cells in which the cardiac cells are so interconnected that when one of these cells becomes excited, the action potential spreads to all of them. This latticework gives it a characteristic branched appearance. Cardiac muscle is involuntary striated muscle.

55. b. An electrocardiogram (ECG) is a quick, low-risk and relatively low-cost investigation that is invaluable in diagnosing acute myocardial infarction (AMI). There are a number of ECG changes that are indicative of an AMI and should be treated with thrombolysis or primary percutaneous coronary intervention. At least one of the following changes should be accompanied by chest pain lasting less than 12 h: ST segment elevation >1 mm in two or more contiguous limb leads, ST segment elevation >2 mm in two or more contiguous chest leads, new-onset left bundle branch block, and posterior infarct (dominant R waves and ST depression in V_1 to V_3). The area affected by an AMI can be deduced by noting which leads have changed, and knowledge of cardiac anatomy gives an indication of the artery involved (see table below).

Heart surface	ECG leads	Coronary artery involved
Inferior wall	II, II, aVF	Right – 90% Circumflex – 10%
Septal	V1–V3	Left anterior descending
Anterior	V1–V4	Left anterior descending
Anterolateral	V1–V6	Left common
Lateral	I, aVL, V4–V6	Circumflex
Posterior	V1–V3 (reciprocal changes)	Posterior descending (right or circumflex)

56. a. The stroke volume is the volume of blood pumped from the ventricle in one beat. It is calculated by subtracting the end-systolic volume from the end-diastolic volume of the ventricle. Men have higher stroke volumes than women. Increasing preload can increase stroke volume by ventricle muscular stretching (Frank–Starling law). An increase in afterload can reduce stroke volume, such as in aortic stenosis.

57. a. Inotropes are substances that alter the inotropic state of the heart. Positive inotropes increase the strength of myocardial contractility, whereas negative inotropes reduce it. Inotropes are either endogenous (from the adrenal medulla) or exogenous (synthetic derivatives of endogenous inotropes). Adrenaline acts mainly on β receptors but is a mild α agonist, whereas noradrenaline is predominantly an α agonist with mild β-stimulating properties. Noradrenaline causes peripheral vasoconstriction and increases systemic vascular resistance. It is used to increase blood pressure in patients with resistant shock.

58. b. Noradrenaline is a catecholamine and a phenethylamine that acts as a stress hormone and, among other roles, a neurotransmitter. Noradrenaline can be given as an exogenous drug to primarily act on α-adrenergic receptors to vasoconstrict the microvasculature in an attempt to increase peripheral vascular resistance. Noradrenaline also acts weakly on $β_1$ receptors. However, any smooth muscle relaxation brought on by β receptor activation is overcome by α receptor activation. The increased vascular resistance results in increased venous return to the heart, increased preload and, consequently, increased end-diastolic volume. The increased end-diastolic volume leads to an increased stroke volume and therefore cardiac output in accordance with the Frank–Starling law. Problems with noradrenaline relate to the fact that the physiological effects increase cardiac strain, and if given in high enough doses, it can cause limb ischaemia.

59. d. The effect of adrenaline in the blood and by noradrenaline released from sympathetic nerve endings is both excitatory and inhibitory. This is due to the different cell membrane receptors. The two major classes of these receptors are alpha and beta, and these are further differentiated into α_1, α_2, β_1 and β_2. The different activation or inhibition caused by these receptors is explained by the 'flight or fight' or 'rest and digest' response. During the flight response the heart has increased inotropy and chronotropy. This is because the cardiac muscle has predominantly β_1 receptors. The smooth muscle of the respiratory tract has a predominance of β_2 receptors and allows bronchioles to dilate owing to smooth muscle relaxation. The liver has α_1 and β_1 receptors allowing for glycogenolysis and secretion of glucose. Blood vessels dilate with α_1 control and constrict with β_2 control. The uterine smooth muscle does not have β_2 receptors.

60. a. The end point of blood coagulation is the formation of fibrin from fibrinogen by thrombin. The clotting cascade involves two separate pathways: intrinsic and extrinsic. These two pathways result in the activation of factor X, beyond which is the final common pathway where prothrombin is converted to thrombin. Thrombin then catalyzes the conversion of fibrinogen to fibrin, eventually forming a cross-linked fibrin clot. The intrinsic pathway involves normal blood components and requires clotting factors VIII, IX, X, XI and XII. The extrinsic pathway requires tissue thromboplastin, which is released from damaged cells, and clotting factors VII and X.

61. b. Stroke volume falls on standing; therefore, there is an increase in systemic vascular resistance and heart rate to maintain blood pressure. On standing there is a fall in pulse pressure, causing a reduction in carotid baroreceptor stimulation. This reduces vagal and increases sympathetic stimulation of the heart, leading to increased heart rate, vasoconstriction to increase the systemic vascular resistance, and some venoconstriction to limit the amount of venous pooling. Arterial pressure = cardiac output × systemic vascular resistance. Cardiac output = heart rate × stroke volume.

62. c. Erythropoiesis is the production of erythrocytes from stem cells in the bone marrow. This process is stimulated by erythropoietin, which is mainly secreted from the kidneys. Erythropoietin secretion, in turn, is stimulated mainly by low tissue PO_2 levels. Vasodilatation would increase blood supply to the tissues and hence allow more oxygen supply.

63. a. Myoglobin is a single-chain globular protein of 153 or 154 amino acids (16.7 kDa) containing a haem (iron-containing porphyrin) group with eight alpha helices and a hydrophobic core. Being monomeric, it has instant binding with oxygen rather than the cooperative binding seen in haemoglobin. It has a hyperbolic dissociation curve. Its function is to store oxygen in muscle tissues for rapid release during times of need, as is demonstrated by its very high concentration in the muscles of diving mammals that need to hold their breath for long periods.

64. c. A high pulse pressure can be seen in aortic regurgitation, with a low pulse pressure in aortic stenosis. A narrow pulse pressure is a clinical sign of blood loss or significant dehydration. It is normal for the pulse pressure to increase during exercise. Angiotensin-converting enzyme inhibitors are effective at reducing pulse pressure.

65. d.   The majority of fetal haemoglobin is HbF, which has a higher affinity for oxygen than adult haemoglobin. By 6–8 months, 80–90% has become the adult form HbA. HbS represents sickle cell haemoglobin. HbE causes a mild haemolytic anaemia.

66. d.   Central venous catheter (CVC) lines are mainly used in high-dependency units and intensive care units and have several uses. Central venous pressure (CVP) monitoring is useful to assess the intravascular fluid status. Certain drugs are best administered via a CVC line, such as amiodarone and total parental nutrition (TPN) feeds, as they can cause phlebitis in peripheral veins. Dialysis can be carried out via a central line while patients wait for a permanent atrioventricular fistula formation surgically. Central lines are not useful during emergency fluid resuscitation in trauma as peripheral lines are quicker and safer to insert and achieve higher flow rates.

67. d.   The sinoatrial (SA) node is located in the right atrium near the entrance of the superior vena cava. It receives parasympathetic supply from the vagus and sympathetic fibres from T1–T4. Its blood supply is mainly from the right coronary artery. The SA node normally initiates the cardiac contraction.

68. c.   During vigorous exercise, cardiac output increases, with an increase in heart rate, stroke volume and cardiac contractility. The Central venous pressure (CVP) remains unchanged, but if there is prolonged exercise leading to dehydration, then the CVP may drop. The end-systolic volume increases with a small increase in end-diastolic volume.

69. d.   The ejection fraction (EF) is the fraction of blood expelled from the ventricle relative to its end-diastolic volume. The proportion of blood expelled from the ventricle against a given afterload depends on the strength of the ventricular contraction. For a healthy 70 kg man who has stroke volume of approximately 70 mL and an end-diastolic volume of 120 mL, the EF is 70/120, giving 58%. Normal individuals have an EF of around 60% in resting conditions. During exercise, more blood is ejected per beat as the end-diastolic volume increases. The increased end-diastolic volume increases the stroke volume of the heart, but the EF is relatively constant for a range of end-diastolic volumes. Athletes, while exercising, have an increased stroke volume, but also increased inotropy, and can reach an EF of 90%.

70. d.   The baroreceptors are stretch receptors in the walls of the heart and blood vessels. The afferent nerve fibres from the carotid sinus form a distinct branch of the glossopharyngeal nerve: the carotid sinus nerve (or Hering's nerve). The afferent fibres from the baroreceptors of the aortic arch form a branch of the vagus nerve: the aortic depressor nerve. Increased baroreceptor discharge inhibits the tonic discharge of sympathetic nerves and excites the vagal innervation of the heart. These neural changes produce vasodilation, venodilation, hypotension, bradycardia and a decrease in cardiac output.

71. c.   Renin is an enzyme produced in the juxtaglomerular apparatus in response to a decrease in arterial blood pressure, sodium levels or sympathetic activity. It stimulates the system to produce angiotensin II and ultimately aldosterone, which aids in increasing reabsorption of salt and water. The Anrep effect is an autoregulation method in which myocardial contractility increases with afterload. The Bowditch effect is an increase in myocardial contractility in response to an increase in heart rate. Conn syndrome is a primary cause of hyperaldosteronism.

72. d. Addison's disease is a rare condition of chronic adrenal insufficiency, with lack of glucocorticoid and mineralocorticoid. Typically, there is a raised level of adrenocorticotropic hormone (ACTH) and cortisol levels are reduced. Biochemically, the patient may have low sodium, with raised serum potassium, raised urea and low blood glucose, and increased plasma renin activity with normal or reduced aldosterone. Clinically, the patient will have symptoms of dehydration and hypotension because of the mineralocorticoid deficiency. He may also have vomiting, loss of appetite, weight loss, lethargy, hypoglycaemia and postural hypotension due to glucocorticoid reduction. If the adrenal glands are non-functioning, an increase in ACTH can also increase melanocyte-stimulating hormone (MSH) levels, causing increased skin and mucosa pigmentation.

73. b. The heart pumps blood to all organs in the body, including itself. Left ventricular systolic contraction results in high-pressure outflow of blood into the aorta. The papillary muscles contract prior to ventricular contraction to close the mitral and tricuspid valves to prevent regurgitation of blood into the atria. Coronary perfusion, however, occurs mainly during diastole as intramyocardial arteries are compressed during systole. Coronary blood flow is normally about 250 mL/min at rest, and this can rise to 1 L/min during strenuous exercise.

Note:

$$\text{Cardiac out (CO)} = \text{heart rate (HR)} \times \text{stroke volume (SV)}$$

$$\text{Cardiac index (CI)} = \text{CO/body surface area (BSA)}$$

74. e. There are two broad types of lymphatic vessels:

1. Initial lymphatics
   a. Valveless
   b. No smooth muscle in walls
   c. Located in skeletal muscle/intestinal walls
   d. Fluid is transported due to massage from muscular contractions
2. Collecting lymphatics
   a. Valves
   b. Smooth muscle in walls
   c. Contract via peristalsis

The normal lymph turnover is 2–4 L in 24 h.

75. c. Oedema is defined as excess accumulation of fluid in the extravascular space. Typically an exudate is a consequence of increased capillary permeability secondary to an inflammatory process. Nephrotic syndrome results in a transudate due to reduced colloid osmotic pressure from loss of plasma proteins and albumin via the glomerulus. Increased capillary permeability due to inflammatory mediators (serotonin, histamine, bradykinin, PGE2) results in the formation of an exudate. Exudates are rich in fibrinogen and protein, in contrast to transudates.

76. c. The pressure of nail-bed capillaries at the arteriolar end is roughly 32 mmHg. The pressure of nail-bed capillaries at the venous end is roughly 15 mmHg. The pulse pressure of nail-bed capillaries at the arteriolar end is roughly 5 mmHg. The pulse pressure of nail-bed capillaries at the venous end is 0 mmHg.

77. d. Hartmann's solution – Na 131 mmol/L, K 5 mmol/L, Ca 2 mmol/L, Cl 111 mmol/L, HCO_3 29 mmol/L, osmolality – 278 mosmol/L; normal saline – Na 154 mmol/L, K 0 mmol/L, Cl 155 mmol/L, osmolality – 308 mosmol/L; 5% dextrose – osmolality – 278 mosmol/L.

GASTROINTESTINAL SYSTEM

78. d.   Gallstones are most commonly formed in the gallbladder. Several conditions predispose to the formation of gallstones and are linked with a higher incidence, including female gender, obesity, fatty diet, haemolytic diseases and geographical distribution, with a higher incidence in developed countries. There are three main types of stones: mixed type (80%) consisting of cholesterol, bile pigment and calcium; cholesterol stones (10%) consisting of pure cholesterol; and pigment stones (10%) composed of calcium bilirubinate. There are several pathological consequences of gallstones: these are mainly acute cholecystitis, chronic cholecystitis, obstructive jaundice, acute pancreatitis and gallstone ileus. A fistula formed between the gallbladder and duodenum can allow a stone to pass through and impact at the terminal ileum. These can also spontaneously pass through and appear in the stool.

79. a.   Bile is secreted by hepatocytes, with hepatic ducts adding to its fluid content – approximately 1 L of bile is produced each day. Essential amino acids are those which cannot be endogenously synthesized by the body – the liver is responsible for synthesis of all non-essential amino acids. Glycogenolysis involves the breakdown of glycogen stores to glucose, occurring in early starvation; conversely, ketone bodies are produced from fatty acids during starvation via beta-oxidation. The cytochrome P450 system of the liver is involved in the degradation of peptide and steroid hormones, in addition to various drugs; phenytoin acts to increase the effect of the system, rendering possible concomitant medications such as warfarin and the oral contraceptive pill (OCP) less effective.

80. a.   Parietal cells of the stomach produce gastric acid and intrinsic factor, and are regulated by histamine vagal nerve stimulation and gastrin. The enzyme hydrogen potassium ATPase is unique to parietal cells and is responsible for the transportation of hydrogen ions. Intrinsic factor is required for vitamin B_{12} absorption. In pernicious anaemia, autoantibodies are directed against parietal cells or intrinsic factor. Chief cells produce pepsinogen and are present in the fundus of the stomach.

81. d.   Gastrin is released by G-cells of the stomach, duodenum and pancreas. Its role is to stimulate gastric acid production from parietal cells. Gastrin production is increased with stomach distension, vagal nerve stimulation and the presence of partly digested proteins in the duodenum. Gastrin production is inhibited by the presence of acid in the duodenum.

82. b.   Gastrin is released by G-cells of the stomach, duodenum and pancreas. Its role is to stimulate gastric acid production from parietal cells. Gastrin production is increased with stomach distension, vagal nerve stimulation and the presence of partly digested proteins in the duodenum. Gastrin production is inhibited by the presence of acid in the duodenum.

83. b.   G-cells secrete gastrin and are found in the glands of the pylorus – gastrin stimulates HCl production by parietal cells. HCl secretion is inhibited by secretin (produced by the duodenum), cholecystokinin and somatostatin. Chief cells secrete pepsinogen (precursor of pepsin). Parietal cells secrete HCl and intrinsic factor and are found in the glands on the fundus. Gastric secretion amounts to 1–1.5 L/day.

84. c.   Oxyntic gland is composed of three cell types: (1) mucous neck cells, which secrete mainly mucus; (2) peptic (or chief) cells, which secrete large quantities of pepsinogen; and (3) parietal (or oxyntic) cells, which secrete hydrochloric acid and intrinsic factor. Hydrochloric acid is formed at the villus-like projections inside these canaliculi and is then conducted through the canaliculi to the secretory end of the cell. Intrinsic factor is essential for absorption of vitamin B_{12} in the ileum.

85. a.   The severity of pancreatitis can be assessed according to several physiological parameters. A scoring system (Glasgow scale) has been established to monitor the changes in these parameters on admission, and subsequently. Patients with increasing severity may require admission to a high-dependency unit for closer monitoring. Corrected calcium levels <2 mmol/L are usually associated with a more severe pancreatitis. Loss of insulin production from the pancreas raises blood glucose levels.

86. a.   Daily secretion of saliva normally ranges between 800 and 1500 mL. Saliva has a pH between 6.0 and 7.0, which is a favourable range for the digestive action of ptyalin. The bactericidal action of saliva results from the presence of thiocyanate ions and lysozyme, which attack the bacteria. The thiocyanate ions, on entering the bacteria, become bactericidal. The concentration of bicarbonate ions is 50–70 mEq/L, which is about two to three times that of plasma.

87. c.   Approximately 2–3 L of fluid is ingested each day; 9–10 L of fluid is absorbed and 7–8 L is secreted into the gastrointestinal tract (GIT), but only 100 mL is excreted in the faeces. Clearly, huge fluid shifts occur and the absorption is dependent on the osmotic gradient established by the absorption of nutrients and electrolytes. Below is a table summarizing the absorption and secretion within the GIT.

	Absorption	Secretion/ingestion
Mouth	Nil	2.5 L fluid ingested 1.5 L saliva secreted
Stomach	Lipid-soluble molecules	2.5 L gastric juices secreted
Gallbladder	Absorbs water concentrating bile	500 mL bile secreted
Pancreas	Nil	1.5 L pancreatic juices secreted
Small intestine	8–9 L fluid absorbed	1.5 L intestinal secretions
Large intestine	1 L fluid absorbed	100 mL excreted in faeces

88. d.   The process of chewing helps food to be broken down and for it to be mixed with saliva. Saliva helps the food bolus to be swallowed more easily but also exposes the bolus to the enzyme amylase. The function of amylase is to digest starch. Oral amylase (ptyalin) works most efficiently in the mouth's neutral pH environment, acting to cleave some of the bonds between adjacent glucose molecules. Oral amylase, in comparison with pancreatic amylase, does not contribute a great deal to digestion. This is because most people do not chew their food long enough for the enzyme to work, and once inside the stomach the acid pH denatures the enzyme.

89. e.   Vomiting is a reflex action of expulsion of gastric/duodenal contents through the mouth. It is controlled by higher centres of the brain on the floor of the fourth ventricle, known as area postrema. There are several causes that can trigger vomiting including severe pain, motion sickness, raised intracranial pressure, infection of the gastrointestinal tract and stimulation of the chemoreceptor trigger zone by chemicals (drugs). Vomiting is usually preceded by pallor, sweating and dizziness. Excessive vomiting can lead to metabolic alkalosis due to loss of H^+ ions. Aspiration pneumonia generally occurs in those who have lost their gag reflex (e.g. secondary to coma, alcohol or anaesthesia).

90. a.   Pyloric stenosis classically affects male infants between 4 and 6 weeks. They present with projectile vomiting, persistent hunger and weight loss. The biochemical disturbance seen is hypokalaemic hypochloraemic alkalosis associated with hypovolaemia and haemoconcentration. The urine is acidic. Treatment involves correction of the biochemical disturbances and pyloromyotomy.

91. c.   Jaundice is yellow discoloration of skin and sclera caused by raised bilirubin levels in the blood. It can be classified according to pre-hepatic, hepatic and post-hepatic (cholestatic) causes. Bilirubin is produced from red cell breakdown in an unconjugated (water-insoluble) form. This is bound to albumin and enters the liver, where it is conjugated with glucuronic acid and becomes water soluble. It is secreted into the gut with bile and is excreted in urine and faeces. Pre-hepatic jaundice is caused by excessive red cell breakdown resulting in increased concentrations of unconjugated bilirubin. Hepatic jaundice is usually caused by liver disease such as cirrhosis or liver cancer. Post-hepatic jaundice is caused by obstruction to bile outflow resulting in increased concentrations of conjugated bilirubin entering the blood circulation but not the gut, leading to pale stools and dark urine. Bile salts are deposited in the skin in cholestatic jaundice, causing pruritus.

92. e.   There is net absorption of water and sodium in the colon, with net secretion of potassium and bicarbonate. The colon has an indirect role in the synthesis of vitamin K and B vitamins via production from its inherent bacterial flora – important fatty acids are also produced in this manner. Mass action contraction involves simultaneous contraction of smooth muscle over a long length. The result is transportation of material from one area of the colon to another in one movement. It normally occurs one to three times a day.

93. b.   Pancreatic resection can cause several physiological effects. There is loss of proteolytic and lipolytic enzyme secretion, leading to poor digestion and absorption of protein and fat. This in turn causes weight loss and malabsorption of fat-soluble vitamins A, D, E and K. Furthermore, a pancreatic resection may lead to malabsorption of vitamin B12 but a true deficiency is rare. Loss of alkaline pancreatic secretion causes failure to neutralize gastric chyme, and subsequently malabsorption of essential minerals such as Ca^{2+}, Fe^{2+} and PO_4^-. This can lead to anaemia and osteoporosis.

94. a. The pancreas has an important exocrine role. A bicarbonate (alkaline) secretion, rich in enzymes, is released into the duodenum to neutralize the gastric acidity and allow digestion of the chyme. Two types of cells contribute to the exocrine secretions – acinar cells and duct cells. The acinar cells respond to cholecystokinin and acetylcholine to release enzymes and Cl^-. The duct cells respond to secretin (released from the mucosa of the duodenal and upper jejunum) to release a HCO_3^- rich fluid. Several enzymes are secreted by the pancreas and include trypsin and lipase. They act on proteins and triglycerides, respectively. The ratio of different enzymes varies with diet. A diet rich in carbohydrates will lead to a rise in amylase, whereas a diet high in protein will lead to trypsin being released.

95. a. Glasgow criteria include:

- PO_2 <8 kPa
- Age >55 years
- Neutrophils >15 × 10^9/L
- Corrected calcium <2.0 mmol/L
- Urea >16 mmol/L
- Albumin <32 g/L
- Glucose >10 mmol/L
- AST >125 units/L
- LDH >600 units/L

96. c. Within the small intestine two major contractions take place: peristalsis and segmentation. Peristalsis in the small intestine is much weaker than in the oesophagus and stomach, and consequently the major contractile activity is segmentation. This term describes the back-and-forth movement of the chyme when the alternate ring-like segments of bowel contract simultaneously. Segmentation occurs at 9–12 contractions per minute. The frequency of contraction decreases down the length of the small intestine. The large bowel has a contraction frequency of three to four per minute. The small bowel has an intrinsic nervous system that allows autonomic contractions. The rhythm of the contractions is paced by graded depolarizations called slow waves. Parasympathetic activity increases the amplitude and duration of the slow waves, resulting in increased intestinal activity. Peristalsis is stimulated in part by intrinsic stretch reflexes related to a bolus of chyme, but it is also thought to be stimulated by the hormone serotonin.

97. e. There are three main phases to swallowing:

- Oral/voluntary phase (± oral 'preparatory' phase, i.e. formation of food bolus)
- Pharyngeal phase
- Oesophageal phase

The pharyngeal and oesophageal phases are involuntary. The pharyngeal phase of swallowing is the shortest. Contraction of the superior constrictor prevents velopalatal insufficiency.

98. e.   The gastrointestinal tract is both an endocrine organ and a target for the action of a large number of hormones. Gastric inhibitory peptide, as well as glucagon-like peptide-1, stimulate the secretion of insulin. Gastrin stimulates parietal cells to secrete hydrogen chloride and stimulates chief cells to secrete pepsinogen. Guanylin stimulates intestinal secretion of chloride. Cholecystokinin stimulates intestinal motility, contraction of the gallbladder and secretion of pancreatic enzymes, but inhibits gastric motility and secretion. Secretin stimulates water and bicarbonate secretion in pancreatic juice and enhances the actions of cholecystokinin on the pancreas. The table below summarizes the more common hormones.

Hormone	Secreting organ	Effect
Gastrin	Stomach	Stimulates parietal cells to secrete HCl Stimulates chief cells to secrete pepsinogen
Gastric inhibitory peptide	Small intestine	Inhibits gastric motility and secretion Stimulates secretion of insulin from pancreatic islets
Cholecystokinin	Small intestine	Stimulates intestinal motility and contraction of gallbladder Stimulates secretion of pancreatic enzymes Inhibits gastric motility and secretion
Secretin	Small intestine	Stimulates water and bicarbonate secretion in pancreatic juice Enhances actions of cholecystokinin on pancreas
Glucagon-like peptide-1	Ileum and colon	Inhibits gastric motility and secretion Stimulates secretion of insulin from pancreatic islets
Guanylin	Ileum and colon	Stimulates intestinal secretion of chloride

99. a.   The liver produces and secretes between 250 and 1500 mL of bile per day. Bile is mainly composed of bile pigment (bilirubin, a derivative of haemoglobin metabolism), bile acids, phospholipids, cholesterol and inorganic ions. Free bilirubin is transported in the blood bound to albumin. In the liver it is conjugated with glucuronic acid so that it can be excreted in the bile. Bile is secreted continuously by the liver and fills up the gallbladder while the sphincter of Oddi is closed. When the intestinal mucosa detects fat, it secretes secretin and cholecystokinin, which stimulate the gallbladder to contract. Bacteria in the intestinal lumen convert conjugated bilirubin into urobilinogen. Urobilinogen is further broken down into stercobilin and urobilin, which colour faeces and urine, respectively. Only about 50% of urobilinogen is secreted in the faeces. The rest is absorbed and undergoes enterohepatic circulation or is secreted by the kidney. Bile acids are the derivatives of cholesterol and aid lipid absorption.

100. c.   Pepsin is a peptic enzyme of the stomach. It is most active at a pH of 2.0 to 3.0 and is inactive at a pH above about 5.0. One of the important features of pepsin digestion is its ability to digest the protein collagen, an albuminoid type of protein that is affected little by other digestive enzymes. Pepsin initiates the process of protein digestion, usually providing only 10–20% of the total protein digestion to convert the protein to proteoses, peptones and a few polypeptides.

101. d.   The myenteric plexus or Auerbach's plexus is part of the enteric nervous system. It consists mostly of a linear chain of many interconnecting neurons that extends the entire length of the gastrointestinal tract. Its stimulation causes increased tonic contraction and gut peristaltic waves associated with rhythmic contractions.

102. a.   Swallowing takes part in three phases: oral, pharyngeal and oesophageal. The tongue forms a bolus of food; on transition of the bolus touch receptors are stimulated activating swallowing reflexes. Sensation at this stage is provided by cranial nerve (CN) V, with CN XII controlling involuntary motor functions. The next stage of the swallowing takes part in the pharynx. The soft palate is elevated and the vocal cords pulled together; during this stage there is a brief inhibition of breathing. The upper oesophageal sphincter relaxes and the bolus is propelled by the superior constrictor muscle. CN IX receives sensory information with CNs V, IX and X for autonomic motor control. The oesophageal phase consists of peristaltic actions under autonomic muscular control (CNs V, IX, X) with sensation from CN X. The rate of peristalsis is 5 cm/s.

103. a.   On transit of food through the oesophagus, receptors ahead of the bolus allow relaxation of the lower oesophageal sphincter (LOS), allowing food to enter the stomach. If food remains in the oesophagus, the subsequent distension causes secondary peristalsis to occur above the food bolus so as to push the food down. Relaxation of the LOS is initiated by inhibitory neurons of the myenteric plexus.

   Several cranial nerves are involved in swallowing:

- *Trigeminal nerve:* Sensory supply to anterior two-thirds of tongue; motor to chewing muscles
- *Facial nerve:* Sensory to taste; motor to lips, cheek and stylohyoid
- Glossopharyngeal nerve: Innervates salivary glands; sensory to soft palate, posterior tongue and upper pharynx; motor to stylopharyngeus and superior constrictors
- *Vagus nerve:* Sensory to posterior and lower pharynx and larynx; motor to palatoglossus, cricopharyngeus and intrinsic muscles of larynx
- *Accessory nerve:* Motor to palatopharyngeus, levator veli palatine and uvula
- *Hypoglossal nerve:* Motor to all muscles of tongue except palatoglossus

104. b.   The rate of primary peristalsis is 5 cm/s. Receptors ahead of the food bolus allow relaxation of the lower oesophageal sphincter (LOS), allowing food to enter the stomach. If food remains in the oesophagus, the subsequent distension causes secondary peristalsis to occur above the food bolus, so as to push the food down. Relaxation of the LOS is initiated by inhibitory neurons of the myenteric plexus.

105. a.   Metabolic complications of parenteral nutrition include:

- Hyperglycaemia/hypoglycaemia
- Hyperlipidaemia
- Essential fatty acid deficiency
- Hyperchloraemic metabolic acidosis
- Hyperammonaemia

106. e.   Vitamin K is necessary for the liver for formation of five important clotting factors: prothrombin, factor II, factor VII, factor IX, factor X and protein C. In the absence of vitamin K, a subsequent insufficiency of these coagulation factors in the blood can lead to serious bleeding tendencies.

107. a.   The secretion of gastric acid is highly regulated by the autonomic nervous system and by several hormones. Parasympathetic stimulation via the vagus nerve acts to stimulate gastric acid secretion, while gastrin stimulates the parietal cells to produce gastric acid. Gastric acid secretion is inhibited by hormones such as cholecystokinin and secretin. Nausea acts to inhibit histamine-stimulated gastric acid secretion by multiple mechanisms including sympathetic innervation. Pepsinogen is a zymogen that is then converted to enzyme pepsin within an acidic environment, which is important for proteolysis.

RENAL SYSTEM

108. e. Intravesical pressure is approximately 3 cm H_2O. The volume inside the bladder needs to reach 200–300 mL before there is much change in the intravesical pressure and the desire to urinate occurs. As the volume increases, so does the pressure and the desire to urinate. The changes in volume are detected by stretch fibres within the bladder wall. The parasympathetic nervous system (PNS) acts via the S2–S4 nerve roots to increase contraction of the detrusor muscle and decrease contraction of the internal urethral sphincter. Parasympathetic nerves also innervate the external urethral sphincter via the pudendal nerve. Sympathetic nerves run via the hypogastric plexus (L1–L2) and decrease contraction of the detrusor and increase contraction of the internal urethral sphincter. Micturition is therefore initiated via the PNS and the impulses of the sympathetic nervous system (SNS) are inhibited by the brainstem.

109. d. Serum potassium levels are controlled by uptake into cells, renal losses and extra-renal losses (e.g. gastrointestinal). The most common causes of chronic hypokalaemia are diuretic usage and hyperaldosteronism. Acutely, hypokalaemia may be caused by potassium-free intravenous fluid replacement and redistribution into cells. Uptake of potassium into cells is stimulated by insulin, β-adrenergic stimulation and use of theophylline. Aldosterone stimulates renal excretion of potassium and hydrogen ions in exchange for sodium. Renal failure leads to hyperkalaemia.

110. b. Filtrate from the glomerulus enters the proximal convoluted tubule. Here, around 70% of the filtered sodium is reabsorbed, with water following the osmotic gradient. The reabsorption of sodium relies on the energy-dependent ATP pump. Filtrate then enters into the descending limb of the loop of Henle, which is permeable to Na^+ and water. High osmolality of the surrounding medulla causes water to be reabsorbed and Na^+ to be passively added into the descending limb. This results in a highly concentrated filtrate at the end of the descending loop. The ascending limb is permeable to Na^+ but impermeable to water. There is active reabsorption of Na^+ into the surrounding medulla and this maintains its high osmolality. The filtrate at the end of the ascending limb will be more diluted as it enters the distal tubule and collecting ducts for further water and Na^+ reabsorption. Furosemide and thiazide diuretics work in different parts of the nephron to produce a higher urine volume by inhibiting Na^+ reabsorption.

111. d. The loop of Henle is part of a nephron. The descending loop is permeable to water and solutes, and given the high medullary osmolality, water moves out osmotically from the descending loop, whereas Na^+ and Cl^- are added. As a result, the tubular filtrate becomes increasingly more concentrated distally. The ascending limb is impermeable to water. Both Na^+ and Cl^- are actively transported out of the ascending limb into the medulla, and tubular filtrate becomes increasingly less concentrated as it ascends.

112. c. The kidney regulates bicarbonate levels. The proximal convoluted tubule reabsorbs 90% of bicarbonate and the distal nephron reclaims very little. The proximal convoluted tubule contains more carbonic anhydrase than the distal segments. Most hydrogen ions are secreted in the distal tubule segments. The hydrogen ions are actively secreted into the tubular lumen in exchange for sodium ions, allowing the bicarbonate to bind with a hydrogen ion, forming carbonic acid. Carbonic anhydrase converts carbonic acid into carbon dioxide and water, which can rapidly enter the cell.

113. d. The physiological daily requirement of sodium is 1 mmol/kg. Sodium is the major extracellular cation – 5% is intracellular, 50% is extracellular, 45% is within bone. Atrial natriuretic peptide is secreted by the cardiac atria following cardiac wall distension (i.e. an increase in circulating volume) – it has the opposite effect as antidiuretic hormone (ADH) (arginine vasopressin) and increases sodium excretion. ADH is produced by the posterior pituitary gland and increases water absorption at the renal collecting duct.

114. a. The history is of a prolonged transurethral resection of prostate (TURP), involving continuous irrigation of the bladder. Although blood loss occurs, observations show that he is haemodynamically stable. In this case the diagnosis of TURP syndrome can be made with a low sodium, which usually causes restlessness and headache, leading to respiratory distress and hypoxia. The TURP syndrome consists of pulmonary oedema, cerebral oedema and hyponatraemia. Treatment is with furosemide and fluid restriction.

115. e. The anion gap = $(Na^+ + K^+) - (HCO_3^- + Cl^-)$. If there is a high anion gap, there is an unmeasured anion present in increased quantities. This can be seen in ketoacidosis and lactic acidosis. A normal anion gap can still be seen in metabolic acidosis. This implies that HCl is being retained, or that $NaHCO_3$ is being lost. In this case, plasma HCO_3^- is replaced with chloride to maintain electroneutrality. This can lead to hyperchloraemic acidosis. Examples of this are seen in diarrhoea, ileostomy and renal tubular acidosis. A fall in albumin level can lead to a decrease in the anion gap.

116. e. Renin is released in response to a drop in blood pressure. This activates the renin–angiotensin–aldosterone (RAA) system to increase blood pressure. Renin secretion tends to be inhibited by hyperkalaemia and stimulated by hypokalaemia. This is opposite and independent of the effects of potassium on aldosterone secretion. Beta-blockers also inhibit secretion of renin. In the kidneys, β_1-adrenergic receptors are present in the juxtaglomerular apparatus, which when stimulated releases renin. Aldosterone inhibits renin via a negative feedback mechanism. Salt depletion reduces blood pressure and hence stimulates renin.

117. b. Atrial natriuretic peptide (ANP) is a protein that is released by cardiac myocytes in the atria in response to high blood pressure and an increase in extracellular fluid (ECF), causing the atria to stretch. The function of ANP is to increase water and sodium loss through the kidneys, lowering the blood pressure and ECF. ANP also inhibits the secretion of renin and thus the renin–angiotensin–aldosterone system.

118. b. The renin–angiotensin–aldosterone system is activated in response to a loss of blood volume or a drop in blood pressure. The juxtaglomerular cells of the kidney secrete renin in response to low blood flow. Renin converts plasma angiotensinogen to angiotensin I, and this is then converted to angiotensin II in the lungs by the enzyme angiotensin-converting enzyme (ACE). Angiotensin II stimulates the release of aldosterone and antidiuretic hormone (ADH). As well as causing arterial vasoconstriction. This results in reduced Na^+ and water loss from the kidney and increased blood pressure.

119. c. Antidiuretic hormone (ADH). Acts at the collecting duct to increase its permeability to water allowing reabsorption. ADH is produced in the supraoptic nucleus in the hypothalamus but released by the posterior pituitary when the body is dehydrated. Secretion occurs in response to a high plasma osmolality and a reduction in plasma volume. The release of ADH causes the kidney to conserve water and excrete more concentrated urine.

120. c. The adrenal gland consists of the cortex and medulla. The cortex can be divided into the zona glomerulosa, zona fasciculata and zona reticularis. The zona glomerulosa is responsible for mineralocorticoid (aldosterone) production, and the zona fasciculata for glucocorticoid (cortisol) production. The zona reticularis is responsible for androgen production. The zona glomerulosa lies superficial to the fasciculata and reticularis. Adrenocorticotropic hormone (ACTH) released by the anterior pituitary gland stimulates cortisol production. The medulla produces adrenaline and noradrenaline.

121. e. The respiratory centre regulates the H^+ concentration by removal of CO_2 (i.e. H_2CO_3) from the extracellular fluid. The respiratory system acts within a few minutes to eliminate CO_2 and H_2CO_3 from the body. The kidneys excrete either acid or alkaline urine, thereby readjusting the extracellular fluid H^+ concentration toward normal during acidosis or alkalosis. The chemical acid–base buffer systems combine immediately with acid or base to prevent excessive changes in H^+ concentration.

122. d. In order to establish the efficacy of the kidney to filter substances (glomerular filtration rate [GFR]) one must use a substance that, once filtered, is neither excreted nor absorbed during its passage through the kidney. If the substance is neither excreted nor absorbed, the volume of substance filtered by the glomeruli per unit time will be the same as the volume of substance in the urine per unit time. Unfortunately, no endogenous substances in the body have these criteria. Plants such as garlic and onions possess a suitable substance called inulin, a derivative of fructose. Inulin is injected and then the concentration of inulin is measured in the urine. If one also knows the urine output, one is able to work out the rate of inulin excretion. Creatinine is used clinically as a rough measure of GFR. Creatinine is a decent substitute because it is released into the blood at a constant rate and its excretion closely matches that of the GFR. However, it is slightly secreted by the renal tubules and so any measurement will always slightly overestimate the actual GFR.

123. c. The pH of blood is carefully controlled between 7.35 and 7.45. Homeostasis is maintained by the compensation mechanism of the lungs for carbon dioxide and the kidneys for bicarbonate. Carbon dioxide is produced by tissues during respiration, transported to the lungs and expired. Acids, such as lactate and ketone bodies, release hydrogen ions into the blood. Under normal conditions the body's major buffering mechanism (bicarbonate) is able to mop up the excess ions according to the equation

$$HCO_3^- + H^+ \rightarrow H_2CO_3 \rightarrow H_2O + CO_2$$

This equation is maintained by the kidney's ability to produce bicarbonate and its ability to excrete H^+. Disturbances in acid–base are caused by a lack or excess of HCO_3^- or H^+. The table below summarizes the different primary disturbances prior to any compensation.

Disturbance	HCO_3^-	CO_2	Cause
Metabolic acidosis	Low	Normal	Increase in acids, e.g. lactate Loss of HCO_3^- in diarrhoea
Metabolic alkalosis	High	Normal	Vomiting, hypokalaemia
Respiratory acidosis	Normal	High	Hypoventilation
Respiratory alkalosis	Normal	Low	Hyperventilation

124. a. The blood gas shows that he has a respiratory alkalosis and the only cause in the list for this is postoperative pain. Adequate analgesia will settle his hyperventilation and therefore the respiratory alkalosis. Pulmonary embolism typically causes a type I respiratory failure, which is defined as hypoxia without hypercapnia. Type II respiratory failure is characterized by hypoxia and hypercapnia. This can be caused by either reduced breathing effort or a reduction in lung surface area for gas exchange. Pneumonia can be grouped into either type I or II respiratory failure. Diabetic ketoacidosis produces an acidotic blood gas. There may be an element of respiratory compensation resulting in hypocapnia.

125. a. Metabolic acidosis can be caused by either:

- Too much acid production – lactic acidosis as a result of anaerobic respiration, e.g. pancreatitis, crush injury, salicylate poisoning
- Diabetic ketoacidosis
- Inability to rid the body of acid, e.g. renal failure

A normal anion gap is between 10 and 18 mmol/L. It is calculated using Na, K, HCO_3 and Cl ions. Causes of metabolic acidosis with a normal anion gap include renal tubular acidosis. An increased anion gap is caused by diabetic ketoacidosis, lactic acidosis and salicylate poisoning.

126. c. The correct answer demonstrates a metabolic acidosis with a raised lactate caused by poor tissue perfusion. The body tries to compensate the acidosis by increasing the respiratory rate to reduce carbon dioxide levels. Answer a is a normal arterial blood gas (ABG). Answer b shows a patient who is unable to oxygenate properly, perhaps an acute asthma attack. Answer d could represent this patient at the initial stage of his injury, where the body is overcompensating for metabolic acidosis and creates a respiratory alkalosis. Answer e is incompatible with life and could be seen in a patient who is in asystole following cardiac arrest.

127. c. Acid–base homeostasis is vital to normal body functions because of the sensitivity proteins have toward changes in pH. An acidosis is an excess of H^+ ions in the blood or a deficit of base, and with an alkalosis the reverse. The homeostatic mechanisms keep the blood pH between 7.35 and 7.45. The respiratory and renal systems help compensate for changes in pH. The respiratory system can act quickly by increasing respiratory rate, but the renal system compensation mechanisms or active excretion or reabsorption acts slowly. A buffer consists of a weak base and its conjugate weak base. The most important buffer in the blood is the carbonic acid–bicarbonate equilibrium. This equilibrium allows excess H^+ ions to be captured with HCO_3^- and released as H_2O and CO_2: $H^+ + HCO_3^- \leftrightarrow H_2CO_3 \leftrightarrow H_2O + CO_2$. This buffering mechanism is powerful in its own right but is particularly beneficial when combined with the homeostatic mechanisms of the lungs and kidneys.

128. b.   Water, electrolytes and metabolites are conserved while wastes are eliminated in the urine. This tubular reabsorption and secretion of substances help maintain body fluid homeostasis. Most of the sodium that is filtered is reabsorbed, that is 25,850 mmol out of 26,000 mmol filtered in 24 h (99.4%). Hence, sodium concentrations are lower in urine in a normal physiological state.

129. e.   Vasoconstriction or dilatation of afferent arterioles affects the rate of blood flow to the glomerulus and in turn affects the glomerular filtration rate (GFR), close control of the GFR is important to ensure that the kidney is able to eliminate wastes and regulate blood pressure, but not so high so that excess water is lost. Sympathetic activity constricts afferent arterioles causing a decrease in GFR. The decreased GFR reduces urine production and therefore helps to preserve blood volume. When sympathetic stimulation is experimentally removed, one can observe that the GFR remains relatively constant over a mean arterial pressure range of 70–180 mmHg. This ability of the kidney is called renal autoregulation. Autoregulation is achieved via locally released chemicals, which affect the afferent and, less importantly, the efferent arterioles. When the blood pressure drops the afferent arterioles dilate, and vice versa. GFR can then remain relatively constant within the autoregulatory range of blood pressure values.

130. d.   In a resting adult, the kidneys receive 1.2–1.3 L of blood per minute, or just under 25% of the cardiac output. The renal artery enters the kidney through the hilum and then branches progressively to form the interlobar arteries, arcuate arteries, interlobular arteries (also called radial arteries) and afferent arterioles, which lead to the glomerular capillaries, where large amounts of fluid and solutes (except the plasma proteins) are filtered to begin urine formation.

131. a.   An appropriate solute needs to be freely filtered by the kidney, not absorbed or secreted; detectable in plasma and urine, not altered renal blood flow; and non-toxic. Although creatinine (produced endogenously) does suffer from tubular secretion, it meets most of the requirements and is therefore most often used. Inulin is a natural storage carbohydrate, which is usually extracted from chicory plants in order for it to be used in humans. Inulin does not suffer from secretion but does require intravenous injection as it is not produced by humans, showing that the solute does not need to be produced endogenously.

ENDOCRINE SYSTEM (INCLUDING GLUCOSE HOMEOSTASIS)

132. a.   Human growth hormone (GH) is a large peptide secreted in response to growth hormone–releasing hormone (GHRH), which is released by the hypothalamus. Hypoglycaemia is a potent stimulator of GH secretion by stimulating the release of GHRH from the hypothalamus. The secretion of GH follows a circadian pattern with higher levels secreted during periods of deep sleep. Other factors that promote GH secretion include trauma, haemorrhage, fever, pain and exercise. Somatostatin inhibits the secretion of GH. During the growing years, GH stimulates skeletal growth by promoting mitosis within the epiphyseal plates in the bones. In adulthood, GH has metabolic functions, including an anti-insulin role (inhibits glucose uptake into cells), promoting glycogenolysis and lipolysis.

133. c.   Cortisol (glucocorticoid) is produced in the adrenal glands, in the zona fasciculata. It has widespread actions but is mainly released as a response to stress (trauma, infection, fear, pain, surgery). It acts to increase blood glucose levels (gluconeogenesis) by counteracting insulin action. It also stimulates lipolysis in response to stress and increased anxiety. Cortisol also dampens the body's immune response by inhibiting complement and preventing the proliferation of T-cells. There is a diurnal variation of normal cortisol levels in the blood, with highest levels found in the morning and lowest levels around midnight.

134. e.   Aldosterone stimulates sodium reabsorption in the distal convoluted tubule (DCT), collecting duct, gut, salivary and sweat glands in exchange for K^+. Pituitary osmoreceptors are stimulated following a rise in Na^+, leading to increased secretion of vasopressin (antidiuretic hormone [ADH]), leading to water retention. Aldosterone may lead to a metabolic alkalosis as H^+ in the plasma may be exchanged for reabsorbed Na^+. Increased K^+ is a stimulus for aldosterone production. Atrial natriuretic peptide (ANP) has an inhibitory effect on renin release – this in turn results in decreased aldosterone synthesis.

135. c.   Hyperaldosteronism is caused by excessive aldosterone production by the zona glomerulosa. It can be primary, where there is autonomous hypersecretion of aldosterone, such as in Conn syndrome, characterized by an adrenal cortical adenoma, or secondary, caused by increased production of angiotensin II followed by activation of the renin–angiotensin system. Secondary hyperaldosteronism may be precipitated by congestive cardiac failure, hepatic failure and cirrhosis. The biochemistry seen in hyperaldosteronism shows raised sodium and low potassium. Plasma renin is reduced in Conn syndrome but raised in secondary hyperaldosteronism. Hypertension is found in both disorders.

136. e.   The anterior pituitary gland secretes thyroid-stimulating hormone, growth hormone, luteinizing hormone, follicle-stimulating hormone, adrenocorticotropic hormone and prolactin. The posterior pituitary gland secretes oxytocin and antidiuretic hormone (vasopressin). Thyrotropin-releasing hormone is produced in the hypothalamus and stimulates thyroid-stimulating hormone release from the pituitary gland.

137. e. Atrial natriuretic peptide (ANP) causes epithelial cells of the collecting duct to increase the synthesis of water channels. The renin–angiotensin system will predominate over the ADH system if there are conflicting interests in blood tonicity and volume (i.e. physiologically it is more important to maintain blood volume and end-organ perfusion than to eliminate water if the blood is hypotonic). Aldosterone causes increased absorption of sodium in the distal convoluted tubule of the nephron. Erythropoietin is secreted in response to chronic hypoxia and results in erythrocyte proliferation. The kidney is involved in the hydroxylation of 25-hydroxycholecalciferol to its active form 1,25-dihydroxycholecalciferol.

138. e. Insulin is secreted by beta cells in the islets of Langerhans within the pancreas. It plays a very important role in the regulation of plasma glucose levels. Insulin secretion is influenced by several factors, but mainly the level of plasma glucose itself. Increased glucose stimulates the secretion of insulin, which increases uptake of glucose into cells in order to reduce plasma levels. However, brain cells can freely take up glucose without insulin. Other factors that stimulate secretion of insulin include fatty acids, ketone bodies, parasympathetic stimulation, gastrin, secretin, cholecystokinin and prostaglandin. Sympathetic stimulation inhibits insulin secretion. Insulin also stimulates protein synthesis and inhibits protein breakdown; it also inhibits lipolysis. Insulin has a very short half-life (5–10 min) and is rapidly broken down in the liver and kidney.

139. b. Approximately 98% of the body's potassium is intracellular. Aldosterone promotes the excretion of potassium in the distal convoluted tubule in exchange for the reabsorption of sodium. Insulin encourages potassium uptake into cells and is involved in the treatment for hyperkalaemia. Addison's disease (primary adrenal insufficiency) is a result of destruction of the adrenal cortex, resulting in decreased synthesis of glucocorticoids, mineralocorticoids and sex hormones. It is thus associated with hyperkalaemia (due to aldosterone deficiency, and decreased sodium absorption/potassium excretion). Conn syndrome (primary hyperaldosteronism) is characterized by increased aldosterone secretion from the adrenal glands, suppressed plasma renin activity, hypertension and hypokalaemia.

140. c. Cholecalciferol (also known as vitamin D_3) is produced after 7-dehydrocholesterol is exposed to ultraviolet light from the sun. Cholecalciferol is converted to 25-hydroxy-cholecalciferol in the liver before being converted to 1,25-dihydroxy-cholecalciferol by 1-α-hydroxylase in the kidney. Parathyroid hormone regulates the action of this enzyme. 1,25-Dihydroxy-cholecalciferol acts to increase calcium levels by increasing calcium absorption via the gut.

141. d. Antidiuretic hormone (ADH), also known as vasopressin, is released by the posterior pituitary gland. It functions mainly in the distal tubule and collecting duct by increasing permeability to water, hence retaining water from being excreted. This results in the production of low-volume concentrated urine during periods of dehydration. Lack of production of ADH causes cranial diabetes insipidus, whereas the inability of the kidneys to respond to ADH causes nephrogenic diabetes insipidus. ADH is inhibited by alcohol. All these conditions lead to the production of high-volume dilute urine.

142. b. The physiological effects of the hormones listed are:

- Growth hormone: Secretion of Insulin-like growth factor 1, resulting in various anabolic effects
- Prolactin: Milk production, breast development
- Oxytocin: Uterine contraction, milk secretion
- Vasopressin: Water retention
- Adrenocorticotropic hormone: Glucocorticoid and mineralocorticoid secretion

143. e. This man has a pituitary adenoma producing Adrenocorticotropic hormone (ACTH) causing raised cortisol known as Cushing disease. Cushing syndrome is characterized by high cortisol from any cause such as ectopic ACTH production or an adrenal adenoma causing a high cortisol level with a low, suppressed ACTH. With dexamethasone suppression in Cushing syndrome ACTH levels may be normal or elevated, with cortisol suppressed only with high-dose dexamethasone. With adrenal adenoma ACTH is low and cortisol is not suppressed. With ectopic ACTH production, ACTH level is high but cortisol is not suppressed. Pro-opio-melanocortin (POMC) is cleaved to produce both MSH and ACTH. ACTH increases cortisol production.

144. d. Ectopic Adrenocorticotropic hormone (ACTH) production from, in this case, lung malignancy would result in a high ACTH level, stimulating cortisol production. Therefore, both ACTH and cortisol would be high.

145. a. Systemic complications of severe burns include:

- Burn shock – hypovolaemic shock due to plasma loss
- Electrolyte disturbance – hyperkalaemia, hypocalcaemia
- Hypothermia
- Systemic inflammatory response syndrome – can lead to multiorgan dysfunction
- Gastric ulceration (stress response)
- Coagulopathy – disseminated intravascular coagulation
- Haemolysis

146. b. Calcium gluconate can be used to antagonize the effects of high magnesium levels on cardiac and neuromuscular function. Diuretics can also be used to treat hypermagnesaemia by promoting magnesium excretion. High magnesium levels are usually associated with a high potassium and high calcium level. Chronic renal failure leads to impaired magnesium excretion resulting in hypermagnesaemia. Other causes included hypothyroidism, Addison's disease and the intake of laxatives. A high magnesium level can cause cardiovascular, neurological and eventually respiratory depression, which may require artificial ventilation.

147. a. The causes of hypomagnesaemia include malnutrition, diarrhoea, excessive alcohol, loop diuretics and acute pancreatitis. An electrocardiogram will show a prolonged QT interval with some broad, flattened T waves. Signs and symptoms include irritability, carpopedal spasm and confusion. Low magnesium levels may be associated with low potassium or calcium levels. Treatment consists of replacement therapy as appropriate.

148. c. The normal serum level of magnesium is 0.7–1.0 mmol/L. The total body magnesium is 25 g, with 65% located in bone. Hypermagnesaemia can lead to bradycardia and sluggish tendon reflexes. The main causes of hypomagnesaemia are renal losses secondary to diuretics, alcoholism and gastrointestinal tract losses such as diarrhoea or malabsorption. Electrocardiogram changes with hypomagnesaemia include a prolonged PR interval and widened QRS complex.

149. b. The normal level of serum potassium lies between 3.5 and 5.0 mmol/L. Approximately 98% of the total body potassium is intracellular with a concentration of 150 mmol/L. Hypokalaemia can be caused by increased losses from the body via either the gastrointestinal tract (vomiting, diarrhoea, enterocutaneous fistulae) or the renal system (Conn and Cushing syndromes or diuretics). Symptoms of hypokalaemia include muscle weakness and lethargy with a risk of arrhythmias. Electrocardiogram changes include small/inverted T waves, U waves, prolonged PR interval and ST depression. A wide QRS complex is seen with hyperkalaemia together with tall tented T waves and small P waves.

150. e. The minimum level of energy required to exist is the basal metabolic rate (BMR) and accounts for about 50–70% of the daily energy expenditure in most individuals. Average BMR is 65–70 kcal/h in a 70 kg man. Skeletal muscle, even under resting conditions, accounts for 20–30% of the BMR. Thyroxine can increase BMR by up to 50 times the normal level. Prolonged malnutrition can decrease the metabolic rate by 20–30%. BMR is low during sleep because of skeletal muscle relaxation and decreased activity in the central nervous system.

151. e. Adrenaline has numerous metabolic effects. It has direct effects on adipose tissue inducing hormone-sensitive lipases, thereby promoting lipolysis and releasing fatty acids into the bloodstream. Increased glycogenolysis in the liver releases large amounts of glucose into the bloodstream. Glycogen synthesis in the liver and in muscles is inhibited. Glycogenolysis in muscles does not increase blood glucose as the glucose generated remains within the muscles for rapid metabolism. Adrenaline is not known to increase insulin secretion, although rising blood glucose levels owing to glycogenolysis in the liver do increase serum insulin levels and inhibit glucagon.

152. d. The adrenal gland consists of the cortex and medulla. The cortex can be divided into the zona glomerulosa, zona fasciculata and zona reticularis. The zona glomerulosa is responsible for mineralocorticoid (aldosterone) production, and the zona fasciculata for glucocorticoid (cortisol) production. The zona reticularis is responsible for androgen production. The zona glomerulosa lies superficially with the fasciculata and reticularis lying deeper, respectively. Adrenocorticotropic hormone (ACTH) released by the anterior pituitary gland stimulates cortisol production. The medulla produces adrenaline and noradrenaline.

153. c. Below are the actions of hormones in the body's response to trauma:

Adrenocorticotropic hormone – glucocorticoid release
Glucocorticoids – protein converted to glucose and glucose to glycogen
Aldosterone – reabsorption of Na and secretion of K
Antidiuretic hormone – increased water absorption
Insulin – low in ebb phase, levels increase in the flow phase, although
    hyperglycaemia remains due to continued resistance
Glucagon – stimulates glycogenolysis, gluconeogenesis
Serotonin – causing vasoconstriction and bronchoconstriction
Growth hormone – stimulating protein synthesis, lipolysis and glycogenolysis

154. c. The actions of cortisol include:

Metabolic effects – breakdown of proteins, lipolysis
Cardiovascular effects – increase vascular tone with vasopressors
Central nervous system – euphoria
Immunosuppressive effects – decrease T-cell number and function and B-cell
    expansion

Other actions include the permissive effects on the activity of aldosterone, antidiuretic hormone and an increase in the effect of triiodothyronine (T_3) in maintaining body temperature.

155. e. Hydrocortisone (cortisol) and other glucocorticoids are secreted by the adrenal cortex in response to Adrenocorticotropic hormone (ACTH). Secretion of ACTH from the anterior pituitary gland is in response to a stress stimulus. Prolonged starvation and exercise are perceived by the body as stressors and so increase cortisol release. The effects of cortisol can be wide ranging, from increasing glucagon and decreasing insulin secretion to promoting lipolysis and ketogenesis. Cortisol increases protein breakdown from muscle. The increased plasma levels of amino acid allow the liver to perform gluconeogenesis; however, it also leads to increased nitrogen excretion. Prolonged elevated levels of cortisol, whether endogenous or exogenous, result in the numerous clinical symptoms and signs of glucocorticoid excess: moon face, thin skin etc.

156. e. Histamine is released by mast cells and basophils by fragments of C3a and C5a in response to inflammation and allergy. Histamine binds to the H1 receptors in the smooth muscle of bronchioles to stimulate constriction. In blood vessels, histamine causes dilatation and increased permeability. This has the beneficial consequence of allowing leukocytes to reach affected areas more easily. Histamine is released by enterochromaffin-like cells in the stomach, where it acts as a paracrine regulator to stimulate the parietal cells to secret hydrochloric acid.

157. a. The zona glomerulosa is involved in the production of mineralocorticoids and is the most superficial layer of the adrenal cortex. The zona fasciculata and reticularis (middle and deepest layers, respectively) produce glucocorticoids, oestrogens and androgens; progestogens are produced as precursors to the synthesis of other hormones.

158. c. Below is a table summarizing the normal temperature of commonly used body areas. These differences are important to bear in mind when taking a temperature reading. In addition, peripheral body sites will vary depending on the degree of peripheral vasoconstriction. The most accurate readings of temperature are taken from the core, and accessible sites are the oesophagus and rectum. Core temperature should be taken when warming a patient from hypothermia. Oral temperature can be reliable, but it is important not to confound the temperature reading by taking it after the imbibitions of hot or cold drinks.

Body site	Normal temperature (°C)
Oral	37
Tympanic	37.5
Axillary	36
Oesophageal	37
Rectal	37

159. c. During an acute phase of injury, the body enters a catabolic phase. The glycogen stores are broken down to increase blood glucose levels. Insulin levels fall as glucose levels rise. The body also releases cortisol in response to stress. Cortisol counteracts insulin and contributes to hyperglycaemia by stimulating gluconeogenesis in the liver. Increased sympathetic activity also mobilizes fat from adipose tissue.

160. c. One percent of total body calcium is free; 99% is stored in bone in the form of hydroxyapatite. Forty percent of free calcium is bound to albumin – the remaining 60% of unbound calcium is the form that is of physiological importance. Acidosis dissolves bone through activation of osteoclasts, releasing ionized calcium into the blood. The normal serum calcium level is 2.2–2.6 mmol/L.

161. c. Angiotensin II produces arteriolar constriction and a rise in systolic and diastolic blood pressure. It acts directly on the adrenal cortex to increase the secretion of aldosterone. Through its effects on the subfornical organ and the organum vasculosum of the lamina terminalis angiotensin II causes an increase in water intake (dipsogenic effect). It also facilitates the release of noradrenaline by a direct action on post-ganglionic sympathetic neurons.

162. e. Vasopressin is secreted by the neurohypophysis. Adrenocorticotropic hormone acts on the zona fasciculate. Growth hormone is produced by the adenohypophysis. Dopamine stimulates prolactin production from the adenohypophysis. Oxytocin initiates parturition and stimulates uterine contraction and milk secretion.

163. e. The renin–angiotensin–aldosterone system involves complex communication between hormones and organs to control the extracellular fluid volume with additional effects on the vascular system and blood pressure. A decrease in blood volume is detected by the juxtaglomerular complex (made up of granular cells and the macula densa), which is found between the afferent arteriole (granular cells) and the thick ascending limb of the loop of Henle (macula densa). The complex releases renin, which converts angiotensinogen into angiotensin I. Angiotensin I is then catalyzed to angiotensin II by the angiotensin-converting enzyme, found mainly in the lungs. Angiotensin II stimulates the zona glomerulosa in the adrenal cortex to secrete aldosterone. Aldosterone then acts in the cortical collecting duct of the kidney to increase Na^+ reabsorption and K^+ excretion. Consequently, Na^+ is retained in the blood and increases blood volume. The macula densa is found within the thick ascending limb of the loop of Henle and is part of the juxtaglomerular complex. When an increased concentration of Na^+ is detected by the macula densa, it inhibits renin secretion from the granular cells.

164. a.   Sodium serum concentration is carefully controlled; however, a number of different conditions can decrease its concentration via different mechanisms. In hypervolaemic hyponatraemia, both the body's sodium and water content increase but the water gain is greater; examples include liver cirrhosis, congestive heart failure and nephrotic syndrome. In euvolaemic hyponatraemia, the total body water increases but the body's sodium concentration remains stable; examples include hypothyroidism, glucocorticoid deficiency and syndrome of inappropriate antidiuretic hormone (SIADH). In hypovolaemic hyponatraemia, both the body's water and sodium content decrease but the sodium loss is greater; examples include prolonged diarrhoea or vomiting, Addison's disease and congenital adrenal hyperplasia.

Hyponatreamia can also be classified by the plasma osmolality. A cause of hypertonic hyponatraemia is mannitol and hyperglycaemia administration. A cause of an isotonic hyponatraemia is tansurethral resection of prostate (TURP) syndrome. A common example of a hypotonic hyponatraemia is diuretic use.

NERVOUS SYSTEM

165. b.   Hemisection of the spinal cord leads to a lesion of the three main neural systems within the spinal cord: the corticospinal tract, dorsal columns and spinothalamic tract. The corticospinal tract carries nerve impulses to the skeletal muscle and the fibres decussate in the medulla. Therefore, a lesion of this tract produces spastic paralysis and hyperreflexia below the level of the lesion on the ipsilateral side. The dorsal column carries fine touch, vibration and proprioception impulses up the ipsilateral side until the medulla where decussation occurs. Therefore, the dorsal column lesion will produce ipsilateral loss of fine touch, vibration and proprioception. The spinothalamic tract carries crude touch, pain and temperature impulses up the contralateral side of the body due to immediate decussation. Therefore, this lesion will lead to loss of pain and temperature sensation on the contralateral side of the body below the level of the lesion.

166. e.   Tissue oedema will occur in relation to inflammation following an operation. Placing a cast or bandage tightly around the area of inflammation may lead to constriction producing similar effects to compartment syndrome. With this patient, the pain originates from the relative hypoxia of the muscle and the nerve compression, in this case the median nerve. The nerve is suffering from a neuropraxia. At this stage, the best management is to split the bandages down to the skin and then elevate the arm. Analgesia can also be given, but a high dose could potentially mask an impending compartment syndrome. A return to theatre should be considered if splitting the bandages, elevating the arm and judicious analgesia do not settle the patient's symptoms. Compartment syndrome can be identified through the use of dedicated pressure monitors, but this can be unreliable and diagnosis remains a clinical one; exquisite pain on a passive stretch of the muscles within the affected compartment is the most sensitive clinical sign.

167. d.   An ulcer within the gastrointestinal tract following head trauma is known as a Cushing's ulcer. The ulcer may occur in relation to other stressful events on the brain such as operations or strokes. The ulcers occur more commonly in the stomach compared to the duodenum and are usually asymptomatic. The precise cause of the ulcer is unknown, but treatment will involve reducing acid production with the use of a proton pump inhibitor. Punched-out ulcers are related to arterial disease in the foot. Curling's ulcer is a stress ulcer related to burns. Marjolin's ulcer is a type of squamous cell carcinoma which develops from a chronic wound. A neuropathic ulcer is caused by localized trauma to the foot (e.g. a stone in a shoe) from a lack of sensitivity caused by diabetes.

168. a.   The gag reflex is stimulated by touching the back of the throat and tongue. The afferent limb is the glossopharyngeal nerve and the efferent limb is the vagus nerve. The afferent limb to different reflexes is supplied by the following nerves:

- Cough reflex – vagus nerve
- Blink reflex – ophthalmic division of the trigeminal nerve
- Sneeze reflex – mandibular division of the trigeminal nerve
- Jaw jerk reflex – maxillary division of the trigeminal nerve

169. d. The fight or flight (or freeze) response is a physiological response to perceived stress actioned by the sympathetic nervous system and hormones. The response is initiated by the amygdala. This leads to the release of Adrenocorticotropic hormone (ACTH) via activation of the hypothalamus and the pituitary gland. ACTH then stimulates the adrenal medulla to release cortisol and catecholamine hormones. The affect is to produce a wide variety of responses which prime the body for violent muscular action. These responses include tachycardia, decreased lacrimation and salivation, sweating, increased peripheral vascular resistance, sphincter relaxation (bladder), decreased gastric motility and mydriasis (pupil dilitation).

170. b. Following such major head trauma, further brain injury must be minimized by preventing hypoxia and hypotension and controlling ventilation to prevent hypercapnia. Although mannitol and anticonvulsant therapy may have a role in the management of head injury, preventing hypoxia/hypotension/hypercapnia is the primary aim as these parameters greatly influence the cerebral perfusion pressure and hence oxygen delivery to the brain.

171. c. The heart is supplied by the autonomic nervous system. Both the sympathetic and parasympathetic supply play an important role in ensuring effective contraction and adequate blood supply to the rest of the body. β_1-Adrenergic receptors predominate the heart and, when stimulated by catecholamines, have a positive inotropic and chronotropic effect on the heart. β_2 Receptors predominate the vascular smooth muscles and when stimulated cause vasoconstriction and increased systemic vascular resistance. β-Adrenergic stimulation enhances Ca^{2+} influx into cardiac myocytes, activating those cells. Parasympathetic supply is mainly to the sinoatrial and atrioventricular nodes via the M_2 muscarinic receptors. Under basal conditions of the body, the parasympathetic nervous system (inhibitory effects) predominantly affects the heart functions, in contrast to the excitatory effects of the sympathetic nervous system. As a result, the heart rate and contractions are just enough for basal metabolic activities.

172. a. Cerebral perfusion pressure (CPP) = mean arterial pressure (MAP) – intracranial pressure (ICP). Rising ICP causes reduced CPP and hence cerebral ischaemia. The resulting response (known as Cushing's reflex) is caused by a combination of autonomic imbalance, hypothalamic overactivity as well as vasomotor ischaemia. Hypothalamic sympathetic stimulation increases cardiac contractility and vasoconstriction, increasing blood pressure. Raised blood pressure is detected by baroreceptors, triggering a vagal response to reduce heart rate. Initially, there may be pupillary constriction owing to a 3rd cranial nerve compression; however, at a later stage there may be pupillary dilatation secondary to coning.

173. a. Conservative management of raised intracranial pressure involves sedation and intubation keeping intracranial pressure (ICP). At 10 mmHg and maintaining Cerebral perfusion pressure (CPP) at 60–70 mmHg. CPP is maintained by a phenomenon called autoregulation. Autoregulation is impaired in head injury patients and CPP <70 mmHg is associated with a poor outcome. Therefore, the priority is to maintain CPP as these patients are susceptible to brain injury caused by hypotension. Cerebral perfusion pressure can be calculated using mean arterial pressure (MAP) and intracranial pressure: CPP = MAP – ICP. MAP is calculated using the formula 1/3 (pulse pressure) + diastolic pressure = MAP.

174. d. Cerebral blood flow accounts for 15% of the cardiac output. The rate of flow remains fundamentally constant due to local autoregulation, of which there are two basic mechanisms:

- Vasodilator 'washout'
- Myogenic response

Hypoxia produces cerebral vasodilatation. Cerebral perfusion pressure is the difference between mean arterial pressure and intracranial pressure – for adequate perfusion it must remain above 70 mmHg. Hypercarbia produces cerebral vasodilatation.

175. c. The volume of cerebrospinal fluid (CSF) is 150 mL. It is produced at a rate of 500 mL/day. CSF is produced by the choroid plexus and blood vessels lining ventricular walls; the order of flow is as follows:

- Lateral ventricle
- Foramen of Monro
- 3rd ventricle
- Aqueduct of Sylvius
- 4th ventricle
- Foramen of Monro and two lateral foramen of Luschka
- Subarachnoid space
- Foramen magnum
- Arachnoid villi (CSF absorption)

176. d. Resting membrane potential is maintained between –70 and –95 mV for different types of cells by the prevention of the free movement of certain types of ions. Potassium ions at rest have almost free permeability, while the movement of all other ions is restricted to gated channels. At a temperature of 37°C, with intracellular potassium concentrations of about 170 mmol/L and extracellular potassium concentrations of about 5 mmol/L, the resting membrane potential is about –70 mV (negative inside). This potential difference is maintained by the Na^+/K^+ ATPase pump, and the repulsion of negative ions from the outside of the membrane because of the high intracellular negative charge on protein molecules. During an action potential, the voltage-gated sodium channels are open, causing a large influx of sodium ions neutralizing the resting membrane potential.

177. e. Axons have a resting membrane potential of between –70 and –95 mV. The initial depolarization is caused by a rapid influx of sodium ions, raising the membrane potential to +40 mV. This leads to the opening of voltage-gated potassium channels allowing potassium to flow down a concentration gradient and the membrane repolarizes. Myelinated fibres have a conduction velocity of 50–100 m/s compared to 1 m/s for unmyelinated fibres. Large α motor fibres have a diameter of 15–20 μm, compared to 0.5–1 μm for the smaller unmyelinated fibres.

178. d. Action potentials allow nerves to transmit information and the electrical signals are described as 'all or none'. Nerve axons have a resting potential of about –70 mV, caused by the relative concentration of extracellular Na^+ and intracellular K^+ across the membrane. The resting potential is maintained by the constant activity of Na^+/K^+ pumps, which transport out three Na^+ for every two K^+ they bring in. Once a sufficient stimulus decreases the membrane potential over the 'threshold', (approximately = 55 mV) the axon depolarizes. The action potential results from an explosive increase in Na^+ permeability and causes a rapid (a few tenths of a millisecond) reversal of the membrane potential to around +40 mV. After a short delay the voltage-gated K^+ channels open and K^+ rapidly (but relatively more slowly compared with the speed of the Na^+ movement) leaves the cell. After depolarization, the cell repolarizes to return the cell membrane potential to normal.

179. e. Brainstem reflexes are absent:

- Pupils are fixed
- No corneal reflex
- Absent vestibulo-ocular reflex
- No motor response
- Absent gag reflex
- Absent respiratory movements once disconnected from the mechanical ventilator

Medical criteria:

- No sedation
- No muscle relaxants
- Normothermic
- Normal electrolyte levels
- Normoglycaemic

180. b. The brain receives approximately 10–15% of the cardiac output. Cerebral blood flow is controlled by three mechanisms: myogenic, neural and local. Autoregulation maintains the cerebral perfusion pressure between 60 and 160 mmHg. Myogenic autoregulation can be impaired by hypoxia, ischaemia, trauma, tumour and infection. The cerebral circulation receives sympathetic vasoconstrictor and parasympathetic vasodilator innervations. Increases in PCO_2 are associated with an increase in cerebral blood flow due to marked cerebral vasodilatation with a fall leading to vasoconstriction. Increases in PO_2 can cause a mild cerebral vasoconstriction.

181. d. When the spinal cord is suddenly transected in the upper neck owing to trauma, all cord functions immediately become depressed and sometimes absent (spinal shock). At the onset of spinal shock, the arterial blood pressure falls instantly, sometimes to as low as 40 mmHg. The pressure ordinarily returns to normal within a few days. All skeletal muscle reflexes integrated in the spinal cord are blocked during the initial stages of shock. However, some reflexes may be hyperexcitable, particularly if a few facilitatory pathways remain intact between the brain and the cord while the remainder of the spinal cord is transected.

182. d. The tight junctions between capillary endothelial cells in the brain, and between the epithelial cells in the choroid plexus, effectively prevent proteins from entering the brain in adults and slow the penetration of smaller molecules. This uniquely limited exchange of substances into the brain is referred to as the blood–brain barrier. Water, CO_2 and O_2 penetrate the brain with ease, whereas proteins and polypeptides do not. The neurons are dependent on the concentrations of K^+, Ca^{2+}, Mg^{2+}, H^+ and other ions in the fluid bathing them. Even minor variations have far-reaching consequences. Hence the blood–brain barrier helps maintain the normal milieu.

183. e. Cerebrospinal fluid lies in the subarachnoid space. The total volume is 130–150 mL with a daily rate of production of 500 mL. The fluid is produced by the choroid plexus in the lateral, third and fourth ventricles. The fluid flows from the lateral ventricles to the third ventricle via the interventricular foramina, then to the fourth ventricle through the cerebral aqueduct. From here the fluid flows into the subarachnoid space via the foramen of Luschka and Magendie. The normal cerebrospinal fluid pressure is approximately 0.5–1.0 kPa.

184. d. There are two major types of glial cells in the nervous system: microglia and macroglia. Microglia are scavenger cells that resemble tissue macrophages and carry out phagocytosis. Three main types of macroglia are oligodendrocytes, Schwann cells and astrocytes. Oligodendrocytes and Schwann cells are involved in myelin formation around axons in the central nervous system and peripheral nervous system, respectively. Astrocytes are the most common type of macroglial cell in the central nervous system. They have a support function, holding the multitude of nerves together, but their role also involves maintaining the brain's internal environment and managing the blood–brain barrier.

185. a. Pre-ganglionic fibres are myelinated and are located in the lateral horns of the spinal grey matter (i.e. a thoracolumbar distribution – T1 to L2); a large diameter results in a more rapid transmission of action potential. In summary, pre-ganglionic cells of both the sympathetic and parasympathetic nervous systems secrete acetylcholine (ACh) (acting on nicotinic receptors); post-ganglionic cells differ between the two systems, in that noradrenaline is the neurotransmitter for the sympathetic nervous system (SNS) (acting on α and β receptors) and ACh is for the parasympathetic nervous system (acting on muscarinic receptors). The adrenal medulla is composed of chromaffin cells, which receive direct innervation from pre-ganglionic sympathetic fibres; stimulation results in catecholamine release – in this sense, the chromaffin cells are comparable to post-ganglionic cells of the SNS.

186. c. A motor unit is defined as a motor neuron and all the muscle fibres that it innervates. As a muscle is stimulated, graded contractions of whole muscles are made possible by variations in the number of motor units activated. Not all motor units are of the same size, and some muscles have a variety of innervation ratios (the number of muscle fibres per motor neuron). For example, the extraocular muscles have approximately 23 motor units per neuron, whereas the gastrocnemius has a range of 100:1 to 2000:1. This difference in motor units indicates the level of muscle control possible, with finer control offered with a lower innervation ratio. During muscle contractions of gradual increasing strength, larger motor units are sequentially activated in a process known as recruitment.

187. a. The endoneurium surrounds the peripheral nerve and is composed of collagen-containing capillaries and lymphatics. This layer protects from stretching forces. The perineurium is made up of dense connective tissue forming a strong mechanical barrier. The diffusion layer protects the nerve fibre from large ionic fluxes. The epineurium is the most peripheral layer, functioning to join fascicles together to form a thick protective coat. This can form the majority of the cross-sectional area of the nerve comprising a higher proportion over joints. Panneurium and transneurium are not layers of the peripheral nerves.

188. d. Her Glasgow Coma Scale (GCS) is 8: she scores 4 for motor responsiveness (withdrawing to pain), 2 for eyes (only opening to pain) and 2 for voice (for making noises to pain). The GCS offers a reliable, reproducible quantitative assessment of a patient's level of consciousness. It is measured on three scales, with the lowest possible score being 3 and the highest 15.

Eye opening

- 4 – spontaneously
- 3 – to speech
- 2 – to pain
- 1 – not at all

Motor response

- 6 – obeys commands
- 5 – localizes pain
- 4 – withdraws from pain
- 3 – abnormal flexion to pain
- 2 – extension to pain
- 1 – no response

Verbal response

- 5 – orientated
- 4 – confused conversation
- 3 – inappropriate words
- 2 – incomprehensible sounds
- 1 – no verbalization

189. b. GCS:

Eye opening

- 4 – spontaneously
- 3 – to speech
- 2 – to pain
- 1 – not at all

Motor response

- 6 – obeys commands
- 5 – localizes pain
- 4 – withdraws from pain
- 3 – abnormal flexion to pain
- 2 – extension to pain
- 1 – no response

Verbal response

- 5 – orientated
- 4 – confused conversation
- 3 – inappropriate words
- 2 – incomprehensible sounds
- 1 – no verbalization

190. c. Nerve fibres are divided into types A and C. Type A fibres are further subdivided into α, β, γ and δ fibres. Type C fibres are the small unmyelinated nerve fibres that conduct impulses at low velocities. The C fibres constitute more than one-half of the sensory fibres in most peripheral nerves as well as all the post-ganglionic autonomic fibres.

THYROID AND PARATHYROID

191. d.   Synthesis of thyroid hormones includes trapping of iodide absorbed from the plasma by the iodide pump against its electrical gradient. Iodide is converted to iodine by the enzyme thyroid peroxidase. Iodine is secreted into the colloid where iodine is added onto tyrosine by the enzyme iodinase. Thyroid-stimulating hormone (TSH) causes the substance to be transported back into the thyroid follicular cell. T_3 and T_4 are released by proteolysis. Both T_3 and T_4 are secreted into the bloodstream with T_4 in higher concentration. Approximately 99% of T_3 and T_4 is bound to proteins such as thyroid-binding protein and albumin.

192. b.   The widespread effects of thyroid hormones in the body are secondary to stimulation of O_2 consumption (calorigenic action). They have a catabolic effect on muscle tissue, increasing protein breakdown. They also help regulate lipid metabolism and increase the absorption of carbohydrates from the intestine.

193. e.   The thyroid gland produces three hormones:

1. Tetraiodothyronine (T4/thyroxine): The principle hormone
2. Triiodothyronine (T3): Shorter duration, but more potent than T_4
3. Calcitonin: Produced by parafollicular C-cells; involved in calcium balance

The steps in the production of T_4 and T_3 can be summarized as follows:

- An active pump concentrates iodine into the thyroid follicular cells.
- Iodine is oxidized into its active form (by peroxidase).
- Iodine binds with tyrosine, to form tyrosyl units (organification).
- Tyrosyl units bind to a protein core, to form thyroglobulin.
- Tyrosyl units combine while bound to the protein core to form either T_3 or T_4.
- Thyroglobulin molecules are stored as colloid in follicles.
- TSH stimulates the release of T_3 and T_4 into the blood.

194. a.   This is a tricky question – while the actions of parathyroid hormone (PTH) are to increase calcium reabsorption from the distal renal tubule and to increase phosphate excretion from the proximal tubule, one may expect that hyperparathyroidism would result in increased renal calcium reabsorption. In actual fact, the plasma concentration of calcium often overwhelms the renal tubules, and calcium excretion is actually increased. PTH acts on bone to cause calcium resorption (i.e. liberation of calcium into the bloodstream through the action of osteoclasts). PTH indirectly increases calcium absorption in the gut, by increasing the formation of vitamin D.

195. d.   Large doses of thyroid hormones result in decreased peripheral resistance; the slight raise in core body temperature results in peripheral vasodilation as a homeostatic compensatory mechanism. Hypothyroid patients are found to have elevated cerebral spinal fluid protein levels; however, as with hyperthyroidism, cerebral blood flow, oxygen extraction and glucose concentrations are normal. Thyroid hormones result in increased formation of hepatic low-density lipoprotein (LDL) receptors, which results in increased hepatic removal of cholesterol from the circulation.

196. e.   Thyroid receptors (TRs) are intranuclear; hormone–receptor complexes subsequently bind to Deoxyribonucleic acid (DNA) via zinc fingers, leading to increased/decreased expression of various genes. TRβ2 is found solely in the brain. TRα2 and TRβ1 are widely distributed throughout the body. The TRα2 is unable to bind T_3. T_3 is more potent (approximately three to five times) and has a more rapid mode of action than T_4.

197. b.   Osteoclasts are large phagocytic, multinucleated cells (as many as 50 nuclei), derivatives of monocytes or monocyte-like cells formed in the bone marrow. The osteoclasts are normally active on less than 1% of the bone surfaces of an adult. Factors that inhibit osteoclasts are calcitonin, oestrogen and prostaglandin (PGE2). Only corticosteroids inhibit osteoblasts. Parathyroid excess leads to loss of calcium from bone by activating osteoclasts.

198. c.   Parathyroid glands produce parathyroid hormone (PTH), which acts to increase calcium levels. It is released from chief cells from within the gland. PTH acts in the bone, gut and kidney via cell surface receptors resulting in an increase in cyclic Adenosine monophosphate (AMP) production. This causes an overall increase in calcium and decreased serum phosphate in response to low calcium levels. PTH increases bone resorption by stimulating osteoclastic activity.

199. b.   Primary hyperparathyroidism is where there is excessive parathyroid hormone production by the parathyroid glands, usually owing to an adenoma or hyperplasia of the gland. Biochemistry shows a raised parathyroid hormone level resulting in raised calcium, low phosphate, mild acidosis, normal vitamin D levels and raised 24 h urinary calcium secretion.

200. d.   Secondary hyperparathyroidism has excessive parathyroid hormone (PTH) in response to a low calcium, for example in renal failure and malabsorption. Typical biochemistry includes normal or low calcium, high PTH and high phosphate. Increased bone resorption by the stimulation of osteoclasts occurs because of a reduction in 1,25-dihydroxy-vitamin D synthesis and reduced calcium reabsorption.

201. a.   Tertiary hyperparathyroidism is usually caused by a chronic overstimulation of the parathyroid gland causing a hypersecreting adenoma. This results in a high parathyroid hormone (PTH) level, raised calcium with symptoms of hypercalcaemia and increased bone resorption.

202. a.   Calcitonin is produced by the parafollicular thyroid C-cells and acts to reduce the level of serum calcium. Calcitonin levels rise when serum calcium levels are high and acts to inhibit osteoclastic bone resorption and increase renal excretion of calcium and phosphate.

203. b.   Calcitonin is a 32–amino acid protein, with a molecular weight of 3500. Plasma calcitonin levels are directly proportionate to calcium levels; other factors that increase calcitonin secretion include:

- β adrenergic agonists
- Glucagon
- Gastrin

- Cholecystokinin
- Oestrogens

Gastrin is elevated in pernicious anaemia and Zollinger–Ellison syndrome, in which calcitonin levels are elevated accordingly. The half-life of calcitonin is less than 10 min.

204. b. Thyroid stimulation hormone (TSH), also known as thyrotropin, is an anterior pituitary hormone. TSH increases all the known secretory activities of the thyroid glandular cells. It increases the rate of 'iodide trapping' in the glandular cells through increased activity of the iodide pump. The most important early effect after administration of TSH is to initiate proteolysis of thyroglobulin, which causes the release of thyroxine and triiodothyronine into the blood within 30 min. The other effects require hours or even days and weeks to develop fully.

205. d. Hypocalcaemia may be characterized by tetany, circumoral numbness and a prolonged QT interval on an electrocardiogram. Chvostek's sign is positive when there is contraction of the facial muscles by tapping near the angle of the jaw, whereas Trousseau's sign is abnormal wrist flexion and fingers drawn together in extension after a blood pressure cuff is inflated on the arm for 3 min.

206. d. Calcium is regulated by two hormones, parathyroid hormone (PTH) and calcitonin. PTH is produced in the parathyroid glands and acts to increase serum calcium levels. Calcitonin is secreted by C-cells within the thyroid gland and acts to reduce calcium levels. Clinically raised calcium levels can cause several features; however, tetany is usually caused by hypocalcaemia. Low calcium levels increase the permeability of neuronal membranes to sodium, increasing the ease with which action potentials are initiated, causing involuntary contraction of muscles.

207. c. Low calcium levels stimulate parathyroid hormone (PTH) production. PTH increases serum calcium concentration by indirectly increasing osteoclastic activity. This raises the level of bone resorption. It also increases calcium reabsorption from the distal tubules and thick ascending limb of the kidney, while also reducing phosphate reabsorption from the proximal tubule. PTH upregulates enzymatic 1-hydroxylation of 25-hydroxy vitamin D, increasing intestinal absorption of calcium.

208. a. The clinical features of hypercalcaemia include 'stones, bones, abdominal groans and psychic moans' (renal stones, bone pain, abdominal pain and psychosis). Hyperparathyroidism and malignancy account for about 90% of all cases and other causes are listed below:

Abnormal parathyroid function

- Primary hyperparathyroidism – adenoma, hyperplasia, carcinoma, multiple endocrine neoplasia (MEN) syndrome
- Lithium use

Malignancy

- Solid tumours – breast, lung, squamous cell carcinoma
- Haematological – multiple myeloma, lymphoma, leukaemia

Vitamin D disorders

- Hypervitaminosis D

High bone turnover

- Hyperthyroidism
- Thiazide diuretics
- Paget's disease

Renal failure

- Severe secondary hyperparathyroidism
- Milk alkali syndrome

Pancreatitis is a known cause of hypocalcaemia.

209. e. Following surgery or trauma, circulating levels of T_3 and T_4 drop and are inversely related to the increased sympathetic activity; the levels usually normalize over a few days.

210. b. Many clinically unwell patients, particularly after major trauma or surgery, have deranged thyroid function tests. Sick euthyroid syndrome is characterized by a clinically euthyroid patient with low T_3 levels, normal T_4 and thyroid stimulating hormone (TSH). TSH levels may be slightly higher than the normal range but are usually not as elevated as patients who are hypothyroid. These patients do not require thyroid hormone supplementation.

211. e. A significant interaction exists between levothyroxine, iron, calcium, proton pump inhibitors, statins and oestrogen. Glucocorticoids and histamine receptor antagonists have been found to have no effect.

212. d. The parathyroid gland contains two types of cell: oxyphil and chief cells. The chief cells are responsible for parathyroid hormone production. No specific function has been found for the oxyphil cells. The parafollicular cells produce calcitonin with the follicular cells producing thyroid hormones.

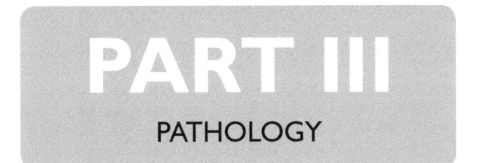

PART III

PATHOLOGY

CHAPTER 5
PATHOLOGY

Questions

INFLAMMATION

1. A patient presents to the colorectal clinic with a perianal abscess. Which of the following statements regarding abscesses is false?
   a. Abscesses only occur in patients with poor personal hygiene.
   b. Small abscesses can sometimes be treated with antibiotics on their own.
   c. Prompt management is required in diabetic patients.
   d. Abscesses are usually painful.
   e. Abscesses can cause septicaemia if treated incorrectly.

2. A 36-year-old male presents to the surgical team with a purulent discharge from the natal cleft. On examination, there is no evidence of any localized collection in the natal cleft; however, there are several pits visible. Which of the following statements defines a sinus?
   a. A blind ending tract
   b. An abnormal connection between two epithelial surfaces
   c. A physiological connection between two epithelial surfaces
   d. A collection of pus
   e. A membranous cavity containing fluid

3. Which of the following forms of necrosis is characteristic of tuberculosis?
   a. Coagulative
   b. Caseous
   c. Colliquative
   d. Gangrenous
   e. Fibrinoid

4. All of the following are free radicals except:
   a. Superoxide
   b. Hydrogen peroxide
   c. Hydrogen chloride
   d. Hydroxyl ions
   e. Nitric oxide

5. Acute inflammation caused by the contraction of the endothelial cell cytoskeleton associated with acute inflammation results in which of the following?
   a. Delayed transient increase in permeability
   b. Early transient increase in permeability
   c. Delayed permanent increase in permeability
   d. Early permanent increase in permeability
   e. None of the above

6. Concerning inflammation, which of the following statements is correct?
   a. The predominant cell involved in acute inflammation is the lymphocyte.
   b. IL-2 causes pyrexia.
   c. There is a decrease in capillary permeability in the acute phases.
   d. Complement is a component of the innate immune system.
   e. Fibrin is converted to fibrinogen, which forms a fibrinous meshwork, limiting the spread of pathogens.

7. Which of the following are the main cells involved in chronic inflammation?
   a. Macrophages
   b. Eosinophils
   c. Neutrophils
   d. Plasma cells
   e. Basophils

8. Which of the following chemical messengers of acute inflammation is correctly paired with its role?
   a. Interleukin-1 – differentiation of B-cells
   b. Interferon – activation of macrophages and natural killer cells
   c. Tumour necrosis factor – vasodilatation
   d. Histamine – fever
   e. Interleukin-2 – neutrophil adhesion

9. All of the following are chemical mediators of inflammation except:
   a. Histamine
   b. Prostaglandins
   c. Chemokines
   d. 5-Hydroxytryptamine
   e. Telomerase

10. All of the following features are noted in an acute inflammation except:
    a. Redness
    b. Swelling
    c. Pain
    d. Loss of function
    e. Calcification

11. Which of the following is true regarding reversible cell injury under light microscope?
    a. Cellular swelling is present.
    b. Fatty change of cells.
    c. Amorphous densities are present in the mitochondria.

   d. Both a and b.

   e. None of the above.

12. A 37-year-old male is recovering well after an omental patch repair for a perforated duodenal ulcer. On day 9 the patient presents with a swinging pyrexia, feeling generally unwell, with nausea and pain felt across his upper abdomen. On further questioning he is poor at localizing the pain, but reports pain in his right shoulder tip. Which of the following is the most likely diagnosis?

   a. Gallstones

   b. Chest infection

   c. Pelvic abscess

   d. Subphrenic abscess

   e. Perforated gallbladder

CELLULAR INJURY OTHER THAN BY INFECTION

13. A 23-year-old female was rescued from a house fire 5 days ago, from which she suffered 27% third-degree burns. Which of the following types of ulcers is usually associated with major burns?
    a. Cushing ulcer
    b. Curling ulcer
    c. Marjolin ulcer
    d. Venous ulcer
    e. Arterial ulcer

14. Morphological changes of irreversible cell injury include which of the following?
    a. Amorphous densities in mitochondria
    b. Swelling of the cell membrane
    c. Disruption of lysosomes
    d. All of the above
    e. b and c only

15. All eukaryotic cells have membrane-bound organelles. Which one of the following organelles is self-replicating?
    a. Golgi body
    b. Mitochondrion
    c. Smooth endoplasmic reticulum
    d. Rough endoplasmic reticulum
    e. Lysosome

16. Which one of the following pigments is associated with ageing cells?
    a. Melatonin
    b. Lipofuscin
    c. Melanin
    d. Eosin
    e. Reticulin

17. A young man presents to the accident and emergency department with a gunshot wound to the abdomen. Which of the following statements is false regarding gunshot wounds?
    a. The injury is dependent on the relationship between kinetic energy, mass and velocity.
    b. There may be high- or low-velocity wounds.
    c. Different bullets may cause different injuries.
    d. Exit wounds normally have a well-defined appearance.
    e. High-velocity projectiles induce cavities of approximately 30 times their size.

WOUNDS AND WOUND HEALING

18. An 82-year-old male sustains a Colles fracture following a fall onto an outstretched hand. Regarding bone healing at a fracture site, the following statements are true except:
    a. A haematoma usually forms at the fracture site.
    b. Osteoblasts form a callus.
    c. Lamella bone is replaced by woven bone.
    d. Interposition of soft tissue may affect bone healing.
    e. An internal callus is found in the medullary cavity of the bone.

19. A 57-year-old male undergoes an elective laparoscopic cholecystectomy for chronic cholecystitis. He is reviewed in clinic 4 weeks later and has made an excellent recovery. His wounds are healing well. All of the following statements regarding wound healing are true except:
    a. Hypertrophic scars extend beyond the original wound.
    b. Type III collagen predominates during the early stages of wound healing.
    c. It is affected by the use of steroids.
    d. Macrophages play a key role.
    e. Type I collagen is stronger than type III.

20. A 67-year-old male presents to the emergency department with abdominal pain and sepsis. There is clinical and radiological evidence of a sigmoid perforation; therefore an emergency Hartmann's procedure is performed. The consultant asks you to close the abdomen. Which of the following statements regarding concepts relating to mass closure of the abdominal wall with a continuous suture is incorrect?
    a. The length of suture should be four times the length of the incision.
    b. Sutures should be placed 1 cm apart.
    c. Sutures should be placed 1 cm from the wound edge.
    d. The assistant should ensure that the sutures are tight.
    e. Delayed closure can be performed if intra-abdominal contents cannot be reduced.

21. A 50-year-old victim of a road traffic incident is brought into the accident and emergency department on a spinal board. Due to multiple other trauma cases attending the department, you are on your own when assessing this patient. Which of the following injuries to your patient should receive attention first?
    a. Open fracture of hand and wrist
    b. Open abdominal wound with slight haemorrhage
    c. Massive orofacial trauma
    d. Tension pneumothorax
    e. Cardiac tamponade

22. Which one of the following statements regarding wound healing is correct?
    a. In secondary intention the wound edges are closely apposed.
    b. A wound with extensive tissue loss heals by secondary intention.
    c. In primary intention, the wound fills with granulation tissue.

    d. There is increased risk of scarring with primary intention.

    e. Contraction of myofibroblasts in granulation tissue causes an increase in the size of the wound.

23. Which one of the following statements regarding keloid scars is correct?
    a. They are less common in pigmented skin.
    b. They extend beyond the previous borders of the wound.
    c. Re-excision reduces the risk of recurrence.
    d. They occur more commonly on the extensor surfaces.
    e. Steroid injections have no effect on cosmesis.

24. A 50-year-old man is seen 5 days post-laparotomy for a perforated segment of small bowel with significant contamination. The wound was left open to heal by secondary intention. Wound review reveals granulation tissue and wound contraction. At which of the four stages of wound healing is he currently at?
    a. Coagulative
    b. Exudative
    c. Inflammatory
    d. Remodelling
    e. Proliferative

25. A 45-year-old obese man with diabetes has a periumbilical hernia repair. Ten days after the operation you check the wound and notice that the left lateral third has not healed. The wound is discharging fluid and you see a stitch protruding from the wound. Which of the following factors is likely to have lead to his poor wound healing?
    a. Obesity
    b. Diabetes
    c. Local infection
    d. All of the above
    e. b and c only

VASCULAR DISORDERS

26. A 32-year-old female is admitted under the surgical team with a diagnosis of alcohol-induced pancreatitis. She remains haemodynamically unstable despite aggressive resuscitation, and she is therefore transferred immediately to the intensive care unit. To optimize her management, a central line is required. Which of the following is not a recognized immediate complication of central line insertion?
    a. Haemothorax
    b. Chylothorax
    c. Cardiac tamponade
    d. Infection
    e. Arrhythmias

27. A middle-aged man presents to the hospital with severe chest pain. He is clinically shocked with asymmetrical pulses and blood pressure in the upper limbs. An initial chest X-ray shows a widened mediastinum. Which of the following is not a recognized predisposing factor for aortic dissection?
    a. Marfan syndrome
    b. Pregnancy
    c. Mitral valve prolapse
    d. Bicuspid aortic valve
    e. Pseudoxanthoma elasticum

28. Lymphoedema is an accumulation of tissue fluid as a result of dysfunction of the lymphatic system. Which one of the following statements regarding primary lymphoedema is incorrect?
    a. Primary lymphoedema can be congenital.
    b. Primary lymphoedema can be defined as praecox.
    c. Primary lymphoedema can be defined as tarda.
    d. Milroy disease is an example of primary lymphoedema.
    e. It is always characterized by pitting oedema.

29. An 80-year-old female smoker presents to the vascular clinic with a short history of leg ulceration. Following a focused history and examination, you conclude that these are likely to be arterial ulcers. Which of the following comments regarding arterial ulcers is correct?
    a. They are typically punched-out lesions.
    b. There is a normal capillary refill on examination.
    c. They have a sloping edge.
    d. They are often found in the gaiter area.
    e. They are usually painless.

30. A 53-year-old insulin-dependent diabetic male is referred to the clinic by his general practitioner with persistent diabetic ulcers. Which of the following statements regarding diabetic ulcers is correct?
    a. They are found in the gaiter area.
    b. They typically have reduced capillary refill.
    c. They commonly have reduced or absent peripheral pulses.

d. They are painless.

e. They are associated with lipodermatosclerosis and haemosiderin deposits.

31. Risk factors for deep vein thrombosis (DVT) include all but which one of the following?

a. Increasing age

b. Female

c. Malignancy

d. Thrombocytopenia

e. Protein C deficiency

32. A 28-year-old man presents to your clinic with bilateral calf pain, which is exacerbated by walking over the past few months. His claudication distance is now only 100 m. He has no personal or family history of diabetes or ischaemic heart disease. He is a builder by trade, smokes 30 cigarettes a day and drinks minimal alcohol. On examination you find his foot pulses weak, but present, and the feet are cool. You also note that there is a small painful ulcer developing over the distal aspect of his great toe on the right. Which one of the following is the correct diagnosis?

a. Kawasaki disease

b. Buerger disease

c. Takayasu disease

d. Giant cell arteritis

e. Atherosclerosis

33. Which of the following is not a common cause of transudate ascites?

a. Budd–Chiari syndrome

b. Thoracic duct obstruction

c. Pseudomyxoma

d. Hypothyroidism

e. Protein losing enteropathy

34. Which of the following is not a form of acquired aneurysm?

a. Mycotic aneurysm

b. Arteriovenous aneurysm

c. Atheromatous aneurysm

d. Berry aneurysm

e. Dissecting aneurysm

35. A 72-year-old man day 4 post left hemicolectomy develops a low-grade pyrexia of 37.7°C, is tachycardic with a pulse rate of 107 bpm and has a respiratory rate of 24 with oxygen saturations of 88%. His electrocardiogram (ECG) shows sinus tachycardia with a right bundle branch block. Which one of the following is the most likely diagnosis in this presentation?

a. Pulmonary embolism (PE)

b. Anxiety

c. Urinary tract infection

d. Wound infection

e. Pain

DISORDERS OF GROWTH, DIFFERENTIATION AND MORPHOGENESIS

36. Stratified squamous epithelium can be found in which of the following structures?
    a. Epididymis
    b. Colon
    c. Trachea
    d. Cornea
    e. Uterus

37. A 47-year-old male undergoes a colonoscopy and polypectomy. The pathology report describes the polyp as being dysplastic. Regarding dysplasia, the following statements are true except:
    a. It is a potentially premalignant condition.
    b. It is characterized by increased mitotic activity.
    c. It is an irreversible condition.
    d. There is a high nuclear–cytoplasmic ratio.
    e. There is decreased cellular differentiation.

38. Which one of the following statements is a definition of metaplasia?
    a. It is an increase in the size and number of cells.
    b. It is an increase in the size of cells.
    c. It is a decrease in the number of cells.
    d. It is a reversible transformation of one type of terminally differentiated cell into another fully differentiated cell type.
    e. It is an irreversible transformation of one type of terminally differentiated cell into another fully differentiated cell type.

39. Which one of the following pigments is associated with ageing cells?
    a. Melatonin
    b. Lipofuscin
    c. Melanin
    d. Eosin
    e. Reticulin

40. A 69-year-old male is referred to the surgical team with a gangrenous left leg. Which one of the following statements regarding gangrene is correct?
    a. Wet gangrene usually has a low number of organisms compared with dry gangrene.
    b. Wet gangrene occurs when both venous and arterial obstruction are present.
    c. Putrefaction is more severe in dry gangrene than wet gangrene.
    d. Pulses are usually absent in diabetic gangrene.
    e. Dry gangrene is a primary infection of healthy tissue characterized by *Clostridium perfringes*.

41. Which of the following statements concerning metabolic diseases of the liver is correct?
    a. Haemochromatosis is caused by a mutation on chromosome 15.
    b. Haemochromatosis commonly affects the kidneys, lungs and liver.
    c. Heterozygotes with α1-antitrypsin deficiency are often severely affected.
    d. Wilson's disease is an autosomal dominant condition.
    e. Wilson's disease is caused by a mutation on chromosome 13.

42. Which of the following syndromes is not correctly matched with the affected gene?
    a. Von Hippel–Lindau – VHL
    b. Multiple endocrine neoplasia (MEN) – RET
    c. Familial polyposis coli – APC
    d. Retinoblastoma – Rb1
    e. Li–Fraumeni – BRCA1

43. Which of the following teratogens is incorrectly paired with its effect?
    a. Folic acid – heart defects
    b. Rubella – microphthalmia
    c. Warfarin – facial abnormalities
    d. Alcohol – microcephaly, abnormal facies
    e. Thalidomide – rudimentary limbs, heart, kidney abnormalities

44. The following chromosomal abnormalities are autosomal dominant except:
    a. α_1-Antitrypsin deficiency
    b. Polycystic kidney disease
    c. Achondroplasia
    d. Marfan syndrome
    e. Hereditary spherocytosis

45. Concerning blastomas, which of the following statements is correct?
    a. A high cytoplasm–nucleus ratio is characteristic.
    b. Hypochromatic nuclei are characteristic.
    c. Metastasis is rare.
    d. Both alleles of the Rb gene must be abnormal within a cell for it to continually proliferate into a retinoblastoma.
    e. They most often occur in the elderly.

46. Concerning Down syndrome, which of the following statements is correct?
    a. Translocation accounts for the majority of cases.
    b. Mosaicism accounts for the majority of cases.
    c. Non-disjunction typically occurs in mothers under 40 years old.
    d. All cells have trisomy 21 in mosaicism.
    e. All cells have trisomy 21 in non-disjunction.

47. Which of the following is not an example of a pathological giant cell?
    a. Oocyte
    b. Warthin–Finkeldy cell

   c. Reed–Sternberg cell
   d. Skeletal muscle cell
   e. Osteoblast

48. Concerning cell damage, which of the following statements is correct?
   a. Infarction is an abnormal reduction in blood supply or drainage to a tissue.
   b. Failure of the cellular sodium/potassium ATPase channel occurs early in ischaemic cell injury.
   c. Ischaemic injury becomes irreversible for neurons after 1–2 h.
   d. There is preservation of tissue architecture in caseous necrosis.
   e. Heterolysis refers to cell degradation by intracellular enzymes.

49. A 65-year-old male presents to the surgical department with lower abdominal pain. He states that he has recently been diagnosed with amyloidosis. Which of the following statements regarding amyloid deposition is correct?
   a. The P protein is the variable component of amyloid.
   b. Localized amyloidosis can be seen with papillary carcinoma of the thyroid.
   c. Amyloidosis associated with chronic inflammation consists of amyloid light-chain (AL) protein as the variable component.
   d. Amyloid fibrils are arranged in B pleats.
   e. Amyloid stains green with Lugol's iodine solution.

50. Which of the following statements about apoptosis is incorrect?
   a. Induction of apoptosis involves either physiological or pathological stimuli.
   b. No inflammatory response is initiated.
   c. Cell shrinkage and fragmentation occur.
   d. Cell membrane integrity is lost.
   e. The dead cells are phagocytosed by neighbouring cells.

51. Which one of the following is a type of apoptosis?
   a. Histoplasmic
   b. Cytotoxic
   c. Morphogenetic
   d. Hypertrophic
   e. Kinetic

52. Which of the following statements is correct regarding apoptotic bodies?
   a. They are called Civatte bodies in lichen planus.
   b. In melanocytic lesions they present as Kamino bodies.
   c. Councilman bodies are associated with acute viral hepatitis.
   d. All of the above.
   e. a and b only.

53. The following statements regarding growth are true except:
   a. Hyperplasia is reversible when the stimulus is removed.
   b. Hyperplasia of the bone marrow occurs at high altitude.

c. Myocardial hypertrophy is an example of pathological hypertrophy.
d. Hypertrophy is irreversible even after the stimulus is removed.
e. Hypertrophy is an increase in cell size without cell replication.

54. Which of the following statements is true regarding necrosis?
   a. Necrosis and apoptosis are essentially the same process.
   b. Coagulative, colliquative and fat are all different types of necrosis.
   c. Gangrene is not necrosis.
   d. Fibrinoid necrosis is the most common form.
   e. Coagulation necrosis is induced by the action of lipases that catalyze decomposition of triglycerides to fatty acids.

NEOPLASIA

55. Concerning the stages of the cell cycle, the following are true except:
    a. G1: Gap phase, following completion of mitosis
    b. S: DNA synthesis
    c. M: Nuclear and cytoplasmic division
    d. G0: Mitotic phase
    e. G2: Premitotic phase

56. The following conditions have a potential for malignancy except:
    a. Basal cell naevus syndrome
    b. Actinic keratosis
    c. Necrobiosis lipoidica
    d. Peutz–Jeghers syndrome
    e. Balanitis xerotica obliterans

57. Which one of the following is the incorrect association of an oncogenic virus?
    a. Human papilloma virus and cervical cancer
    b. Epstein–Barr virus and Burkitt lymphoma
    c. Herpes virus and lung carcinoma
    d. Hepatitis B virus and hepatocellular carcinoma
    e. Human T-lymphotropic virus-1 and leukaemia

58. Which of the following is an example of a malignant tumour of skeletal muscle (mesenchymal) origin?
    a. Osteoma
    b. Rhabdomyosarcoma
    c. Leiomyosarcoma
    d. Lipoma
    e. Adenoma

59. Which chemical carcinogen is commonly associated with the oesophagus and stomach?
    a. Aromatic amines
    b. Vinyl chloride
    c. Nitrosamine
    d. All of the above
    e. None of the above

60. A 25-year-old female presents to the breast clinic with a 2 cm mobile lump in the upper outer quadrant of the left breast. The lump clinically and radiologically appears benign. Which of the following is most likely to reduce the risk of developing breast cancer?
    a. Early menarche
    b. Nulliparity
    c. Hormone replacement therapy
    d. Breastfeeding
    e. Late menopause

61. Which one of the following tumour markers is incorrectly paired with the conditions it is associated with?
    a. Carcinoembryonic antigen (CEA) – colorectal cancer
    b. Ca 19-9 – uterine cancer
    c. Ca 125 – ovarian cancer
    d. β-Human chorionic gonadotrophin (hCG) – seminoma
    e. α-Fetoprotein – teratoma

62. Regarding adenomas, the following statements are true except:
    a. They are commonly found in the liver.
    b. They have malignant potential.
    c. They can be villous in nature.
    d. They can result in paraneoplastic syndrome.
    e. They can exert a mass effect.

63. Which one of the following statements regarding carcinoma of the prostate is true?
    a. It is common in young adults.
    b. It is a transitional cell carcinoma.
    c. It is can spread via lymphatics.
    d. It is not associated with a higher risk if a first-degree relative is affected.
    e. It is usually found in the anterior region of the gland.

64. The following tumours are correctly paired with the virus that they are most implicated with except:
    a. Hepatocellular carcinoma – hepatitis B virus
    b. Cervical cancer – human papilloma virus
    c. Burkitt lymphoma – herpes simplex virus
    d. Kaposi sarcoma – human immunodeficiency virus
    e. T-cell lymphoma – human T-cell leukaemia type 1 virus

65. Male breast cancer is much rarer than female breast cancer. Which one of the following is the most common form of breast cancer in males?
    a. Invasive ductal carcinoma
    b. Papillary
    c. Invasive lobular carcinoma
    d. Lymphoma
    e. Sarcoma

66. The following conditions are malignant in nature except:
    a. Lymphoma
    b. Hepatoma
    c. Melanoma
    d. Seminoma
    e. Papilloma

67. The following conditions can predispose to the development of oesophageal cancer except:
    a. Smoking
    b. Gastro-oesophageal reflux disease

c. Oesophageal webs
d. Oesophageal varices
e. Coeliac disease

68. The following viruses are known to be carcinogenic except:
    a. Cytomegalovirus (CMV)
    b. Human papilloma virus (HPV)
    c. Epstein–Barr virus (EBV)
    d. Human immunodeficiency virus (HIV)
    e. Hepatitis B virus (HBV)

69. The following microorganisms are associated with malignancy except:
    a. *Helicobacter pylori*
    b. *Bacillus cereus*
    c. *Aspergillus flavus*
    d. *Schistosoma*
    e. *Clonorchis sinensis*

70. The following familial cancer syndromes are paired with their associated affected genes except:
    a. Breast cancer – BRCA 1
    b. Multiple endocrine neoplasia (MEN) – RET
    c. Li–Fraumeni syndrome – TP53
    d. Retinoblastoma – RB1
    e. Von Hippel–Lindau – myc

71. The following can be a paraneoplastic effect of malignancy except:
    a. Cushing syndrome
    b. Syndrome of inappropriate secretion of antidiuretic hormone (SIADH)
    c. Hyperparathyroidism
    d. Dermatomyositis
    e. Membranous glomerulonephritis

72. The following statements concerning cancer screening programmes are true except:
    a. There must be an effective treatment for the type of cancer being screened.
    b. The tests used must be highly sensitive and specific.
    c. Breast cancer screening is carried out in those between 25 and 64 years old.
    d. Cervical cancer screening is carried out by exfoliative cytology.
    e. Breast cancer screening is repeated every 3 years.

73. Which of the following cancer types is unlikely to spread via the transcoelomic route?
    a. Ovarian cancer
    b. Stomach cancer
    c. Bronchial cancer
    d. Colon cancer
    e. Prostate cancer

74. A Krukenberg tumour arises from which of the following histological tumour types?
    a. Adenocarcinoma
    b. Melanoma
    c. Basal cell carcinoma
    d. Squamous cell carcinoma
    e. Lymphoma

75. Which of the following is a benign tumour of smooth muscle?
    a. Adenoma
    b. Lipoma
    c. Chondrosarcoma
    d. Rhabdomyosarcoma
    e. Leiomyoma

76. Which of the following is a recognized risk factor for colorectal cancer?
    a. Low-protein diet
    b. Low vitamin C + E intake
    c. Irritable bowel syndrome
    d. Turner syndrome
    e. Low-fat diet

77. Which of the following statements about primary malignant bone tumours is correct?
    a. Osteosarcoma is the most common primary tumour of bone.
    b. Osteoclastomas have high malignant potential.
    c. Chondrosarcomas are fast-growing tumours arising from chondroblasts.
    d. Myelomas are very common before 50 years of age.
    e. Osteosarcomas spread via the lymphatics to the lungs.

78. An 85-year-old male has recently been diagnosed with oesophageal carcinoma. He presents to the surgical outpatient clinic to discuss his diagnosis further. Which of the following statements regarding oesophageal cancer is correct?
    a. The most common malignant tumour is squamous cell carcinoma.
    b. Most cancers are found in the upper third.
    c. Barrett's oesophagus refers to dysplasia of the distal oesophagus.
    d. Carcinoembryonic antigen (CEA) may be used as a screening tool.
    e. Plummer–Vinson syndrome is associated with the development of squamous cell carcinoma.

79. Concerning carcinogenesis, the following carcinogens and neoplasms are correctly paired except:
    a. B-Naphthylamine: Bladder carcinoma
    b. Asbestos: Pulmonary mesothelioma
    c. Nickel: Carcinoma of the larynx

d. Vinyl chloride: Hepatocellular carcinoma

e. Arsenic: Carcinoma of the bronchus

80. Concerning familial inheritance of colorectal carcinoma, which of the following statements is correct?
    a. Familial polyposis coli (FAP) is autosomal recessive.
    b. Hereditary non-polyposis colorectal cancer (HNPCC) is autosomal recessive.
    c. The p53 gene is located on chromosome 17.
    d. The APC gene is located on chromosome 18.
    e. The mutL gene is located on chromosome 5.

81. A concerned 78-year-old female presents to the rapid assessment upper gastrointestinal (GI) clinic with progressive dysphagia and weight loss. Risk factors for gastric cancer include all of the following except:
    a. Excess salt intake
    b. Excess alcohol consumption
    c. *Helicobacter pylori* infection
    d. Male gender
    e. Blood group B

82. The pathological report of a colorectal specimen from a 54-year-old female is discussed during the multidisciplinary meeting. Which of the following statements regarding Dukes classification of colorectal cancer is correct?
    a. In class B, there is breach of muscularis propria.
    b. In class A, the 5-year survival rate is approximately 75%.
    c. In class C2, the apical node is –ve.
    d. In class C1, the 5-year survival rate is approximately 65%.
    e. In class D, the 5-year survival rate is approximately 25%.

83. The following tumour markers are correctly paired with an associated neoplasia with one exception:
    a. Liver cirrhosis: α-Fetaprotein
    b. Colorectal cancer: carcinoembryonic antigen (CEA)
    c. Seminoma: β human chorionic gonadotropin (hCG)
    d. Breast cancer: Ca 15-3
    e. Teratoma: Carcinoembryonic antigen (CEA)

84. As part of her triple assessment, a 55-year-old woman undergoes a fine-needle aspiration (FNA) of her breast lump. The cytology comes back as 'C3'. Which one of the following describes C3?
    a. Insufficient sample
    b. Breast cancer
    c. Equivocal
    d. Suspected breast cancer
    e. Benign

85. A 48-year-old woman undergoes a triple assessment for a left upper outer quadrant breast lump. The results of the clinical assessment show the lump to be 4.5 cm in diameter cancer, with mobile lymph nodes on the same side and no evidence of distant metastases. Which of the following is her TNM classification?
    a. T1N3M0
    b. T2N2M0
    c. T3N1M0
    d. T2N3M1
    e. T2N1M0

86. Gastric carcinoma is one of the most common cancers worldwide. The risk factors include all of the following except which one?
    a. Blood group A
    b. Pickled foods
    c. *Helicobacter pylori* infection
    d. Pernicious anaemia
    e. Increased vitamin C consumption

87. A 70-year-old man comes to see you in clinic complaining of progressive lower back pain with increasing tiredness. He has mentioned in the last few days that his legs have become discoordinated. Emergency scans diagnose lytic bone lesions and spinal cord compression. Prostate-specific antigen (PSA) levels are normal. Which one of the following is the most likely diagnosis in this gentleman?
    a. Acute myeloid leukaemia
    b. Non-Hodgkin lymphoma
    c. Multiple myeloma
    d. Prostate cancer
    e. Lung cancer

88. A 60-year-old woman is admitted with abdominal pain complaining of absolute constipation for 5 days with a 2-day history of vomiting. An initial abdominal X-ray shows dilated large bowel loops. Which of the following tumour markers most likely suggests a malignancy of the colon?
    a. α-Fetoprotein (AFP)
    b. Cancer antigen (Ca) 19-9
    c. Cancer antigen (Ca) 125
    d. Human chorionic gonadotrophin
    e. Carcinoembryonic antigen (CEA)

89. A 60-year-old man is admitted with a 3-month history of weight loss, with reduced appetite and more recently upper abdominal pain that eases on sitting forward. He has a history of heavy smoking and diabetes. Which of the following markers is most likely to be elevated?
    a. α-Fetoprotein
    b. Ca 19-9
    c. Ca 125
    d. Human chorionic gonadotrophin
    e. Carcinoembryonic antigen

90. Which of the following viruses has been shown to be associated with Kaposi sarcoma?
    a. Human herpes virus 8
    b. Human T-cell leukaemia virus type 1
    c. Epstein–Barr virus
    d. Hepatitis B virus
    e. Human papilloma virus

91. Which of the following is a recognized premalignant condition?
    a. Crohn disease
    b. Xeroderma pigmentosum
    c. Paget disease of the bone
    d. Cirrhosis of the liver
    e. All of the above

SURGICAL IMMUNOLOGY

92. The following types of hypersensitivity reaction are matched according to their specific Gell and Coombs classification except:
    a. Hay fever – type I
    b. Systemic lupus erythematosus (SLE) – type II
    c. Post-streptococcal glomerulonephritis – type III
    d. Rheumatoid arthritis – type III
    e. Contact dermatitis – type IV

93. Virus-laden cells are specifically killed by which of the following?
    a. T-cells
    b. Neutrophils
    c. Complement
    d. Natural killer cells
    e. Erythrocytes

94. All of the following contribute toward innate immunity except:
    a. Mucosal epithelium
    b. Lactoferrin
    c. Calcitonin
    d. C-reactive protein
    e. Mannose-binding lectin

95. Which one of the following immunoglobulins is the first to be produced by B lymphocytes after primary encounter with antigen?
    a. Immunoglobulin A (IgA)
    b. Immunoglobulin E (IgE)
    c. Immunoglobulin G (IgG)
    d. Immunoglobulin M (IgM)
    e. Immunoglobulin F (IgF)

96. IgA deficiency is associated with which of the following conditions?
    a. Mucosal infections
    b. Rickets
    c. Chondrocalcinosis
    d. Bleeding diathesis
    e. Scurvy

97. Which of the following statements about hypersensitivity is correct?
    a. Type I response is immunoglobulin E mediated.
    b. Antibody against cell surface antigens is responsible for type II reactions.
    c. Type III response is caused by immune complex deposition.
    d. Contact dermatitis is a type IV response caused by cell-mediated immunity.
    e. All of the above.

98. Which of the following statements regarding renal transplant rejection is correct?
    a. Hyperacute rejection is caused by pre-existing complement-fixing antibodies.
    b. Accelerated rejection is mediated by pre-existing non-complement-fixing anti-human leukocyte antigen (HLA) antibodies in sensitized patients.
    c. A combination of cellular and vascular rejection represents acute rejection.
    d. Chronic rejection may reflect antibody responses to antigen mismatches that are not suppressed by immunosuppressive agents.
    e. All of the above.

99. Patients with primary antibody deficiency are predisposed to which one of the following?
    a. Osteoporosis
    b. *Salmonella* osteomyelitis
    c. *Mycoplasma* arthritis
    d. Rheumatoid arthritis
    e. Psoriasis

100. Which of the following is not a recognized tumour of the thymus gland?
    a. Teratoma
    b. Hodgkin disease
    c. Carcinoid
    d. Non-Hodgkin disease
    e. Sarcoma

101. Concerning the complement cascade, which of the following is correct?
    a. The classical pathway is activated by antibody–antigen complexes.
    b. The alternative pathway is activated by bacterial exotoxins.
    c. C3 is a component of the final common pathway.
    d. The alternative pathway is part of the specific immune system.
    e. C5 is a component of the classical pathway.

102. The following immunodeficiencies and immune components affected are correctly paired except:
    a. Acquired immunodeficiency syndrome: T-cell deficiency
    b. Di George syndrome: B-cell deficiency
    c. Leukocyte adhesion deficiency: Neutrophil defects
    d. Selective immunoglobulin A deficiency: B-cell deficiency
    e. Wiskott–Aldrich syndrome: Combined T- and B-cell deficiency

103. Concerning classification of hypersensitivity, which of the following statements is correct?
    a. Myaesthenia gravis is an example of a type III reaction.
    b. Immunoglobulin E antibodies interact with cell surface antigens in a type II reaction.
    c. Contact dermatitis is an example of a type IV reaction.

d. Basophil degranulation with histamine release characterizes a type I reaction.

e. Hyperacute allograft rejection is an example of a type III reaction.

104. In granulomatous chronic inflammation which type of leukocyte becomes activated?
    a. Basophil
    b. Eosinophil
    c. Lymphocyte
    d. Monocyte
    e. Neutrophil

105. Which of the following is an endogenous pyrogen?
    a. Interferon-γ (IFN-γ)
    b. Interleukin-1 (IL-1)
    c. Nitric oxide
    d. Interleukin-12 (IL-12)
    e. Interleukin-6 (IL-6)

106. Which of the following primarily acts as a chemoattractant of neutrophils?
    a. Substance P
    b. Complement 3b (C3b)
    c. Bradykinin
    d. Histamine
    e. Interleukin-8 (IL-8)

107. A 7-year-old boy is given intravenous flucloxacillin for severe cellulitis. Rapidly, he developed urticaria, stridor, respiratory distress and shock. Which of the following pathological processes is the likely cause of this reaction?
    a. Type I hypersensitivity
    b. Type II hypersensitivity
    c. Type III hypersensitivity
    d. Type IV hypersensitivity
    e. None of the above

SURGICAL HAEMATOLOGY

108. A 35-year-old female with known sickle cell disease presents to the acute surgical assessment unit with lower abdominal pain. A diagnosis of acute appendicitis is suspected. Which of the following statements describe the clinical features of haemoglobin S (HbS)?
    a. Severe anaemia
    b. Vaso-occlusive crises
    c. Chronic hyperbilirubinaemia
    d. All of the above
    e. None of the above

109. Which of the following endothelial cell products has a prothrombotic effect?
    a. Prostacyclin (PGI$_2$)
    b. Nitric oxide (NO)
    c. von Willebrand factor (vWF)
    d. Thrombomodulin
    e. Tissue plasminogen activator (tPA)

110. Low-molecular-weight heparin (LMWH) is used commonly in surgical patients. When compared with unfractionated heparin, which of the following statements is incorrect?
    a. LMWH has less effect on thrombin than heparin.
    b. LMWH has less effect on factor Xa than unfractionated heparin.
    c. Heparin acts by binding to antithrombin III.
    d. Protamine can be used as a reversal agent.
    e. LMWH can be a once or twice daily dose subcutaneously.

111. Which of the following tests of coagulation assesses the intrinsic pathway?
    a. Platelet count
    b. Bleeding time
    c. Thrombin time
    d. Activated partial thromboplastin time
    e. Prothrombin time

112. A 23-year-old female with menorrhagia is diagnosed to have iron deficiency and treated with oral ferrous sulphate. Her peripheral blood film at diagnosis is likely to show which of the following results?
    a. Macrocytic anaemia
    b. Hypochromic microcytic anaemia
    c. Ring sideroblasts
    d. Sickle-shaped cells
    e. Spherocytosis

113. The following blood film microscopy appearances are linked with the condition it is usually associated with except:
    a. Target cells – thalassaemia
    b. Howell–Jolly bodies – post-splenectomy
    c. Auer rods – chronic lymphocytic leukaemia

    d. Hairy cells – hairy cell leukaemia

    e. Basophilic stippling – lead poisoning

114. Which of the following is most likely to reduce the risk of developing a deep vein thrombosis?

    a. Preoperative dehydration

    b. Oral contraceptive pill

    c. Malignant disease

    d. Prolonged surgery

    e. Pneumatic calf compression

115. A 40-year-old woman in theatre recovery post-splenectomy receives her first unit of blood transfusion. Seconds after starting the transfusion, she becomes hypotensive, spikes a very high temperature and complains of severe abdominal pain. Which one of the following is the likely reaction taking place?

    a. Incompatibility of white cells

    b. ABO incompatibility

    c. Adverse reaction to transfused platelets

    d. Graft versus host disease

    e. Transfusion-related lung injury (TRALI)

116. A 75-year-old male presents to the preoperative assessment clinic in preparation for a total hip replacement. He states that he has taken warfarin for the past 10 years for atrial fibrillation. Concerning warfarin, the following statements are true except:

    a. It inhibits the activity of factors II, VII, IX and X.

    b. It prevents formation of thrombi.

    c. Metronidazole can increase the effect of warfarin.

    d. It can be used during the first trimester of pregnancy but avoided in the later stages.

    e. Lifelong warfarin therapy may be required for patients with protein C deficiency.

117. A 65-year-old female is diagnosed with a deep vein thrombosis following a total abdominal hysterectomy. The following statements regarding thrombosis are true except:

    a. Arterial thrombosis can result from atherosclerotic disease.

    b. The most common cause of venous thrombosis is an increase in the viscosity of blood.

    c. The lines of Zahn are a common appearance on the surface of thrombi.

    d. Artificial heart valves increase the risk of thrombosis.

    e. A large pelvic mass may disrupt normal lamina blood flow, increasing the risk of thrombosis.

118. Regarding embolism, the following statements are true except:

    a. The majority of venous thromboembolisms arise from lower limb veins.

    b. Arterial thromboembolism may arise from the venous system.

    c. Gas must be in solution in the bloodstream to embolize.

d. Death from amniotic fluid embolism is most commonly caused by disseminated intravascular coagulation (DIC).

e. Fat embolism can pass from pulmonary circulation into systemic circulation.

119. Idiopathic thrombocytopenic purpura (ITP) is characterized by all but which one of the following?
    a. Low platelet count.
    b. Autoantibodies to platelet antigens.
    c. Megakaryocytes in the bone marrow can be at normal or slightly increased levels.
    d. Symptoms include development of bruises and epistaxis.
    e. ITP is another name for Evans syndrome.

120. Which one of the following statements is true regarding vitamin B_{12} deficiency?
    a. There is a microcytic anaemia.
    b. Bone marrow is hypocellular.
    c. It is associated with reduced red cell haemolysis.
    d. It is not associated with terminal ileal disease.
    e. It can lead to myelin degeneration in the posterior and lateral columns of the spinal cord.

121. An 80-year-old man is admitted to the ward with right iliac fossa tenderness. He is found to be anaemic and, upon further investigation, has a large caecal carcinoma. He mentions that he has had small amounts of altered blood in his stool for some time. Which one of the following comments is correct regarding iron metabolism and iron deficiency anaemia?
    a. Iron is absorbed mainly via the terminal ileum.
    b. There are high numbers of reticulocytes on blood film.
    c. Classically, there is a hyperchromic, microcytic anaemia.
    d. Iron deficiency anaemia can be associated with dysphagia.
    e. Leuconychia is a sign of iron deficiency anaemia.

122. Which comment concerning pernicious anaemia is correct?
    a. Atrophy of the epithelial surface of the vagina and tongue develops.
    b. Red blood cells are macrocytic and hypochromic.
    c. Nervous symptoms are associated with degeneration of the anterior columns of the spinal cord.
    d. Vitamin B_6 deficiency is an aetiological factor.
    e. Pernicious anaemia is associated with gastric mucosa hypertrophy.

123. Regarding leukaemia, which of the following is correct?
    a. Viral aetiological factors include human herpes virus.
    b. Most cases of chronic lymphocytic leukaemia are of T-cell lineage.
    c. Acute myeloblastic leukaemia is the most common form of childhood leukaemia.
    d. Genetic aetiological factors include Down syndrome.
    e. Philadelphia chromosome is found in 50% of cases of chronic myeloid leukaemia.

124. Which statement regarding the natural anticoagulants is correct?
    a. Action of antithrombin III is potentiated by warfarin.
    b. Congenital antithrombin III deficiency is inherited in an autosomal recessive manner.
    c. Protein C degrades factors Va and VIIIa.
    d. Protein C and S synthesis is dependent on vitamin C.
    e. Protein S is a cofactor for antithrombin III.

125. Which of the following is not a cause of thrombocytopenia?
    a. Aplastic anaemia
    b. Viral infections – cytomegalovirus, Epstein-Barr Virus (EBV)
    c. Disseminated intravascular coagulation
    d. Post-transfusion
    e. Chloramphenicol

126. Which of the following is not a commonly recognized cause of disseminated intravascular coagulation?
    a. Septicaemia
    b. Acute pancreatitis
    c. Amniotic fluid embolism
    d. Pulmonary embolism
    e. Trauma

127. The following diseases all result in a hypercoaguable state except:
    a. Protein C deficiency
    b. von Willebrand's disease
    c. Protein S deficiency
    d. Factor V Leiden
    e. Antithrombin III deficiency

128. In iron deficiency anaemia, which of the following statements is correct?
    a. The serum ferritin is high, the serum transferrin is low and the serum iron is low.
    b. The serum ferritin is low, the serum transferrin is low and the serum iron is low.
    c. The blood film shows target cells.
    d. The blood film shows marked rouleaux formation.
    e. The erythrocyte sedimentation rate (ESR) is elevated disproportionately to the degree of anaemia.

129. An inherited mutation of which haemoglobin chain results in sickle cell disease?
    a. Alpha
    b. Beta
    c. Delta
    d. Theta
    e. Omega

130. Haemophilia B is caused by a deficiency of which clotting factor?
    a. V
    b. VII

c. VIII
d. IX
e. X

131. In the haematology laboratory, the serum of a patient requiring a transfusion reacts (agglutinates) with blood from group B and the blood cells of this patient react with the antisera anti-A and anti-D. Which of the following is the blood group of this patient?
    a. A negative
    b. A positive
    c. B negative
    d. B positive
    e. O negative

132. A young man presents to the accident and emergency department in severe pain. He informs you that he is known to have sickle cell anaemia. Which of the following statements regarding sickle cell anaemia is true?
    a. The haemoglobin (Hb) molecule in sickle cell disease (HbS) has one alpha and one beta chain.
    b. It has an autosomal dominant inheritance.
    c. Sickling may be precipitated by infection and fever.
    d. Sickle cell anaemia results in reduced coagulation.
    e. Parvovirus B19 is associated with an aplastic crisis.

133. A patient on the ward suffers a large haemorrhage following an anterior resection. You are asked to see him and prescribe blood products. Which of the following statements are false regarding blood products?
    a. The shelf life of platelets is 2 days.
    b. Rhesus sensitization is possible with platelet transfusion.
    c. Fresh frozen plasma (FFP) is stored at −30°C for up to 12 months.
    d. The dose of FFP is weight dependent.
    e. FFP may be used to reverse the effect of warfarin.

134. Which of the following statements regarding disseminated intravascular coagulation (DIC) is false?
    a. It can present with a non-blanching purpuric rash.
    b. It is defined as the widespread intravascular activation of the clotting cascade leading to bleeding.
    c. Bleeding occurs primarily because of consumption of clotting factors.
    d. Increased activated partial thromboplastin time (APTT) alone is diagnostic of DIC.
    e. Fluid resuscitation is a part of the management of these patients.

Chapter 5 PATHOLOGY: QUESTIONS

247

SURGICAL MICROBIOLOGY

135. Gas gangrene is most commonly caused by which of the following organisms?
    a. *Staphylococcus aureus*
    b. *Streptococcus pyogenes*
    c. *Clostridium tetani*
    d. *Clostridium perfringens*
    e. Mycobacteria

136. Which of the following are not infectious organisms?
    a. Prion
    b. Fungus
    c. Bacteria
    d. Virus
    e. Protozoa

137. Which one of the following statements regarding *Helicobacter pylori* is incorrect?
    a. It produces urease.
    b. Initial infection causes acute neutrophilic gastritis.
    c. It commonly affects the pyloric antrum.
    d. It can lead to intestinal metaplasia.
    e. It can lead to gastric gland hypertrophy.

138. Which of the following classifications is correct?
    a. *Staphylococcus aureus* is a Gram-positive coccus that occurs in chains.
    b. *Streptococcus pyogenes* is a Gram-positive coccus that occurs in clusters.
    c. *Clostridium tetani* is a Gram-positive aerobic sporing bacillus.
    d. *Listeria monocytogenes* is a Gram-positive aerobic non-sporing bacillus.
    e. *Bacillus anthracis* is a Gram-positive aerobic bacillus.

139. Which of the following is not a Gram-negative bacilli?
    a. *Yersinia pseudotuberculosis*
    b. *Proteus mirabilis*
    c. *Clostridium difficile*
    d. *Pasteurella multocida*
    e. *Shigella sonnei*

140. Regarding tetanus infection, which statement is incorrect?
    a. *Clostridium tetani* is an anaerobic Gram-positive bacillus.
    b. Treatment includes benzylpenicillin.
    c. Clinical features include trismus and risus sardonicus.
    d. The neurotoxin blocks the inhibitory activity of spinal reflexes.
    e. Despite supportive treatment, mortality is about 5%.

141. Which statement regarding disinfectants is incorrect?
    a. Formaldehyde has a wide antibacterial and antiviral spectrum.
    b. Glutaraldehyde kills spores slowly.

c. Quaternary ammonium salts have no action against *Pseudomonas*.

d. Boiling water kills tuberculosis.

e. Betadine (povidine-iodine) is bacteriocidal.

142. Which of the following statements regarding macrolide antibiotics (erythromycin) is incorrect?

a. They may potentiate warfarin.

b. They can cause phlebitis when given intravenously.

c. They are valuable against *Campylobacter*.

d. They are nephrotoxic.

e. They are used for respiratory tract infections.

143. Which of the following statements regarding viral hepatitis is incorrect?

a. Hepatitis A has an incubation period of 2–4 weeks.

b. Hepatitis E is a picornavirus.

c. Hepatitis D is spread by the parenteral route.

d. Approximately 90% of children with hepatitis B develop chronic symptoms.

e. Approximately 6 weeks after infection with hepatitis B the surface antigen (HBsAg) appears in the blood.

144. Concerning actinomycosis, which statement is correct?

a. Actinomyces meyeri is the most commonly implicated pathogen.

b. It is easily differentiated from malignancy by history and clinical examination.

c. It has been linked to the usage of the intrauterine contraceptive device.

d. 'Sulphur granules' are pathognomonic.

e. Serology may help to confirm/refute the diagnosis.

145. Which of the following statements regarding clostridia bacteria is correct?

a. It is a Gram-negative organism.

b. It is a saprophytic organism.

c. It is an aerobic organism.

d. Its pathological effects are due to endotoxins.

e. Tetanospasmin binds to peripheral nerve gangliosides.

146. Concerning bacterial toxins, which of the following statements is correct?

a. An endotoxin is a glycoprotein located on the outer wall of a Gram-negative bacteria.

b. An exotoxin is a glycoprotein located on the outer wall of a Gram-positive bacteria.

c. Endotoxins are non-immunogenic.

d. Tetanus is caused by endotoxins.

e. Diphtheria is caused by endotoxins.

147. A 52-year-old patient with known chronic obstructive pulmonary disease (COPD) and type 2 diabetes was admitted to the intensive care unit (ICU) after having an emergency Hartmann procedure for an obstructing colorectal carcinoma. He is currently ventilated on ICU as he suffered a cardiac arrest postoperatively. Five days postoperatively he has a temperature

spike and his inflammatory markers have risen. Blood cultures grow Gram-negative bacilli. Based on this Gram stain, which of the following is the most likely causal organism that will be found/looked for?

a. *Staphylococcus aureus*
b. *Pseudomonas aeruginosa*
c. *Listeria monocytogenes*
d. *Actinomyces israeli*
e. *Moraxella catarrhalis*

148. A patient with a large laceration over the forearm attends his general practitioner to receive a tetanus booster. Which of the following statements is false regarding tetanus?

a. *Clostridium tetani* is a Gram-negative anaerobe.
b. Tetanospasmin is a neurotoxin that is responsible for reducing neuromuscular inhibition.
c. Tetanolysin causes red cell haemolysis.
d. Burns and high-energy wounds are prone to tetanus.
e. Passive immunization with immunoglobulin for high-risk patients may be indicated.

149. You are asked by the medical team to review a patient who they think has necrotizing fasciitis. Which of the following infective agents can be associated with this condition?

a. *Streptococcus pyogenes*
b. *Staphylococcus aureus*
c. *Clostridium perfringens*
d. All of the above
e. a and c only

150. A 47-year-old male presents with a short history of left knee pain and swelling. On examination, he is clinically septic with a swollen knee that is warm to touch with a reduced range of movement. Which is the most common causative agent of septic arthritis in adults?

a. *Neisseria gonorrhoea*
b. *Haemophilus influenzae*
c. *Streptococcus pyogenes*
d. *Staphylococcus aureus*
e. *Escherichia coli*

SURGICAL BIOCHEMISTRY

151. A 17-year-old man attends his general practitioner surgery with a 7-day history of diarrhoea and vomiting and a 3-day history of jaundice. He does not complain of any pain apart from mild abdominal discomfort. Examination of other systems was unremarkable. Blood tests show increased levels of unconjugated bilirubin. Which of the following is the most likely diagnosis?
    a. Crigler–Najjar syndrome
    b. Hereditary spherocytosis
    c. Autoimmune haemolytic anaemia
    d. Gilbert syndrome
    e. Rotor syndrome

152. The following statements regarding hypercalcaemia are true except:
    a. It is associated with paraneoplastic syndromes.
    b. It may be caused by multiple myeloma.
    c. It can be a result of blood transfusion.
    d. It may present with abdominal pain.
    e. It is associated with hyperparathyroidism.

153. A 35-year-old man presents to the accident and emergency department with a gradual onset of generalized abdominal pain, several episodes of vomiting and weight loss. Clinically, he is severely dehydrated, hypotensive and has hyperpigmentation of his skin and buccal mucosa. His blood biochemistry shows low sodium with raised potassium and urea. Which of the following is his most likely diagnosis?
    a. Conn syndrome
    b. Addison disease
    c. Cushing disease
    d. Secondary hyperaldosteronism
    e. Hyperthyroidism

154. Causes of hyponatraemia include all of the following except:
    a. Transurethral resection of prostate (TURP) syndrome
    b. Diabetes insipidus
    c. Addison disease
    d. Nephrotic syndrome
    e. Syndrome of inappropriate antidiuretic hormone secretion

155. Which of the following disorders is correctly paired with a vitamin deficiency?
    a. Beriberi – vitamin B_6
    b. Haemolytic anaemia – vitamin E
    c. Pellagra – vitamin B_1
    d. Dermatitis – vitamin B_3
    e. Neuropathy – vitamin A

CHAPTER 6
PATHOLOGY

Answers

INFLAMMATION

1. a.　Abscesses are more common in patients with certain conditions such as diabetes, with patients more at risk of septicaemia. In certain cases of small abscesses not amenable to drainage, conservative management with antibiotics is a valid option. Abscess cavities should be opened completely with all loculations broken down allowing residual discharge to drain easily and healing to occur from within.

2. a.　A sinus is a blinding ending tract, which in this scenario is formed by the body to drain any underlying infection. A fistula is an abnormal connection between two epithelial surfaces. An abscess is a collection of pus within a cavity lined by granulation tissue. A cyst is an epithelial-lined cavity usually containing fluid.

3. b.　Necrosis is defined as cellular or tissue death in a living organism. Coagulative necrosis involves denaturation of intracytoplasmic proteins and typically occurs in ischaemic injury. Colliquative necrosis is commonly seen in the brain due to lack of supporting stroma. Caseous necrosis is characteristic of tuberculosis. Gangrenous necrosis involves the association with putrefaction of tissues due to certain bacterial infections, and fibrinoid necrosis involves the arteriole smooth muscle wall associated with malignant hypertension.

4. c.　A free radical is a molecule bearing an unpaired electron, making it highly reactive and short lived. They are present in lysosomes and are used by the body to destroy bacteria. They are formed as final products of many cellular processes. Vitamin D and glutathione act as free radical sinks and protect cells against these highly reactive products.

5. b.　Increased vascular permeability leading to the escape of a protein-rich fluid (exudate) into the extravascular tissue is characteristic of acute inflammation. The most common mechanism of vascular leakage is elicited by the release of chemical mediators like histamine, bradykinin, leukotrienes and the neuropeptide substance P. These mediators cause endothelial gaps in venules lasting from

15 to 30 min (immediate transient response). The loss of protein from plasma increases the osmotic pressure of the interstitial fluid. The net increase of extravascular fluid results in oedema.

6. d. The predominant cell involved in acute inflammation is the neutrophil, which phagocytoses pathogens. Interleukin-2 (IL-2) causes differentiation of natural killer (NK) and B-cells. There is an increase in capillary permeability during the acute phase of inflammation. Complement is a component of the innate immune system, consisting of a protein cascade that, when activated, can form a protein complex (membrane attack complex [MAC]) – this perpetuates the inflammatory response to the invading pathogen, by recruiting neutrophils to the affected site (via chemotaxis), and also destroys bacterial cell walls directly. Fibrinogen is converted to fibrin forming a fibrinous meshwork, limiting spread of the pathogen.

7. a. Macrophages arise from the conversion of circulatory monocytes in tissues, which themselves are derived from bone marrow precursor cells. They are an inherent component of the mononuclear phagocyte system and can be activated to form epithelioid cells, or differentiated according to the specific tissue they are present in (i.e. Kuppfer cells in the liver or alveolar macrophages in the lung). The remainder are mainly involved in acute inflammation.

8. b. Acute inflammation requires many messengers for communication and control of the immune response. Cytokines are soluble, biologically active molecules with a variety of functions. The roles of some of these are listed below:

- Interleukin-1 – neutrophil adhesion
- Interleukin-2 – differentiation of B-cells and natural killer cells
- Histamine – vasodilatation, increased capillary permeability
- Interferon – activation of macrophages and natural killer cells
- Tumour necrosis factor – fever, neutrophil adhesion

9. e. Histamine is stored in mast cells and causes vascular dilatation. Prostaglandins are derived from arachidonic acid and potentiate vascular permeability. Chemokines selectively attract various types of leukocytes to the site of inflammation. Mast cells have a high concentration of 5-hydroxytryptamine, which causes vasoconstriction. The enzyme telomerase allows for replacement of short pieces of DNA known as telomeres, which are otherwise shortened when a cell divides via mitosis.

10. e. The essential physical characteristics of acute inflammation were formulated by Celsus (30 B.C.–38 A.D.) using the Latin words *rubor* (redness), *calor* (heat), *tumour* (swelling) and *dolor* (pain). Loss of function was subsequently added by Virchow (1821–1902).

11. d. Reversible cell injury is identified by two patterns of microscopic changes on light microscopy. Cellular swelling is caused by disturbance in the ionic and fluid homeostasis. Fatty change occurs in hypoxic injury and various forms of toxic or metabolic injury. It is manifested by the appearance of small or large lipid vacuoles in the cytoplasm and occurs in hypoxic and various forms of toxic injury.

It is principally encountered in cells involved in, and dependent on, fat metabolism such as the hepatocyte and myocardial cells. Amorphous densities in the mitochondria represent irreversible cell injury.

12. d. A swinging pyrexia is an indication of a deep-seated abscess, in this case a subphrenic abscess, which causes referred pain at the shoulder tip. It normally presents 7–21 days postoperatively with malaise, nausea, pain and, in some cases, local peritonism. Treatment entails drainage of the collection, which can be achieved percutaneously (image guided) or surgically.

CELLULAR INJURY OTHER THAN BY INFECTION

13. b. Curling ulcer is an acute peptic ulcer associated with major burns. Reduced plasma levels lead to hypovolaemic shock, which causes sloughing of the gastric mucosa secondary to ischaemia. It may result in perforation and haemorrhage and have a high mortality rate. A Cushing ulcer is associated with head injury and raised intracranial pressure. A Marjolin ulcer is a squamous cell carcinoma (SCC) that develops within chronic venous ulcers.

14. d. The common causes of cell injury are physical and chemical agents, infectious pathogens, nutritional imbalances and genetic derangements. Following such injurious stimulus the cell undergoes characteristic morphological changes, which are initially reversible. This involves swelling of the cell and its organelles, blebbing of the plasma membrane, detachment of ribosomes from the endoplasmic reticulum and clumping of nuclear chromatin. Transition to irreversible injury is characterized by increasing swelling of the cell, swelling and disruption of lysosomes, the presence of large amorphous densities in swollen mitochondria and disruption of cellular membranes.

15. b. Mitochondria are 0.5–10 μm organelles with a double layer of membrane found in all eukaryotic cells. They have their own DNA and are thought to be symbiotic prokaryotes that have been assimilated into eukaryotic cells in our biological past. They replicate by mitosis to form a clonal population. All the mitochondrial DNA in humans is derived from the clonal population from the ovum and therefore is maternally inherited.

Oxidative phosphorylation (Krebs cycle) occurs in the mitochondrial matrix.

16. b. Lipofuscin is a brown pigment that accumulates in ageing cells. It is mainly formed from old cellular membranes that have become cross-linked as a result of free radical damage and which accumulate in residual bodies without being metabolized. It is also referred to as the age pigment.

17. d. Gunshot exit wounds normally have an irregularly defined edge, sometimes described as stellate in appearance. The injury is dependent on the relationship between kinetic energy, mass of the projectile and velocity. The management of these injuries involves resuscitation according to Advanced Trauma Life Support (ATLS) guidelines.

WOUNDS AND WOUND HEALING

18. c. Bone healing is a proliferative physiological process that can be divided into three phases. The first phase – the reactive phase – occurs initially where a haematoma resulting from ruptured bone and periosteal vessels form around the fracture site. Fibroblasts, macrophages and new vessels invade the area by the first week, forming granulation tissue. The second phase – the reparative phase – involves osteoblasts and chondroblasts developing within the haematoma to form woven bone and fibrocartilage, forming a callus. Internal callus lies within the medullary canal, whereas external callus envelops the fracture site, acting as a 'splint'. Woven bone is subsequently replaced by lamellar bone. The final phase – the remodelling phase – takes place as lamellar bone is replaced by compact bone. Factors that affect bone healing include movement at the site, misalignment, infection, pre-existing bone disease and interposition of soft tissue preventing fracture site union.

19. a. Hypertrophic scars are usually confined within the borders of the wound. They usually develop around 3 weeks after injury. Keloid scars extend beyond the margins of the original wound and may take up to 1 year to develop. Type III collagen is produced during the early stages of wound healing. It is weaker than type I collagen, which predominates during the maturation phase of wound healing. Macrophages carry out phagocytosis of necrotic cells as well as help to repair damaged tissue by recruiting fibroblasts and endothelial cells.

20. d. To close the abdomen using mass closure, a suture four times the length of the wound is used. Bites are usually 1 cm deep and 1 cm apart, taking bites of the rectus sheath for maximum support, without too much tension. Care should be taken to avoid damage to the bowel during suturing and to prevent the sutures from being excessively tight, as this can lead to tissue necrosis. If there is gross peritonitis or if the intra-abdominal contents cannot be reduced, the abdomen can be left open and closed at a later date.

21. c. The ABCDE approach to management should be adhered to in all cases. The injury in this case most likely to cause an airway problem is orofacial trauma. Massive facial trauma is almost always a prelude to airway compromise and therefore should be treated first in this instance.

22. b. In primary intention, the margins of the wound are closely apposed. Secondary intention is where the wound's margins are not apposed, possibly owing to extensive tissue damage, so the tissue defect fills with granulation tissue that contracts, resulting in a scar. Myofibroblasts within the granulation tissue contract bringing together the surrounding matrix, reducing the size of the wound.

23. b. Keloid scars are most common on the sternum and deltoid area, and on the dorsal surfaces. They extend beyond the previous wound, unlike hypertrophic scars, which are confined to the wound. Contraction of the fibrous tissue in keloid scars can occur across the joints. They are more common in pigmented skin. Re-excision leads to recurrence, whereas steroid injections may help with cosmesis.

24. e. There are four stages of wound healing:

Stage 1: Coagulative; occurs immediately post-incision and is characterized by vasoconstriction, platelet adhesion and activation, and fibrin clot formation

Stage 2: Inflammatory stage; occurs up to 3 days post-incision and is characterized by vasodilatation, exudation and phagocytosis

Stage 3: Fibroblastic or proliferative stage; occurs between 3 days and 3 weeks, whereby granulation, contraction and epithelialization are characteristic features

Stage 4: Remodelling phase or maturation stage; takes place between 3 weeks and up to 2 years post-incision. This is characterized by reorganization, regression and scar tissue formation.

25. d. Wounds heal in a step-wise process. The process is complicated and any number of factors can lead to a wound breaking down. The factors responsible can be categorized into local and systemic factors. Examples of each are:

- *Local:* Poor blood supply, local infection, foreign body, haematoma, mechanical stress, poor surgical technique, suture failure
- *Systemic:* Old age, anaemia, drugs (steroids or cytotoxic medications), diabetes, malnutrition, obesity, systemic infection, uraemia

VASCULAR DISORDERS

26. d. Central venous cannulas can be used for measurement of the central venous pressure, fluid resuscitation, drug administration or feeding. Common vessels used for access include the internal jugular vein, subclavian vein and femoral vein. Immediate complications include pneumothorax, haemothorax, air embolism, haematoma, chylothorax (thoracic duct injury), cardiac tamponade (right atrial perforation) and arrhythmias.

27. c. Aortic dissection is a tear in the wall of the aorta causing blood to flow between the layers forcing them apart. It initially commences as an intimal tear, and then propagates along the plane between the inner two-thirds and outer one-third of the media. Patients present with severe stabbing pain, signs of shock and sometimes signs of cardiac tamponade or neurological signs. Risk factors include atherosclerosis, hypertension, aortic valve defects, Turner syndrome, Marfan syndrome, Ehlers-Danlos syndrome and pseudoxanthoma elasticum, which is a genetic disorder that causes fragmentation of elastic fibres within tissues. Investigations include chest X-ray, electrocardiogram (ECG), angiography and CT/MRI imaging.

28. e. Primary lymphoedema can be divided into three stages: congenital is present at birth, praecox such as Milroy disease and tarda affecting 30- to 40-year-olds. Primary lymphoedema is usually unilateral, starting as pitting oedema and then progressing to non-pitting oedema. Milroy disease is a congenital hereditary primary lymphoedema caused by aplasia of the lymph trunks, resulting in progressive swelling of one or both legs. Secondary lymphoedema is where there is a known cause of lymphatic failure, for example surgical excision during axillary dissection.

29. a. Arterial ulcers are punched-out lesions, with poor capillary refill and reduced or absent distal pulses. They are usually painful. Venous ulcers are typically found in the gaiter area, with a sloping edge with a sloughy base and a moderate degree of exudate. It is important to exclude coexisting ischaemia with venous ulcers and treat if present, as the management of venous ulcers is by elevation and four-layer bandaging with regular dressings which can further compromise the blood supply. The surrounding skin can be hyperpigmented with lipodermatosclerosis. Diabetic ulcers occur on pressure-bearing areas, are painless and may have normal blood supply.

30. d. Diabetic foot ulcers develop as a result of peripheral neuropathy, atherosclerotic arterial disease and changes in the bony architecture of the foot. Diabetic ulcers occur on pressure-bearing areas, are painless and may have normal blood supply.

31. d. Risk factors for deep venous thrombosis (DVT) include protein C and S deficiency, antithrombin III deficiency, prolonged surgical procedure, oral contraceptive pill, age, female, previous DVT/pulmonary embolism (PE), malignancy, dehydration, reduced muscle activity and polycythaemia. Virchow's triad of blood stasis, vascular wall damage and hypercoagulability describe the broad three categories that are risk factors for thrombosis. Risk can be reduced using thromboembolic deterrent stockings, prophylactic low-molecular-weight heparin injections and pneumatic calf compression. Thrombocytopenia also reduces risk as it causes a bleeding diathesis.

32. b.   Buerger disease occurs in young men who smoke. It presents with severe claudication and rest pain leading to gangrene. Instead of atheromatous disease there is inflammation of the arteries. Kawasaki disease is a disease of infants affecting the main aortic branch arteries. Takayasu disease is a rare inflammatory disorder of the aorta and proximal branches. It can present with ischaemic symptoms of the arms with loss of arm pulses. Giant cell arteritis mainly affects the arteries in the head and neck, and is rare under the age of 50 years. Vessel occlusion caused by atherosclerosis is unlikely in this case because of his age.

33. c.   Ascites is the abnormal collection of fluid within the peritoneal cavity. Transudate ascites has a lower protein content (<30 g/L) than exudates (>30 g/L). Causes include:

- Transudate
  - *Hydrostatic changes* – right-sided heart failure, Budd–Chiari syndrome, thoracic duct obstruction
  - *Oncotic changes* – liver failure, protein losing enteropathy, starvation, nephritic syndrome
  - *Metabolic changes* – hypothyroidism
- Exudate
  - *Inflammatory* – peritonitis, pancreatitis, irradiation, pseudomyxoma
  - *Iatrogenic* – continuous ambulatory peritoneal dialysis

34. d.   An aneurysm is an abnormal dilatation of an artery. They may be classified as true – involving all three layers of the arterial wall – or false, for example pulsating haematoma where the cavity is in contact with the arterial lumen but not all layers of the wall are involved. Aneurysms can also be classified as acquired or congenital. Acquired aneurysms include atheromatous, mycotic, syphilitic, dissecting and arteriovenous. A Berry aneurysm is an example of a congenital aneurysm caused by a defect in the media at the junction of vessels in the circle of Willis. They are the most common cause of subarachnoid haemorrhages, with an increased incidence in patients with hypertension.

35. a.   Pulmonary embolism (PE) is the most likely diagnosis. It is important to remember that patients with PEs may be asymptomatic, although classically the patient reports pleuritic chest pain with a low-grade pyrexia and a sinus tachycardia. The respiratory rate may be elevated. If a PE is suspected, an arterial blood gas (ABG) is useful, showing a reduced PaO_2 and low PCO_2 occurring as a result of ventilation perfusion mismatch and the patient consequently hyperventilating. The electrocardiogram finding of S1Q3T3 is rarely seen except in instances associated with a large PE causing right heart strain.

DISORDERS OF GROWTH, DIFFERENTIATION AND MORPHOGENESIS

36. d.   Stratified squamous epithelium consists of several layers of epithelial cells arranged upon a layer of basement membrane. The layers can be sloughed off and replaced constantly; hence it is suited for areas with constant insults and abrasions. Stratified squamous epithelium can be divided into keratinized and non-keratinized types, depending on the presence of keratin on its surface. Examples of keratinized types include the skin, tongue and outer lips. Non-keratinized types include the cornea, oesophagus, rectum and vagina. Epididymis and trachea have pseudo-stratified columnar epithelium, whereas the colon and uterus are lined by simple columnar epithelium.

37. c.   Dysplasia is a premalignant condition with increased cell growth and decreased cell differentiation and is characterized by cellular atypia. There is increased mitotic activity with an increase in tissue bulk and hyperchromatic nuclei with a high nuclear–cytoplasmic ratio. It is caused by long-standing inflammation or exposure to carcinogens. In the early stages, it may be reversible if the stimulus is removed.

38. d.   Metaplasia occurs as a tissue response to environmental stress. This causes a reversible transformation of one type of terminally differentiated cell into another fully differentiated cell type, for example glandular metaplasia of lower oesophagus (Barrett's oesophagus).

39. b.   Lipofuscin is a brown pigment that accumulates in ageing cells. It is mainly formed from old cellular membranes that have become cross-linked as a result of free radical damage and which accumulate in residual bodies without being metabolized. It is also referred to as the age pigment.

40. b.   Necrotic tissue is invaded by putrefactive organisms, notably clostridia. The infected tissue can appear to be green or black and can be classified as either wet or dry. Dry gangrene is typically seen with a gradual reduction in arterial flow, such as ischaemia of the toes. Dry gangrene has a slow putrefactive process with small numbers of organisms. Gas gangrene is a primary infection of healthy tissue by *Clostridium perfringens*. In wet gangrene there is venous as well as arterial obstruction present. Infection and putrefaction are more severe than in dry gangrene. Diabetic gangrene of the toes can occur in the presence of palpable peripheral pulses.

41. e.   Haemochromotosis is caused by a mutation on chromosome 6 encoding the protein which regulates iron absorption leading to excess absorption of iron, particularly in the pancreatic islets, myocardium and liver. Wilson's disease is an autosomal recessive condition caused by a mutation on chromosome 13. It is characterized by an accumulation of copper in the liver, brain and cornea. α1-Antitrypsin deficiency results in liver damage commonly in homozygotes – neonatal hepatitis, chronic active hepatitis or cirrhosis. This deficiency also plays a part in the development of emphysema.

42. e. Familial cancer syndromes

Syndrome	Gene affected	Neoplasm
Li–Fraumeni	p53	Breast and ovarian carcinomas, sarcomas
Retinoblastoma	Rb1	Retinoblastoma, osteosarcoma
Familial polyposis coli	APC	Gastrointestinal carcinoma
Von Hippel–Lindau	VHL	Renal carcinoma, phaeochromocytoma
Multiple endocrine neoplasia	RET	Pituitary, parathyroid, thyroid, pancreas and adrenal tumours
Familial breast cancer	BRCA1, BRCA2	Breast carcinoma, ovarian syndrome

43. a. Teratogens and their effects

Teratogen	Teratogenic effect
Irradiation	Microcephaly
Rubella	Microphthalmia, cataracts, microcephaly
Cytomegalovirus (CMV)	Microcephaly
Alcohol	Microcephaly, abnormal facies
Warfarin	Facial abnormalities
Folic acid	Anencephaly, hydrocephalus, cleft lip/palate
Thalidomide	Absent/rudimentary limbs, heart and kidney defects
Irradiation	Microcephaly

AT Raftery, Basic science for the MRCS, Churchill Livingstone 2006.

44. a. α₁-Antitrypsin deficiency is an autosomal recessive condition, in which homozygotes have a tendency to develop emphysema and hepatic cirrhosis (due to failure to digest protease). Polycystic kidney disease is an autosomal dominant condition that occurs in adult life, with individuals developing large bilateral renal cysts, leading ultimately to chronic renal failure. There is an association with Berry aneurysm formation. Achondroplasia is an autosomal dominant condition in which abnormal bone development predisposes to osteoarthritis and increased risk of fracture. Hereditary spherocytosis is an autosomal dominant condition resulting in haemolytic anaemia – increased risk of (pigment) gallstones is associated.

45. d. Blastomas are rare, occurring in childhood, and are typically aggressive tumours with a propensity to metastasize. Examples include Wilms' tumour (nephroblastoma) and retinoblastoma (which requires both alleles of the Rb gene to be abnormal for a cell to enter a state of continual proliferation). A high nucleus–cytoplasm ratio is characteristic, as is hyperchromatic nuclei.

46. e. Non-disjunction refers to an extra copy of chromosome 21 being inherited due to failed disjunction of a gamete during meiosis – it is the most common cause of Down syndrome, and typically occurs in mothers over the age of 40. Translocation is rare, and refers to material from the 21 chromosome being translocated onto another chromosome. Mosaicism is very rare, and refers to non-disjunction as the blastocyst begins to develop. As a consequence, some cells will be normal and others will have trisomy 21.

47. e. Giant cells are defined as a union of similar cells to formulate a multinuclear cell. These can be either physiological or pathological. Physiological examples of giant cells include:

- Osteoclasts
- Skeletal muscle cells
- Syncytiotrophoblasts
- Oocytes
- Megakaryocytes

Pathological examples of giant cells include:

- Warthin–Finkeldy cells (induced by measles virus)
- Reed–Sternberg cells (modified B-lymphocytes seen in Hodgkin's lymphoma)
- Thyroid and adrenal cytomegaly
- Cytomegalovirus - and herpes simplex virus–induced giant cells
- Langerhans cells (seen in sarcoidosis, tuberculosis and Crohn's disease)
- Foreign body reactions
- Touton giant cells (seen in xanthoma)

48. b. Ischaemia is an abnormal reduction in blood supply or drainage to a tissue; infarction refers to the resultant cell damage. The stages of ischemia-related cell injury include:

- Decreased oxidative phosphorylation.
- Decreased ATP synthesis.
- The sodium/potassium channel is ATP dependent and subsequently fails.
- The cell including the mitochondria and the endoplasmic reticulum swell.
- Protein synthesis fails.
- Membrane damage.
- Calcium influx into cell.
- Cell death.

Different cell types have variable resistance to ischaemia: cerebral neurons are comparatively sensitive to ischaemia, and become irreversibly damaged after 3–5 min, whereas cardiac myocytes do so after 1–2 h. Skeletal muscle cells take greater than 4 h. There is preservation of tissue architecture in coagulation necrosis, which is seen in organs supplied by end arteries (i.e. myocardium). Heterolysis refers to cell degradation by enzymes from external sources (i.e. microorganisms). Autolysis refers to degradation from intracellular enzymes.

49. d. Amyloid is a waxy substance deposited in extracellular tissues. Amyloid fibrils are made up of a minor constant component (amyloid P protein) and a major variable component arranged in B pleats. Affected organs stain brown with Lugol's iodine solution. Systemic amyloidosis can be associated either with chronic inflammation, for example Tuberculosis with amyloid A protein (AA) as the variable protein, or with monoclonal plasma cell proliferation, for example myeloma with amyloid light-chain (AL) as the variable component. Localized amyloidosis can be associated with endocrine tumours such as medullary carcinoma of the thyroid gland.

50. d. Apoptosis is an energy-dependent process for the deletion of unwanted cells. Its functions include morphogenesis and the removal of deoxyribonucleic acid (DNA) damage or virally infected cells. The process involves single cells leading to cell shrinkage and fragmentation to form apoptotic bodies. The cell membrane integrity is preserved. No inflammatory response is initiated by this process in comparison with necrosis.

51. c. Apoptosis is a type of individual cell death associated with growth and morphogenesis. Morphogenetic apoptosis occurs during embryological development involved in alteration of tissue form (e.g. interdigital cell death responsible for separating the fingers).

52. d. The morphological hallmark of apoptosis is the apoptotic body, which is eosinophilic and may contain some nuclear debris. It is a result of shrinkage of the cell cytoplasm and nuclear disruption. These apoptotic bodies are taken by surrounding cells and digested. Historically these have been described with specific names: Civatte or colloid bodies in lichen planus, Kamino bodies in melanocytic lesions and Councilman bodies in acute viral hepatitis.

53. d. Growth may occur in response to physiological or pathological stimuli by hypertrophy, hyperplasia or both. Hypertrophy is an increase in cell size without replication, whereas hyperplasia is an increase in cell number owing to cell division. The stimuli for both hypertrophy and hyperplasia are similar and the mechanism is reversed when the stimulus is removed. Physiological growth includes muscle hypertrophy in athletes, bone marrow hyperplasia at high altitude and hypertrophy and hyperplasia of the uterus in pregnancy. An example of pathological growth is myocardial hypertrophy in hypertension.

54. b. Necrosis (abnormal tissue death) and apoptosis (programmed cell death) are very different processes. Gangrene is also a type of necrosis. There are five different types of necrosis: coagulative, colliquative, caseous, fat and fibrinoid. Coagulative necrosis is the most common and can occur due to ischaemia. Fat necrosis is induced by the action of lipases as opposed to coagulation necrosis.

NEOPLASIA

55. d. The cell cycle can be summarized as follows:

- *G0:* Resting phase
- *G1:* First gap phase; presynthetic phase of variable duration
- *S:* DNA synthesis phase
- *G2:* Second gap phase
- *M:* Mitosis phase → G0

56. c. Necrobiosis lipoidica is a necrotizing skin condition that is usually associated with diabetes. The erythematous skin lesions usually appear on the shin and are often bilateral. It is more commonly found in women. It is not known to be premalignant. All the other conditions have the potential for malignancy.

57. c. An oncovirus is a virus that can cause cancer and can be either deoxyribonucleic acid (DNA) or ribonucleic acid (RNA) based. The main DNA viruses associated with human cancers are human papillomavirus (cervical cancer), Epstein–Barr virus (Burkitt lymphoma) and herpes virus (lymphoma). The RNA oncoviruses are human T-lymphotropic virus (T-cell leukaemia) and hepatitis B virus (hepatocellular carcinoma).

58. b. Rhabdomyosarcoma is a skeletal muscle neoplasm. It usually presents in children and adolescents and can occur in any skeletal muscle in the body. It has three variants: embryonal, alveolar and pleomorphic. The rhabdomyoblast – the diagnostic cell in all types – contains eccentric eosinophilic granular cytoplasm rich in thick and thin filaments. The rhabdomyoblasts may be round or elongate; the latter are known as tadpole or strap cells and may contain cross-striations visible by light microscopy. Leimyosarcoma is a malignant smooth muscle tumour. The remainder are benign tumours.

59. c. Nitrosamines are produced from nitrites and secondary amines, which often occur in the form of proteins. Nitrate preservatives used in processed food are converted to nitrites by bacteria. These are known to react with amines, which are postulated to contribute to the induction of gastric carcinoma. In addition to food preservatives, nitrosamine compounds are also present in tobacco products.

60. d. An increase in oestrogen exposure increases the risk of breast cancer. This includes women with early menarche or late menopause. Exposure to hormone replacement therapy or oral contraceptive pills also causes a small increase in risk. Breastfeeding reduces the risk of developing breast cancer. Early age of first pregnancy decreases the risk of developing breast cancer, whereas being nulliparous increases the risk. Other factors such as genetics, family history and environmental factors are also implicated in breast cancer development.

61. b. Tumour markers can be detected in blood, urine or other body tissues. An elevated level of a tumour marker usually indicates cancer; however, they can also be associated with other conditions. Carcinoembryonic antigen (CEA) is associated with gastrointestinal (GI) malignancies, especially colorectal cancer. Ca 19-9 is also associated with colorectal as well as pancreatic cancer. Ca 125 levels are raised in uterine, ovarian or breast cancer. β-Human chorionic gonadotrophin (hCG) can be detected in seminoma, although only in less than 10% of cases; it is also a useful test of pregnancy. α-Fetoprotein (AFP) is raised in teratomas, liver cirrhosis and hepatocellular carcinoma.

62. a. Adenomas are benign tumours of glandular epithelium. They are commonly found in the colon, adrenal, thyroid and pituitary glands. Structurally they can be either tubular, tubulovillous or villous. Although benign, adenomas have the potential for malignant change (adenocarcinoma). This change usually depends on the size, degree of dysplasia and growth pattern of the adenoma. Generally, larger adenomas with a greater degree of dysplasia have a greater malignant potential. Large adenomas can exert a mass effect on nearby structures and can also produce endogenous hormones in an unregulated manner (paraneoplastic syndrome).

63. c. Prostate cancer is a common tumour among elderly men. It is rarely found in men aged less than 50 years. The aetiology is largely unknown, but there is a high risk of tumour developing in men with first-degree relatives in whom the cancer was diagnosed under the age of 50 years. Macroscopically, it is usually found in the posterior region of the prostate, beneath the capsule. Microscopically, prostate carcinoma (adenocarcinoma) is graded on its degree of differentiation and is given a Gleason score. It can spread locally, invading adjacent structures, or by lymphatic spread to sacral, iliac and para-aortic nodes, and haematogenous spread to bones (sclerotic lesions), liver or lungs. The prognosis is variable, depending on the stage of cancer at presentation.

64. c. Several viruses are known to be carcinogenic. Both deoxyribonucleic acid (DNA) and ribonucleic acid (RNA) viruses can cause cancers. It is thought that when a virus infects a cell, it inserts part of its own genome into the cell nucleus, activating a proto-oncogene and causing uncontrolled cellular proliferation. Cervical cancer has a strong association with human papilloma virus type 16 and 18 infection. Epstein–Barr virus is known to cause Hodgkin lymphoma, nasopharyngeal carcinoma, as well as Burkitt lymphoma.

65. a. Male breast cancer accounts for fewer than 1% of all cases of breast cancer. Invasive ductal carcinoma is the most common cancer type in males, followed by papillary tumours. Invasive lobular carcinoma, lymphoma and sarcoma of the male breast remain exceptionally rare.

66. e. Lymphoma is a malignant tumour of lymphoid cells originating in lymph nodes and presents with lymph node enlargement. Hepatoma is malignancy of the liver (hepatocellular carcinoma). Melanoma is a malignant tumour of melanocytes and causes the majority of skin cancer–related deaths. Seminoma is a malignant germ cell tumour of the testis, originating from the germ cell epithelium of seminiferous tubules. Papilloma is a benign epithelial tumour and can be either squamous cell or transitional cell papilloma.

67. d. Gastro-oesophageal reflux disease can result in metaplasia of the oesophageal squamous epithelium into columnar epithelium (Barrett's oesophagus). Oesophageal webs found in Plummer–Vinson syndrome are also associated with squamous cell carcinoma, and women are at a higher risk than men. Patients with untreated coeliac disease are also at risk of developing oesophageal cancer. Tobacco smoking and alcohol usage have shown to increase risk, more so if used together.

68. a. Cervical carcinoma has a strong association with human papilloma virus (HPV) types 16 and 18. Epstein–Barr causes Burkitt lymphoma as well as nasopharyngeal carcinoma. Human immunodeficiency virus (HIV) causes Kaposi sarcoma and hepatitis B virus (HBV) can lead to hepatocellular carcinoma.

69. b. *Helicobacter pylori* has been associated with gastric lymphoma. *Aspergillus flavus* produces aflatoxins and is associated with a high incidence of hepatocellular carcinoma. Schistosomiasis infection has been implicated with bladder cancer and *Clonorchis sinensis* is associated with cholangiocarcinoma. *Bacillus cereus* causes food-borne illnesses.

70. e. Tumour suppressor genes inhibit a cell from developing into cancer. When these genes are mutated, the inhibition is lost and cells progress into cancer formation with other genetic changes. Breast cancer can develop from mutation to BRCA1 and BRCA2 genes. The gene affected in multiple endocrine neoplasia (MEN) is RET, among others. This leads to tumours of the pituitary, parathyroid, pancreas, thyroid and adrenal glands. Li–Fraumeni syndrome, as a result of mutation to p53, causes ovarian and breast carcinomas as well as astrocytomas. Von Hippel–Lindau syndrome is caused by mutation to the Von Hippel–Lindau gene, resulting in renal carcinoma, phaeochromocytoma and haemangioblastoma. Myc is a type of oncogene, which influences a normal cell to turn into a tumour cell.

71. c. Paraneoplastic symptoms are a consequence of the presence of cancer, but not directly caused by cancer cells or metastasis. They are mediated by humoral or immunological factors. Cushing syndrome and syndrome of inappropriate antidiuretic hormone (SIADH) may occur in bronchial carcinoma. Dermatomyositis can result from either breast or bronchial carcinoma, whereas membranous glomerulonephritis can be initiated from various types of underlying malignancy. Hyperparathyroidism can occur in the presence of parathyroid adenoma, which is a direct metabolic effect of the tumour.

72. c. Cancer screening programmes are aimed to detect cancers in an asymptomatic population, in order to reduce the morbidity and mortality related to them. A screening programme should fulfil certain principles: safe, cost-effective and beneficial to society. Breast cancer screening is carried out by mammogram every 3 years on women aged between 50 and 70 years old (to be extended in England to 47–73 in 2016). Cervical cancer screening is carried out by exfoliative cytology on women aged between 25 and 64 years old every 3–5 years.

73. e. Transcoelomic spread is a route of cancer metastasis across a body cavity, such as the peritoneal, pleural and pericardial cavities. Ovarian and colon cancer can spread to the peritoneum, causing ascites. Stomach cancer spreads to the ovaries (Krukenberg tumour). Bronchial carcinoma can spread to the pleura causing pleural effusion. Prostate cancer usually spreads to the bone via the haematogenous route.

74. a. Krukenberg tumours arise as a result of transcoelomic spread of gastric carcinoma to the ovaries; therefore the tumour type is more likely to be adenocarcinoma. Krukenberg tumours are seen in middle-aged to elderly women following menopause. The prognosis of patients with this type of tumour is generally poor.

75. e. Adenoma is a benign tumour of epithelial glandular tissue and lipoma is a benign tumour of adipose tissue. Chondrosarcoma is a malignant tumour of cartilage. Rhabdomyosarcoma is a malignant tumour of voluntary muscle, whereas leiomyoma is a benign tumour of smooth muscle.

76. b. Risk factors for the development of colorectal cancer are:

- Family history
- Adenomatous polyps
- Familial polyposis coli
- Hereditary non-polyposis colorectal cancer
- Ulcerative colitis
- Gardner syndrome
- Previous colorectal cancer
- Low fibre intake
- High carbohydrate and fat intake
- Low vitamin C + E intake

77. a. Osteosarcoma is the most common primary tumour of bone. It is more common in males, usually under the age of 30. They commonly occur in long bones and spread via the bloodstream to the lungs. Osteoclastomas occur in young adults at the end of long bones. Metastases are uncommon. Chondrosarcomas are slow-growing tumours from chondroblasts (may arise from a pre-existing osteochondroma). Myelomas are rare before the age of 50. They have early dissemination with widespread marrow replacement.

78. e. The most common histological type of oesophageal cancer in the United Kingdon is adenocarcinoma. Most cancers are found in the distal oesophagus. Barrett's oesophagus refers to metaplasia of stratified squamous epithelium to simple columnar epithelium. This occurs secondary to gastro-oesophageal reflux of stomach acid and may progress to adenocarcinoma. Carcinoembryonic antigen (CEA) is not sensitive or specific enough to be used as a screening/diagnostic test in the context of oesophageal cancer. Plummer–Vinson syndrome is a nutritional deficiency syndrome comprised of dysphagia (due to pharyngeal/oesophageal web formation), microcytic anaemia (iron deficiency) and splenomegaly. Plummer–Vinson syndrome is associated with the development of squamous cell carcinoma.

79. d. Some common carcinogens and their resultant neoplasms include:

- *B-Naphthylamine:* Transitional cell carcinoma (bladder)
- *Asbestos:* Pulmonary mesothelioma
- *Nickel:* Squamous cell carcinoma of the larynx, bronchus
- *Vinyl chloride:* Hepatic angiosarcoma
- *Arsenic:* Carcinoma of the bronchus, skin

- *Hardwood sawdust:* Nasopharyngeal adenocarcinoma
- *Aflatoxin (produced by Aspergillus flavus):* Hepatocellular carcinoma
- *Cyclophosphamide:* Lymphoma, leukaemia
- *Nitrosamines:* Gastric adenocarcinoma

80. c. Familial polyposis coli (FAP) is an autosomal dominant condition and accounts for 2% of all colorectal carcinomas. Hereditary non-polyposis colorectal cancer (HNPCC) is an autosomal dominant condition and accounts for 5% of all colorectal carcinomas. The most commonly implicated genetic abnormalities include:

- *Chromosome 2:* mutS gene
- *Chromosome 3:* mutL gene
- *Chromosome 5:* APC gene (**Note:** The earliest detectable genetic mutation)
- *Chromosome 17:* p53 gene
- *Chromosome 18:* DCC gene

81. e. Risk factors include:

- Excess salt intake; smoked/pickled foods
- Excess alcohol consumption (especially undiluted spirits)
- *H. pylori* infection
- Male gender (M/F = 3:1)
- Atrophic gastritis (e.g. pernicious anaemia)
- Chronic gastritis
- Familial adenomatous polyposis
- Smoking
- Age (exponential increase in incidence after 50 years)

Studies to date suggest that blood group A is associated with stomach cancer but not necessarily causative or contributory.

82. a.

- *Class A:* 5-year survival = 90–100%; disease limited to muscularis propria
- *Class B:* 5-year survival = 75%; disease breaches muscularis; no lymph node involvement
- *Class C1:* 5-year survival = 30–40%; lymph node involvement, but not the apical node
- *Class C2:* 5-year survival = 25%; apical lymph node involvement
- *Class D:* 5-year survival = <5%; distant metastases

83. c. Examples of tumour markers include:

- *Pituitary:* Adrenocorticotropic hormone (ACTH), human chorionic gonadotropin (hCG), prolactin
- *Adrenal:* Cortisol
- *Carcinoid:* 5-Hydroxyindoleacetic acid (5-HIAA)
- *Oat cell:* adrenocorticotrophic hormone, antidiuretic hormone
- *Prostate:* Prostate-specific antigen (PSA)
- *Hepatic:* alpha-fetoprotein (AFP) (NB: also cirrhosis, pregnancy, hepatitis, neural tube defect)

- *Colorectal:* Carcinoembryonic antigen (CEA) Ca 19-9 (advanced)
- *Testicular teratoma:* β-hCG, CEA, AFP
- *Testicular seminoma:* Placental alkaline phosphatase
- *Breast:* Ca 15-3
- *Pancreatic:* Ca 19-9
- *Thyroid:* Thyroglobulin, calcitonin (medullary carcinoma)
- *Phaeochromocytoma:* Vanillylmandelic acid (VMA)

84. c. Triple assessment of any breast lump includes: (1) history and examination, (2) mammography and ultrasound scan (USS) and (3) fine-needle aspiration (FNA) or preferentially a core biopsy. The lump is aspirated, if possible, and the contents fixed to a slide before being sent to the laboratory. Once the sample is analyzed, the results are graded as

- *C1* – insufficient sample
- *C2* – benign
- *C3* – uncertain
- *C4* – suspected breast cancer
- *C5* – breast cancer

85. e. TNM is a universally used cancer classification system (tumour, node, metastases) and used in breast cancer. The simplified staging system for breast cancer is:

- *T1* – <2 cm in diameter
- *T2* – 2–5 cm
- *T3* – >5 cm
- *T4* – spread to chest wall or skin
- *N0* – no palpable lymph nodes
- *N1* – ipsilateral axillary mobile nodes
- *N2* – ipsilateral axilla fixed nodes or internal mammary nodes
- *N3* – lymph nodes supra- or infraclavicularly/arm lymphoedema
- *M0* – no evidence of distant metastases
- *M1* – presence of distant metastases

86. e. Increased vitamin C consumption is thought to be protective. In addition, risk factors include a diet high in salt-containing foods, preserved foods, previous gastric surgery, advancing age, smoking and atrophic gastritis, and there is a known familial link associated with mutations of the e-cadherin (a cellular adhesion molecule) gene. Patients often present with advanced disease with non-specific symptoms including anaemia, weight loss, dyspepsia and dysphagia. The majority of gastric carcinomas are adenocarcinomas.

87. c. This man has presented with a history and presentation typical of multiple myeloma (MM), which is common in the 65- to 70-year-old age group and more frequent in males. Due to bone marrow infiltration by the myeloma, patients often present with problems of anaemia, infection and bleeding. High paraprotein levels, causing hyperviscosity, lead to renal impairment, amyloidosis and renal infarction. MM is also associated with lytic bone lesions, which can cause spinal cord compression. Urine samples contain Bence–Jones proteins, and serum protein electrophoresis can be diagnostic. Skull X-rays show a typical pepper pot skull.

88. e.   Carcinoembryonic antigen (CEA) is used to monitor treatment and recurrence in cancers of the bowel, lung, pancreas, stomach and ovary; raised concentrations have been noted in smokers. Of note, tumours markers alone are not generally used to diagnose cancer. Note that α-Fetoprotein (AFP) is associated with liver, germ cell, ovarian and testicular cancer; Ca 19-9 is associated with pancreatic cancer but sometimes cancer of the bile ducts or bowel; and Ca 125 is associated with ovarian cancer. Human chorionic gonadotrophin (hCG) is a marker for testicular and trophoblastic cancer.

89. b.   The presentation is one of pancreatic carcinoma, which is often diagnosed late because of non-specific symptoms. Risk factors include age over 60 years, male, smoking, diabetes, obesity, chronic pancreatitis and diets low in vegetables but high in red meat. Ca 19-9 is elevated in 71–93% of pancreatic cancer patients.

90. a.   Human herpes virus 8 (deoxyribonucleic acid virus) has been found in almost all cases of Kaposi's sarcoma in both human immunodeficiency virus (HIV)-positive and HIV-negative patients. Human T-cell leukaemia virus type 1 is a ribonucleic acid virus that is prevalent in the Caribbean and Japan. The virus infects CD4-positive T-cells and causes expression of interleukin-2 and the interleukin-2 receptor leading to T-cell proliferation. The infection predisposes to monoclonal tumour progression via subsequent mutations. Epstein–Barr virus is associated with the development of four cancers: African Burkitt's lymphoma, some B-cell lymphomas in the immunosuppressed, some Hodgkin's lymphomas and some nasopharyngeal cancers. Hepatitis B virus has a high correlation with hepatocellular carcinoma in places where infection is endemic, such as Southeast Asia. Human papilloma virus has 77 subtypes, of which some are associated with malignant or benign lesions. Squamous cell carcinomas of the cervix, vulva, vagina, anus, oral cavity and larynx have been associated with this virus. Cervical carcinoma is stimulated by sexually transmitted human papilloma virus, particularly types 16 and 18.

91. e.   Premalignancy has two aspects: premalignant lesions and premalignant conditions. A premalignant lesion is an identifiable lesion that has an increased risk of progression to a malignant neoplasm. The types of lesions are diverse and range from benign neoplasms that become malignant to *in situ* malignancy (e.g. Bowen disease) and conditions that follow a metaplasia–dysplasia sequence (e.g. Barrett oesophagus).

A premalignant condition is a non-neoplastic condition which is associated with an increased risk of developing malignant tumours. Examples include crohn disease leading to colorectal carcinoma, xeroderma pigmentosum leading to melanoma and basal and squamous cell carcinoma, Paget disease of the bone leading to osteogenic sarcoma and cirrhosis of the liver leading to hepatocellular carcinoma.

SURGICAL IMMUNOLOGY

92. b. Hypersensitivity reaction is an immunological response with a severe and harmful reaction to extrinsic antigens. The four main types of hypersensitivity reactions according to the Gell and Coombs classification are:

Type I – immediate allergic reaction owing to overproduction of immunoglobulin E (IgE)
Type II – antibody (immunoglobulin M or immunoglobulin G)-dependent cytotoxic reaction to antigens on cell surface
Type III – deposition or formation of immune complexes in the tissues
Type IV – cell-mediated immune memory response involving T-lymphocytes

93. d. Natural killer cells form part of the innate immune system. They make up about 10% of the peripheral blood lymphocytes. They have no T-cell receptors; however, they have the ability to kill virally infected cells and tumour cells.

94. c. An innate immune system is formed by physical barriers, such as mucosal epithelium, and secretions with antibacterial activity, such as lactoferrin. Soluble mediators such as C-reactive protein and mannose-binding lectin help to enhance the activity of innate and specific responses to an antigen.

95. d. B-lymphocytes initially produce immunoglobulin (Ig) M antibodies after an encounter with an antigen as they are effective in complement fixation and opsonization. IgM has a short half-life of approximately 5 days. Subsequently, the B-cell undergoes class switch on T-cell recognition of an epitope on the same antigen. The B-cell then produces IgA and IgE at around 1 week and IgG at around 3 weeks.

96. a. Immunoglobulin (Ig) A is secreted onto mucosal surfaces. It prevents the initial adherence or mucosal penetration of bacterial and viral pathogens, thereby contributing to respiratory and gastrointestinal immunity. IgA deficiency along with absence of IgG is noted in primary antibody deficiency (PAD). Patients present with respiratory infections caused by encapsulated bacteria such as *Haemophilus influenza*, *Streptococcus pneumonia* and mycoplasma. Gastrointestinal infections are caused by *Giardia*, *Campylobacter* and *Salmonella*.

97. e. Hypersensitivity refers to excessive reactions produced by the normal immune system. Hypersensitivity reactions require a presensitized state of the host. Hypersensitivity reactions can be divided into four types: I, II, III and IV, based on the mechanisms involved and time taken for the reaction. Type I hypersensitivity is also known as immediate or anaphylactic hypersensitivity and is mediated by immunoglobulin E. Type II hypersensitivity is also known as cytotoxic hypersensitivity. Type III hypersensitivity is also known as immune complex hypersensitivity. Type IV hypersensitivity is also known as cell-mediated or delayed-type hypersensitivity, for example tuberculin, or Mantoux reaction.

98. e. Hyperacute rejection is caused by immunoglobulin G anti-HLA class I or ABO antibodies. Accelerated rejection occurs in <5 days. Acute rejection occurs in <100 days because of T-cell effector function and antibody-mediated endothelial damage. Chronic rejection takes >100 days to manifest, and unlike acute rejection, it cannot be managed with immunosuppression.

99. c. Primary antibody deficiency (PAD) are disorders of B-cell development or function with impaired or absent antibody production. PAD presents with pneumonia, sinus and gastrointestinal infections because of the absence of immunoglobulin (Ig) G and IgA. PAD patients with low IgG levels are susceptible to *Mycoplasma* arthritis. It results in joint destruction and chronic pain. Treatment is a combination of surgery and tetracycline.

100. e. Thymomas are rare tumours with many patients being asymptomatic with lesions detected on chest X-rays or developing secondary to autoimmune disease. Approximately 80% of patients with myasthenia gravis have either thymic hyperplasia or thymomas. A majority of thymomas are benign and well encapsulated with the malignant tumours locally invasive. The thymus gland is also occasionally the site for metastatic spread from either bronchial or breast carcinomas.

The thymus gland can be the site for a number of tumours:

- Thymoma
- Hodgkin disease
- Non-Hodgkin disease
- Carcinoid
- Germ cell tumours – teratoma
- Thymic carcinoma
- Thymolipoma

101. a. The complement cascade can be summarized as follows:

- Classical pathway: Specific immunity
  - Antigen–antibody complex binds C1, 4 and 2.
  - C1, 4, 2 → C4b2a (C3 convertase).
  - C3 is subsequently cleaved to C3a and C3b.
    - C3a: Anaphylaxis, chemotaxis
    - C3b → activates C5 convertase.
- Alternative pathway: Innate immunity
  - Bacterial endotoxin aggregated immunoglobulin.
  - C3 is cleaved to C3a and C3b.
    - C3a: Chemotaxis
    - C3b → activates C5 convertase.
- Final common pathway
  - C5 convertase cleaves C5 into C5a and C5b.
    - C5a: Anaphylaxis, chemotaxis
    - C5b binds to C6, 7, 8 and 9 to form the membrane attack complex.

102. b. Di George syndrome is a primary immunodeficiency disease associated with an increased susceptibility to infections due to a reduced T-cell production and function. Other abnormalities include altered facial characteristics and cardiac defects. The remaining choices are correctly paired.

103. c. The classification of hypersensitivity can be summarized as follows:

Type I: Immunoglbulin (Ig) E on mast cells combines with antigens, with mast cell degranulation and histamine release, resulting in anaphylaxis (e.g. allergic rhinitis, some types of eczema, urticaria).

Type II: Non-IgE antibodies directly bind to cell surface antigens, with subsequent activation of the complement cascade (e.g. hyperacute allograft rejection, myaesthenia gravis, Goodpasture syndrome).

Type III: Circulating antigen–antibody immune complexes deposit in tissues, with activation of the complement cascade (e.g. glomerular nephritis post-streptococcal sore throat, subacute bacterial endocarditis).

Type IV: T-cell mediated (CD8: direct cell damage; CD4: delayed hypersensitivity), for example contact dermatitis, TB.

104. d. Monocytes are part of the cell-mediated immune response and are granulocytes derived from the myeloid cell line with a typical bilobed nucleus on peripheral blood film. They are activated into macrophages on entering the tissues by chemotaxis along concentration gradients of cytokines. They destroy bacteria by direct phagocytosis after binding to bacterial surface antigens that have specific corresponding receptors on the cell membrane. They also opsonize bacteria that are coated with antibodies bound to the bacterial surface antigens from B-cells. After phagocytosis, they present the antigens from lysed bacteria in association with major histocompatibility (MHC) type II complexes onto their own cell membranes where they are recognized by T-helper cells, which then stimulate B-cells to produce a specific antibody. They are part of the chronic immune response and can fuse together to form giant cells to phagocytose large foreign particles.

105. b. Fever (a rise in body temperature of 1–4°C) is one of the criteria for establishing the clinical diagnosis of the systemic inflammatory response syndrome. A rise in core body temperature is a response to the activation by substances called pyrogens. These substances stimulate prostaglandin synthesis in the vascular and perivascular cells of the hypothalamus. Bacterial products such as lipopolysaccharide (an exogenous pyrogen) stimulate leukocytes to release cytokines such as tumour necrosis factor (TNF) and interleukin-1 (endogenous pyrogens). These cytokines upregulate the cyclooxygenases that convert arachidonic acid into prostaglandins. Then, within the hypothalamus, prostaglandins (especially prostaglandin E2 [PGE2]) stimulate the production of neurotransmitters, such as cyclic adensoine monophosphate, whose function is to alter the temperature set point to a higher level.

106. e. In times of acute inflammation, leukocytes extravasate from capillaries and then migrate toward the site of injury by a process called chemotaxis. There are a number of chemoattractants, both exogenous (e.g. lipopolysaccharide) and endogenous. Endogenous chemoattractants include several chemical mediators: (1) complement, especially C5a; (2) products of the lipoxygenase pathway, predominantly leukotriene B_4 (LTB_4); and (3) cytokines, especially those of the chemokine family such as interleukin (IL)-8. The chemokine IL-8 is secreted by activated macrophages, endothelial cells and other cell types and induces activation and chemotaxis of neutrophils. It also has some activity on monocytes and eosinophils. The production of IL-8 is predominantly stimulated by microbial products and the two major cytokines involved in inflammation, which are interleukin-1 and tumour necrosis factor.

107. a. This is a classic presentation of anaphylaxis, a type I hypersensitivity reaction. Anaphylaxis occurs over a matter of minutes when an antigen binds to a previously sensitized immunoglobulin E antibody, which itself is bound to a mast cell. This activates the mast cell to release substances such as histamine, resulting in vasodilation, increased blood vessel permeability and smooth muscle contraction in the bronchus. Type 1 hypersensitivity reactions can be localized or systemic.

SURGICAL HAEMATOLOGY

108. d. Sickle cell disease is a hereditary haemoglobinopathy caused by abnormal haemoglobin (HbS). When deoxygenated, HbS molecules undergo aggregation (polymerization causing deformation of red cells). Sickling of red cells is initially a reversible phenomenon. However, with repeated episodes of sickling, membrane damage occurs and cells become irreversibly sickled, even when fully oxygenated. Vaso-occlusive crises are episodes of hypoxic injury and infarction associated with severe pain in the affected region. The most commonly involved sites are the bones, lungs, liver, brain and spleen. Abnormal red cells are also susceptible to haemolysis. Chronic haemolysis results in moderately severe anaemia associated with striking reticulocytosis and hyperbilirubinaemia.

109. c. Prostacyclin I_2 inhibits platelet aggregation and is a vasodilator. Nitric oxide plays an important role in vasodilatation and reduces platelet adhesion. Thrombomodulin activates protein C, which in itself causes inactivation of clotting factors Va and VIIIa. Tissue plasminogen activator (tPA) causes fibrinolysis. von Willebrand factor (vWF) is a platelet and factor VIII cofactor, making it important in procoagulation.

110. b. Heparin binds to antithrombin III, which inactivates thrombin and factor Xa. Activated thrombin promotes the conversion of fibrinogen to fibrin, thereby promoting clot formation. Factor Xa is an active protease that converts prothrombin to thrombin. By targeting thrombin and factor Xa, the coagulation cascade can be reduced. Low-molecular-weight heparin (LMWH) has the same effect on factor Xa when compared with unfractionated heparin; however, it has less of a direct effect on thrombin. Protamine is used as the reversal agent for heparin. It has slightly better action against unfractionated heparin than LMWH.

111. d. Tests for platelet function – bleeding time or adhesion studies. Prothrombin time – a measure of the extrinsic and common pathways (9–15 s). Activated partial thromboplastin time – a measure of the intrinsic and common pathways (30–40 s). Thrombin time – a measure of the final common pathway.

112. b. Iron deficiency anaemia is the most common cause of hypochromic microcytic anaemia. It can be caused secondary to either reduced oral intake, reduced absorption or increase in loss. The principal cause in premenopausal women is blood lost during menses. Iron deficiency anaemia is characterized by pallor, fatigue and weakness. Hair loss and light-headedness can also be associated with iron deficiency anaemia.

The blood smear of a patient with iron deficiency shows many hypochromatic, small red blood cells and may show poikilocytosis (variation in shape) and anisocytosis (variation in size). With more severe iron deficiency anaemia the peripheral blood smear may show target cells, hypochromic pencil-shaped cells and occasionally small numbers of nucleated red blood cells (reticulocytes).

113. c. Target cells are red cells with a ring of hypodense staining surrounded by a central area of increased staining and a further ring of increased staining at the edge of the cell, giving a bullseye 'target' appearance. They may be found in liver disease, thalassaemia or sickle cell disease. Howell–Jolly bodies are nuclear remnants found in red cells that are usually removed by the spleen; hence they appear post-splenectomy. Auer rods are long granular needles seen in the cytoplasm of leukaemic blast cells. They are found in acute myeloid leukaemia. Hairy cells are abnormal white cells with hair-like projections from the cytoplasm, seen in hairy cell leukaemia. Basophilic stippling is a description of granular bodies within red cells, occurring during periods of accelerated erythropoiesis such as lead poisoning.

114. e. Risk factors for developing a deep vein thrombosis (DVT) include prolonged surgery that can result in a prolonged period of immobility. Other patient factors include a history of cancer and use of the oral contraceptive pill. Pneumatic calf compression is a device used to intermittently compress the calf muscles, encouraging venous drainage. It is used intraoperatively to prevent a DVT from developing.

115. b. This represents an immediate life-threatening haemolytic transfusion reaction most likely precipitated by ABO incompatibility of the transfused blood. Signs include fever, hypotension, bleeding, haemoglobinuria, oliguria and jaundice. Reactions can occur with only 5–10 mL of incorrectly transfused blood. Immediate management should be to stop the transfusion and administer life support treatment as required.

116. d. Warfarin is an anticoagulant drug and is a synthetic derivative of coumarin. Warfarin is used mainly to reduce thrombosis and thromboembolic disease. It prevents the activation of vitamin K–dependent clotting factors such as II, VII, IX and X. As a result, thrombin formation and subsequently fibrin clot generation are affected, preventing blood clots from developing. Warfarin is teratogenic and is able to cross the placenta; therefore it should be avoided in the first trimester of pregnancy. Protein C deficiency is a rare genetic trait that predisposes to the prothrombotic state. Patients suffering from this condition are at a high risk of thromboembolic disease; hence lifelong warfarin is recommended. Commonly used antibiotics such as metronidazole and macrolide can increase the effect of warfarin by reducing the rate at which it is metabolized.

117. b. A thrombus is a solid mass formed in the living circulation from the components of the streaming blood. Thrombosis is the process of thrombus formation and is influenced by three factors (Virchow's triad): the blood flow, the blood constituents and the vessel wall. Changes in vessel wall that may cause thrombosis are atherosclerotic plaques and synthetic grafts, as well as artificial heart valves. The most common cause of arterial thrombosis is atherosclerosis. Changes in normal laminar blood flow may occur with prolonged immobility following surgery or trauma, and proximal occlusion of venous drainage by pregnancy or pelvic masses. The most common cause of venous thrombosis is stasis. During the formation of thrombus, alternate layers of platelets and blood clots (fibrin and red cells) are laid on the thrombus, giving a rippled appearance known as the lines of Zahn.

118. c. An embolus is an abnormal mass of undissolved material passing from one part of the circulation to another, affecting blood vessels too small to allow it to pass. Venous thromboembolism usually arises from veins in the lower limb and can lead to pulmonary embolism via the inferior vena cava and right side of the heart. Arterial thromboembolism arises from within the heart (mural thrombus, valvular thrombus), atherosclerotic plaques, aneurysms and the venous system (patent foramen ovale of atrial septa). Gas must be free within the blood and not dissolved in solution to embolize. An example is nitrogen embolism in divers ascending rapidly. Amniotic fluid embolism is a rare condition that occurs when the placenta is detached from the uterus, and amniotic fluid escapes into maternal circulation, potentially leading to disseminated intravascular coagulation (DIC) and death. Fat embolism is most commonly associated with long bone fractures, causing respiratory distress, confusion and seizures.

119. e. Evans syndrome is an autoimmune disease characterized by the combination of idiopathic thrombocytopenic purpura (ITP) and autoimmune haemolytic anaemia. ITP is characterized by a low platelet count, and autoantibodies to platelet antigens leading to their destruction. The bone marrow may be normal or show a slight increase in megakaryocytes. Initially, symptoms may include easy bruising on the limbs or bleeding from the genitourinary and alimentary tract. Secondary causes must be excluded before the diagnosis of ITP is made.

120. e. Vitamin B_{12} deficiency leads to macrocytic anaemia, and the bone marrow becomes hypercellular with megaloblasts. Defective cells are prematurely destroyed leading to a haemolytic anaemia. Vitamin B_{12} is normally absorbed by binding to intrinsic factor produced by parietal cells in the stomach and absorbed in the terminal ileum. In pernicious anaemia, there are parietal cell antibodies reducing the levels of intrinsic factor and hence vitamin B_{12} absorption. Complications include myelin degeneration in the posterior and lateral columns of the spinal cord, also known as subacute combined degeneration of the cord.

121. d. Most absorption is via the duodenum and upper jejunum in the ferrous form. Deficiency can be caused by blood loss, which can be either pathological or physiological. Other causes include increased requirements in childhood or pregnancy, malabsorption owing to gastrectomy or poor dietary intake. Classically, there are low numbers of reticulocytes, with a hypochromic, microcytic anaemia. Clinical findings include koilonychia. Iron deficiency anaemia is also associated with dysphagia because of the presence of a posterior cricoid web known as Plummer–Vinson syndrome. Leuconychia is seen in hypoalbuminaemia.

122. a. Pernicious anaemia is due to vitamin B_{12} deficiency and is associated with achlorhydria and gastric mucosal atrophy. Changes in the blood include pancytopenia with the red cells showing signs of macrocytosis and normochromia. There is hyperplasia of the bone marrow. Gastric atrophy is caused by an immune reaction against the parietal cell intrinsic factor. Nervous changes include subacute combined degeneration of the posterior and lateral columns of the spinal cord leading to ataxia and spastic paralysis. Atrophy of the epithelial surfaces commonly occurs in the tongue and vagina.

123. d. Leukaemias can be classified as acute or chronic, myeloid or lymphoid. Aetiological factors include human T-cell leukaemia virus-1 and genetic factors such as Down syndrome. The Philadelphia chromosome is found in more than 95% of cases of chronic myeloid leukaemia. Most cases of chronic lymphocytic leukaemia are of B-cell type with less than 5% of T-cell lineage. Acute lymphoblastic leukaemia is the most common form of childhood leukaemia.

124. c. Antithrombin III is an inhibitor of thrombin. Its action is potentiated by heparin. Congenital deficiency of antithrombin III is inherited in an autosomal dominant fashion. Both proteins C and S are synthesized in the liver and dependent on vitamin K. Protein C degrades factors Va and VIIIa promoting fibrinolysis. Protein S is a cofactor for protein C.

125. e. Platelets are non-nucleated cells formed in the bone marrow by fragmentation of the cytoplasm of megakaryocytes. The normal concentration in blood is $160–450 \times 10^9$/L with a mean survival of 8–10 days. Causes of thrombocytopenia are listed below:

- Reduced production
- Aplastic anaemia
- Drugs – alcohol, tolbutamide
- Viral infections
- Myelodysplasia
- Myeloma
- Megaloblastic anaemia
- Decreased platelet survival
- Idiopathic thrombocytopenic purpura (ITP)
- Drugs – heparin, quinine
- Post-transfusion
- Dated intravascular coagulation
- Hypersplenism
- Sequestration of platelets

126. d. Disseminated intravascular coagulation (DIC) results from the simultaneous activation of coagulation and fibrinolytic systems. This leads to the formation of microthrombi in many organs with the consumption of clotting factors and platelets leading to haemorrhage. Common causes include septicaemia, malignancy, trauma, shock, acute pancreatitis and amniotic fluid embolism. Diagnosis is confirmed by thrombocytopenia, decreased fibrinogen and elevated fibrin degradation products. Pulmonary embolism is not a recognized cause of DIC; however, there are cases reports of massive pulmonary embolism inciting DIC.

127. b. von Willebrand's disease refers to a family of bleeding disorders caused by an abnormality of the von Willebrand factor, a large multimeric glycoprotein that functions as the carrier for factor VIII. von Willebrand factor is also required for normal platelet adhesion. In primary haemostasis, von Willebrand factor attaches to platelets by the glycoprotein Ib receptor on the platelet surface, acting as an adhesive bridge between the platelets and damaged subendothelium at the site of vascular injury. In secondary haemostasis, von Willebrand factor protects factor VIII from degradation and delivers it to the site of injury.

128. c. In iron deficiency anaemia:

- Serum iron is low.
- Serum transferrin is raised.
- Serum ferritin is low.
- Blood film shows target cells and pencil cells (elliptocytes).

In anaemia of chronic disease:

- Serum iron is low.
- Serum transferrin is low.
- Serum ferritin is raised.
- Erythrocyte Sedimentation Rate (ESR) is typically elevated disproportionately to the degree of anaemia.
- Blood film shows marked rouleaux formation (i.e. stacking of erythrocytes).

129. b. Sickle cell disease is the result of an inherited single amino acid substitution mutation in the beta-haemoglobin chain that changes glutamine to valine. This increases the propensity of the haemoglobin to sickle under oxidative stress. Sickle haemoglobin is termed HbAS for heterozygous or HbSS in the more severe homozygous form.

130. d. Haemophilia B is an X-linked genetic disease which results in a lack of function or availability of clotting factor IX. It presents in a similar manner to haemophilia A and is also known as Christmas disease. Spontaneous or excessive haemorrhage sites include the joints/muscles, gastrointestinal and genitourinary system. Treatment involves either factor IX concentrate or prothrombin complex concentrate.

131. b. When classified according to the ABO system, blood cells from group A contain type A surface antigen on the red cell membranes and anti-B antibodies in the serum; similarly, group B red cells have type B surface antigen and anti-A serum antibodies, group O red cells have no surface antigens and both anti-A and anti-B serum antibodies, and group AB red cells have type A and type B surface antigens and no serum antibodies. Thus, if the patient's blood agglutinates with antisera anti-A then the red cells must carry the type A surface antigen, making it either group A or AB. The rhesus blood grouping system consists of 50 different surface antigens of which D is the most significant. A D-positive person has D antigens on the red cells, and no antibodies, while a D-negative person has no antibodies unless previously exposed (either during transfusion or placentally). As this patient's blood cells agglutinate with antisera anti-D, he carries the D antigen, making him D or Rh positive. Therefore, this patient's blood type is A positive.

132. c. Normal haemoglobin has two alpha and two beta chains. In sickle cell disease amino acid substitution occurs on the beta chain resulting in HbS being less soluble than HbA. It has an autosomal recessive inheritance. Sickling may be precipitated by infection, cold, hypoxia, dehydration or fever. Clinical presentation includes painful crises, aplastic crises, acute chest syndrome, priapism and focal neurological or ocular events.

133. a. The shelf life of platelets is 5–7 days if sealed in packaging that allows atmospheric oxygenation (promoting aerobic metabolism) and constant agitation at 22–24°C. Problems associated with platelet transfusion include infection, rhesus sensitization and alloimmunization. Fresh frozen plasma has two main components: cryoprecipitate and cryosupernatant, which are a rich source of clotting factors, von Willebrand factor, fibrinogen and other plasma proteins. It can be stored at –30°C for up to 12 months, and is administered in relation to the patient's weight.

134. d. disseminated intravascular coagulation can present with rash and is defined as the widespread intravascular activation of the clotting cascade leading to bleeding. Increased activated partial thromboplastin time (APTT) is one test that may lead to a diagnosis; however, it is not a sensitive test on its own. Many diseases and illnesses are associated with derangement in the APTT and prothrombin time (PT) clotting profile. Diagnosis is often made by clinical history with prolonged APTT and PT times, thrombocytopenia and high concentrations of fibrin degradation products.

SURGICAL MICROBIOLOGY

135. d.   Gas gangrene is a form of spreading tissue necrosis that occurs when spores of Clostridia infect wounds with extensive soft tissue or muscle injury. Palpable crepitus and gas shadows on radiographs may be noted.

136. a.   Prions are not infectious organisms but infectious proteins, and have been indicated in Creutzfeldt–Jakob disease. Fungi are eukaryotic organisms causing systemic or superficial infection. Viruses are intracellular parasites. Bacteria are infectious organisms, which can be divided into Gram-positive and Gram-negative organisms, and anaerobic and aerobic. Protozoa are unicellular eukaryotes that may develop into cysts. The most important protozoan worldwide is *Plasmodium*, which causes malaria.

137. e.   *H. pylori* is associated with chronic gastritis, mainly affecting the pyloric antrum. It colonizes the epithelial surface beneath a thin layer of mucous, causing an initial acute neutrophilic gastritis. The bacteria produce urease to break down urea, producing CO_2 and NH_3. This ammonia protects it from the acid environment of the stomach. The body then mounts an immune response to the presence of the organism resulting in epithelial damage. Persistence of the infection can last for many years, leading to mucin depletion and damage to the underlying epithelium, atrophy of the gastric glands and eventual intestinal metaplasia.

138. e.   *Staphylococcus aureus* is a Gram-positive coccus that occurs in clusters. *Streptococcus pyogenes* is a Gram-positive coccus that occurs in long chains. *Clostridium tetani* is a Gram-positive, anaerobic sporing bacillus. *Listeria monocytogenes* is a Gram-positive anaerobic non-sporing bacillus. *Bacillus anthracis* is a Gram-positive aerobic bacillus.

139. c.   Gram-negative bacilli: *Escherichia coli, Klebsiella, Proteus, Salmonella, Shigella, Yersinia, Serratia, Morganella*; Gram-negative cocci: *Neisseria*; Gram-positive rods: *Clostridium*.

140. e.   Tetanus is a rare condition caused by *C. tetani*, an anaerobic Gram-positive bacillus. The neurotoxin produced enters peripheral nerves travelling toward the spinal cord where the inhibitory activity of spinal reflexes is blocked. Clinical features include trismus (lockjaw) and opisthotonus. Treatment includes antitetanus immunoglobulin and intravenous benzylpenicillin. Despite this, mortality is around 50%.

141. a.   Betadine is bacteriocidal and has a wide antibacterial spectrum together with spores, fungi and viruses. Formaldehyde has a wide antibacterial spectrum and spores but not viruses. Glutaraldehyde has antiviral properties and kills spores slowly. Boiling water kills bacteria including tuberculosis and some viruses.

142. d.   Macrolides are usually used as a second-line drug when patients are penicillin allergic. They are active against Streptococci, Staphylococci, Clostridia and *Campylobacter*. They are used to manage soft tissue and respiratory tract infections. The main side effect when given intravenously is phlebitis. Nephrotoxicity and ototoxicity are seen with aminoglycosides.

143. b.

Virus	Hepatitis A	Hepatitis B	Hepatitis C	Hepatitis D	Hepatitis E
Type	Picornavirus	HepaDNA	RNA Flavivirus	Defective RNA	RNA Calcivirus
Spread	Faeco-oral	Parenteral	Parenteral	Parenteral	Faeco-oral
Incubation (weeks)	2–4	4–20	2–25	6–9	3–9
Chronic disease	No	5% adults, 90% children	Approximately 50%	Co-infection 5%	No
Vaccine	Yes	Yes	No	Protected by HBV vaccine if HBV negative	No

144. c.   *Actinomyces israelii* is the most commonly implicated pathogen. It is a Gram-positive rod bacterium which can live as a commensal organism on the skin, in the vagina and in the colon. The characteristic cause is progressive and indolent. Patients present with pain, fever, weight loss and sometimes a palpable mass. As a result, actinomycosis can be misdiagnosed as malignancy. Dental procedures may lead to cervical actinomycosis, and aspiration can cause pulmonary actinomycosis. The intrauterine contraceptive device (IUCD) has been implicated in the development of genital actinomycosis. Serology has no role in diagnosing actinomycosis. Sulphur granules may be produced from discharging sinuses and are characteristic, but not necessarily pathognomonic, of the disease.

145. b.   Clostridia are saprophytic (found in soil), Gram-positive, spore-producing anaerobic bacilli, with a variable resistance to oxygen. The species exhibits its pathological effects due to the production of exotoxins. The most commonly encountered species in medicine include:

C. difficile
C. difficile colitis results from a disturbance of the normal bacterial flora of the
    colon, colonization with *C. difficile* and release of exotoxins that cause mucosal
    inflammation and damage. The result is diarrhoea and colitis occasionally
    progressing to life-threatening toxic megacolon.
C. tetani
Spores of *C. tetani* produce two toxins: tetanolysin (a haemolysin with no
    recognized pathologic activity) and tetanospasmin.
Tetanospasmin moves from the contaminated site to the spinal cord, where it
    binds gangliosides at presynaptic inhibitory motor nerve endings, preventing
    the release of inhibitory neurotransmitters.
C. perfringens
Ingestion of exotoxin results in diarrhoea and vomiting.
The organism itself causes gas gangrene in the context of deep tissue infection.

C. botulinum

Botulinus exotoxin affects the peripheral nervous system.

146. c.   An endotoxin is a non-immunogenic heat-resistant lipopolysaccharide from the outer wall of the cell. The pathology effects of Gram-negative bacterium include:

- Complement activation
- Clotting cascade activation
- Leukotriene, prostaglandin and nitric oxide formation

An exotoxin is an immunogenic, heat-sensitive protein secreted from bacteria. Cholera, diphtheria and tetanus are all examples.

147. b.   Of those organisms mentioned, *Pseudomonas* is the only Gram-negative bacillus and is typically seen in immunocompromised patients and hospital-acquired infections. It is associated with respirators and drainage tubes. *Listeria* and *Actinomyces* are Gram-positive bacilli. *Moraxella* is a Gram-negative coccus that is seen in atypical pneumonia. *Staphylococcus aureus* is a Gram-positive coccus.

148. a.   *C.tetani* is a Gram-positive obligate anaerobic bacteria. It is found as spores in the soil and often enters the body through external wounds. *C.tetani* produces two toxins: tetanolysin and tetanospasmin. The neurotoxin tetanospasmin is carried by retrograde axonal transport to the central nervous system, where it fixes to gangliosides at the presynaptic junction of inhibitory nerve endings blocking inhibitory impulses. Passive immunization with immunoglobulin for high-risk patients may be required in cases where the risk of contamination is high.

149. e.   Necrotizing fasciitis is a rapidly spreading infection of the deeper layers of the superficial fascia and skin. The infection is commonly associated with *S. pyogenes* (group A streptococcus), *Vibrio vulnificus*, *C. perfringens* and *Bacteroides fragilis*. Group A streptococcus is the most commonly found organism and produces an exotoxin 'superantigen', which, non-specifically, stimulates immune cells. Consequently, there is excessive cytokine release and macrophage accumulation. The stimulated macrophages cause damage to local tissues by generating oxygen-derived free radical species. The infection can spread at an alarming rate and the initial cellulitis is associated with the appearance of dusky purple patches in its centre, which progress to skin necrosis secondary to thrombosis of its blood supply. Subcutaneous crepitus may also be palpated. If supportive measures and radical dissection are not carried out expediently, the infection is often fatal. Methicillin-resistant *S. aureus* has been known to cause monomicrobial infection but is not usually associated with necrotizing fasciitis.

150. d.   Septic arthritis is an inflammation of a synovial joint associated with a suppurative effusion. The aetiology is usually bacterial but viruses, mycobacteria and fungi can also be involved. The infective source is usually elsewhere in the body and the organism is deposited in the joint via haematological spread. *S. aureus* is the most common cause in adults and *Haemophilus influenzae* is the most common cause in children who have not been immunized. *Neisseria gonorrhoea* is found more commonly in young adults and *E. coli* is found more in drug addicts, the elderly and the seriously ill. Diagnosis is essentially clinical with the help of a Gram stain of the joint effusion.

SURGICAL BIOCHEMISTRY

151. d.   Gilbert syndrome is an autosomal recessive inherited metabolic disorder, causing increased levels of unconjugated bilirubin in the blood. It is a common hereditary cause of hyperbilirubinaemia. There is decreased activity of the enzyme glucuronyltransferase, which conjugates bilirubin in the liver. Bilirubin is excreted from the body only in the conjugated form. Typical presentation is painless jaundice during a concurrent illness.

152. c.   There are several causes of hypercalcaemia, but hyperparathyroidism and malignancy are the most common. Renal failure (decreased excretion) and hyperthyroidism (high bone turnover) can also cause hypercalcaemia. Clinical features of hypercalcaemia include 'stones' (kidney stones), 'bones' (bone pain), abdominal 'groans' and psychic 'moans'. Blood transfusion causes hypocalcaemia as high citrate levels bind to calcium.

153. b.   Addison's disease is a rare condition of chronic adrenal insufficiency, with lack of glucocorticoid and mineralocorticoid. Typically, there is a raised adrencorticotrophic hormone (ACTH) level and cortisol levels are reduced. Biochemically, the patient may have low sodium, with raised serum potassium, raised urea, low blood glucose and increased plasma renin activity with normal or reduced aldosterone. Clinically, the patient will have symptoms of dehydration and hypotension because of the mineralocorticoid deficiency. They may also have vomiting, loss of appetite, weight loss, lethargy, hypoglycaemia and postural hypotension due to glucocorticoid reduction. If the adrenal glands are non-functioning, an increase in ACTH can also increase melanocyte-stimulating hormone (MSH) levels, causing increased skin and mucosa pigmentation.

154. b.   Antidiuretic hormone acts in the distal convoluted tubule and collecting duct, causing the retention of water. In Syndrome of inappropriate antidiuretic hormone, retention of water results in dilutional hyponatraemia. Transurethral resection of prostate (TURP) syndrome results in hyponatraemia following the absorption of large volumes of bladder irrigation fluid. Diabetes insipidus may be neurogenic (i.e. deficient production of vasopressin) or nephrogenic (i.e. renal collecting duct insensitive to vasopressin) – the result is hypernatraemia due to excessive diuresis of hypotonic urine. Addison disease results in mineralocorticoid deficiency, with renal water loss, but greater sodium loss (comparatively). Nephrotic syndrome leads to salt retention, but greater water retention (comparatively) leading to dilutional hyponatraemia.

155. b.

- *Vitamin A:* night blindness
- *Vitamin D:* Rickets
- *Vitamin E:* Haemolytic anaemia
- *Vitamin K:* Clotting disorder
- *Vitamin B1:* Beriberi

- *Vitamin B2:* Dermatitis
- *Vitamin B3:* Pellagra
- *Vitamin B6:* Convulsions, anaemia
- *Vitamin B12:* Pernicious anaemia
- *Vitamin C:* Scurvy

PART IV
SYSTEM-SPECIFIC PATHOLOGY

CHAPTER 7
SYSTEM-SPECIFIC
PATHOLOGY

Questions

NERVOUS SYSTEM

1. To diagnose brainstem death, there should be which of the following?
   a. Fixed and unresponsive pupils
   b. Absent corneal reflex
   c. Absent gag reflex
   d. No motor response to face or limbs after supraorbital pressure
   e. All of the above

2. Which of the following statements regarding raised intracranial pressure is correct?
   a. Normal intracranial pressure in the supine position is 10–20 mmHg.
   b. Systemic effects of raised intracranial pressure include neurogenic pulmonary oedema.
   c. Cerebral herniation leads to contralateral pupil dilatation.
   d. Raised intracranial pressure does not lead to a Cushing's response.
   e. Cerebral herniation leads to optic nerve compression.

3. Neurofibromas are characterized by all of the following features except:
   a. The most common form occurs in the skin as cutaneous neurofibroma.
   b. Plexiform neurofibromas may arise around large nerve trunks.
   c. They can arise sporadically or in association with neurofibromatosis.
   d. They may grow to be large and become pedunculated.
   e. Plexiform neurofibromas have no tendency toward malignant transformation.

4. The following statements regarding a fat embolism are true except:
   a. Steroids have a role in the treatment of fat embolism.
   b. It can be a complication of long bone fracture.
   c. It can present as a petechial rash on the trunk.
   d. It may require admission to the intensive treatment unit.
   e. It is associated with osteoporosis.

5. The following statements about Brown–Séquard syndrome are true except:
   a. There is ipsilateral motor paralysis.
   b. There is contralateral loss of pain and temperature.
   c. It is caused by hemisection of the spinal cord.

d. It may arise as a result of invasive neoplasm.

e. There is contralateral loss of vibration sense.

6. A 20-year-old man is brought by ambulance to the accident and emergency department after being hit on the head with a cricket bat. He had loss of consciousness at the scene for 5 min with a lucid interval of recovery. Upon arrival to the hospital, you notice that he is developing an ipsilateral dilated pupil and a progressive hemiparesis. A computed tomography (CT) scan of the head is performed. Which one of the following findings is most likely to fit your diagnosis?

a. Intraventricular blood

b. Lenticular-shaped haematoma between skull and dura

c. Crescent-shaped haematoma between dura and arachnoid membrane

d. Intracerebral haemorrhage

e. Blood crossing the suture lines of the skull

7. A 60-year-old woman presents to the accident and emergency department with a short history of sudden-onset occipital headache, with no associated visual aura; she has had several episodes of vomiting prior to her attendance. She has a history of hypertension for which she takes regular oral medication and has never experienced these symptoms before. On examination she is haemodynamically stable and afebrile. She is drowsy, with neck stiffness and a positive Kernig's sign. She has no focal neurology. Which one of the following is the most likely diagnosis?

a. Subarachnoid haemorrhage

b. Meningitis

c. Subdural haematoma

d. Extradural haematoma

e. Intracerebral haemorrhage

8. With regard to tentorial herniation, which of the following affected structures is incorrectly paired with the clinical manifestation?

a. Occulomotor nerve – ipsilateral papillary dilatation

b. Ipsilateral cerebral peduncle – contralateral hemiparesis

c. Contralateral cerebral peduncle – ipsilateral hemiparesis

d. Midbrain – cortical blindness

e. Cerebral aqueduct – hydrocephalus

9. Which of the following statements regarding extracerebral haemorrhage is correct?

a. Extradural haemorrhage can be caused by bleeding from the bridging veins.

b. Subdural haemorrhage is seen with rupture from berry aneurysms.

c. Subarachnoid haemorrhage is seen with injuries to the middle meningeal artery.

d. Clinical features of extradural haemorrhage include contralateral hemiparesis and a dilated ipsilateral pupil.

e. Fifty percent of patients with a subarachnoid haemorrhage die within 6 months.

10. Concerning paragangliomas, which of the statement is correct?
    a. The jugular bulb is the most common location.
    b. Glomus tympanicum arises from the tympanic membrane.
    c. Lyre's sign is elicited on angiography of the carotid bifurcation.
    d. Approximately 30% are inherited.
    e. The potential for malignant spread is high.

11. A 32-year-old woman was brought into the emergency department after having suddenly collapsed in the street. A computed tomography (CT) of the head confirmed a large subarachnoid bleed secondary to a berry aneurysm. She is currently being monitored on the neurosurgical intensive care unit (ICU) where she suffered a seizure 3 days into her admission. Which of the following complications are not associated with a subarachnoid haemorrhage (SAH)?
    a. Cardiac abnormalities
    b. Rebleeding
    c. Vasospasm
    d. Hydrocephalus
    e. Hypernatraemia

12. A 10-year-old boy is brought to the attention of the surgical team on call after suffering a head injury from a minor road traffic incident. There was no loss of consciousness (LOC) but he has vomited two times and has a Glasgow Coma Scale (GCS) of 15. Which of the following management options are true?
    a. He requires a computed tomography scan immediately.
    b. He should be sent home.
    c. He should be admitted for neuro-observations.
    d. A skull X-ray is needed.
    e. He needs a neurosurgery referral.

13. Which of the following statements about meningitis is true?
    a. Bacterial meningitis is more common than viral meningitis.
    b. It is an infection of the subdural space.
    c. *Haemophilus influenzae* is a frequent cause of bacterial meningitis in the UK.
    d. Bacterial meningitis causes a decrease in glucose levels in cerebral spinal fluid (CSF).
    e. Meningococcaemia can cause a blanching rash.

14. A 30-year-old male is struck by a car travelling at 20 mph. He is unconscious for 5 min, after which his GCS returns to 15. After a further 30 min his GCS falls to 3 and he subsequently dies. A computed tomography scan of his brain before his death shows a biconcave high-density lesion in the left cerebral hemisphere. Which of the following is the most likely cause of death?
    a. Severe concussion
    b. Acute subdural haematoma
    c. Depression fracture of the occipital bone
    d. Acute subarachnoid haemorrhage
    e. Acute extradural haematoma

MUSCULOSKELETAL SYSTEM

15. Which of the following statements is correct with regard to osteochondromas?
    a. They present as slow-growing masses in late adolescence and early adulthood.
    b. They can be solitary or multiple.
    c. They are the most common benign bone tumour.
    d. All of the above.
    e. a and c only.

16. Which of the following conditions are known to be associated with the development of an osteosarcoma?
    a. Paget disease
    b. Bone infarcts
    c. Radiation exposure
    d. All of the above
    e. a and c only

17. Regarding a fat embolism, the following statements are true except:
    a. It may cause agitation and delirium.
    b. It can cause a rise in platelet numbers.
    c. It is associated with a petechial rash.
    d. It may be prevented with steroids.
    e. It is associated with long bone fractures.

18. Which of the following statements regarding upper limb pathology is correct?
    a. Klumpke paralysis may be associated with Horner syndrome.
    b. Poland syndrome is usually caused by a traumatic birth.
    c. Erb's palsy is caused by damage to C8–T1 roots of the brachial plexus.
    d. Klumpke paralysis typically has loss of sensation in the musculocutaneous nerve distribution.
    e. Poland syndrome usually affects patients bilaterally.

19. Which of the following statements regarding upper limb pathology is correct?
    a. Poland syndrome is characterized by muscular atrophy.
    b. The waiter's tip position is a sign of Klumpke paralysis.
    c. Poland syndrome is caused by damage to the upper aspect of the brachial plexus.
    d. Erb's palsy is usually caused by shoulder dystocia during birth.
    e. Syndactyly is a characteristic sign of Erb's palsy.

20. Which one of the following statements regarding rheumatoid arthritis (RA) is correct?
    a. It is associated with polycythaemia.
    b. Felty syndrome is a triad of rheumatoid arthritis, neutropenia and hepatomegaly.
    c. Extra-articular manifestations of RA include Caplan syndrome.
    d. It is an unsymmetrical deforming polyarthropathy.
    e. It is characterized by involvement of the distal interphalangeal joints.

21. Poland syndrome is characterized by all but which one of the following?
    a. There is underdevelopment or absence of the pectoralis muscle.
    b. Deformities are usually bilateral.
    c. There may be syndactyly.
    d. There may be a simian crease on the affected side.
    e. Males are affected more than females.

22. A 9-year-old boy presents with an acute history of pain in the groin radiating to the left knee, causing him to limp when he walks. He recently had an upper respiratory chest infection. An X-ray of the hip and knee is normal. Which of the following is the most likely diagnosis?
    a. Perthes disease
    b. Slipped upper femoral epiphysis (SUFE)
    c. Developmental dysplasia of the hip (DDH)
    d. Irritable hip
    e. Infected hip joint

23. An obese 13-year-old boy presents to your orthopaedic outpatient clinic complaining of pain in the left knee which is preventing him from playing football. On examination you note slight shortening of the left leg which is held in an externally rotated position. Which of the following is the likely pathology?
    a. Perthes disease
    b. Slipped upper femoral epiphysis
    c. Hip fracture
    d. Acute transient synovitis
    e. Septic arthritis

24. A 9-year-old boy was referred to orthopaedic outpatients with a 6-week history of left leg pain. Plain radiographic imaging revealed a large opacity in the femur. Karyotyping reveals chromosomal translocation between chromosomes 11 and 22. Bone biopsy is performed and reveals small round blue cells. Which of the following is the most likely feature on plain radiographic imaging?
    a. Prominent endosteal scalloping
    b. Bony expansion
    c. Layers of reactive bone deposition – 'onion skin' pattern
    d. Opacity between cortex and raised periosteum – Codman's triangle
    e. Epiphyseal involvement

25. A 60-year-old woman was referred to the orthopaedic outpatient department with a 6-month history of left hip pain. X-ray reveals joint space narrowing, osteophyte formation, juxta-articular sclerosis and subarticular bone cysts, but no periarticular erosions. Which of the following pathophysiological features is not typical of her arthritis?
    a. Fibrillation formation in deeper layers
    b. Stretching of collagen network
    c. Chondrocyte population increases
    d. Swelling of hyaline joint cartilage
    e. Remodelling of subchondral bone

26. Which of the following statements regarding calcification is true?
    a. There is one recognized form of calcification.
    b. Orthotopic calcification may be classified into three groups.
    c. Dystrophic calcification is only seen in damaged heart valves.
    d. There are two phases of dystrophic calcification.
    e. Metastatic calcification does not occur in areas where acidic substances are excreted.

27. Which of the following plain radiographic characteristics is consistent with the diagnosis of osteoarthritis (OA)?
    a. Periosteal osteoporosis
    b. Erosions
    c. Soft tissue swelling
    d. Fracture
    e. Subchondral sclerosis

28. An 84-year-old lady falls in the street onto an outstretched arm sustaining a distal radius fracture. Which of the following statements is true regarding fractures of the distal forearm?
    a. A volar backslab is the preferred method to immobilize a Colles fracture.
    b. An above-elbow plaster of Paris (POP) cast is indicated as first-line treatment in comminuted distal ulnar and radial fractures.
    c. Open fractures always need reduction and fixation in theatre.
    d. A haematoma block is the preferred method of analgesia when operating on distal radial fractures.
    e. Open fractures rarely require immediate administration of antibiotics.

29. Which of the following statements is true in first-line treatment of neck of femur fractures in elderly patients?
    a. Operative fixation is the overriding priority.
    b. A thorough history is very important in the identification of the type of fracture.
    c. Intracapsular fractures are best treated with an intramedullary hip screw.
    d. A thorough history (including collateral) is often important in the identification of perioperative risk.
    e. Parenteral analgesia is not required.

30. Which of the following statements is true regarding greenstick fractures of the forearm?
    a. Greenstick fractures usually remodel well.
    b. Immobilization is not indicated.
    c. Greenstick fractures involve a complete break of the cortex.
    d. Vascular compromise is usually present.
    e. Greenstick fractures occur in all age groups.

31. Which one of the following statements is true regarding supracondylar fracture of the humerus?
    a. It is commonly associated with radial nerve palsy.
    b. It occurs most likely from non-accidental injury in children.

c. It can lead to distal vascular compromise.
d. It should not be immobilized prior to theatre.
e. None of the above.

32. A 7-year-old girl presents to the accident and emergency department after a fall onto her arm. The X-ray shows that the capitellum is not transected by the anterior humeral line. Which of the following is the likely diagnosis?
    a. Diaphyseal fracture of the humerus
    b. Fracture of the radius
    c. Fracture of the ulna
    d. Fracture of the olecranon
    e. Supracondylar fracture

33. On your orthopaedic ward round you see a patient who fractured his left tibia 2 days ago. On examination you discover that he has suddenly become tachycardic, tachypnoeic and acutely confused. On closer inspection you see a diffuse petechial rash over his chest and left upper arm. This history and examination supports a diagnosis of which one of the following?
    a. Pulmonary embolism
    b. Fat embolism
    b. Myocardial infarction
    c. Lower respiratory tract infection
    e. Disseminated intravascular coagulation

34. Which of the following statements about Paget's disease of the bone are true?
    a. It is the second most common metabolic bone disease.
    b. It is characterized by excessive and organized bone turnover.
    c. Most patients experience bone pain.
    d. All of the above.
    e. a and c only.

35. Which of the following statements about osteomalacia are true?
    a. It is characterized by inadequate mineralization of osteoid.
    b. It is commonly caused by a deficiency of calcium.
    c. Bone pain is rarely a symptom.
    d. All of the above.
    e. a and b only.

36. Where in the body are osteosarcomas most commonly found?
    a. The mandible
    b. The humerus
    c. The hip
    d. The knee
    e. The ankle

37. When looking at radiographs of joints, which of the following radiological changes are used to diagnose osteoarthritis?
    a. Joint space narrowing
    b. Periarticular erosions
    c. Osteophytes

    d.   All of the above

    e.   a and c only

38. Pseudogout is a form of crystal arthropathy. Which one of the following statements regarding pseudogout is true?
    a.   The crystals are made from sodium urate crystals.
    b.   It has a prevalence of 10–20% in those aged 85 years or older.
    c.   Men and women are equally affected.
    d.   The crystals are negatively birefringent.
    e.   The first metatarsophalangeal joint is most commonly affected.

39. During a hand examination of a patient in your orthopaedic clinic, you identify several features characteristic of rheumatoid arthritis. Which of the following signs are typically associated with this type of arthritis?
    a.   Z thumb deformity
    b.   Heberden's node
    c.   Ulnar deviation of the carpometacarpal joints
    d.   All of the above
    e.   a and b only

40. With respect to rheumatoid arthritis, which of the following statements is true?
    a.   The large joints are usually involved first.
    b.   The disease is associated with human leukocyte antigen (HLA) DR4.
    c.   The presence of rheumatoid factor is diagnostic.
    d.   Rheumatoid factor is an immune complex of immunoglobulin A (IgA).
    e.   Interleukin-4 (IL-4) is an important cytokine in disease progression.

RESPIRATORY SYSTEM

41. The following are known causes of acute respiratory distress syndrome (ARDS) except:
    a. Sepsis
    b. Smoke inhalation
    c. Fat embolus
    d. Acute renal failure
    e. Acute pancreatitis

42. A 35-year-old patient is admitted to the hospital with acute pancreatitis secondary to excessive alcohol consumption. Over the following 6 h, he rapidly deteriorates, and a diagnosis of acute respiratory distress syndrome (ARDS) is made. The following statements regarding ARDS are true except:
    a. It is characterized by a $PO_2:FiO_2$ ratio of <200 mmHg change.
    b. There are bilateral pulmonary infiltrates on chest X-ray.
    c. It is commonly managed in a general ward.
    d. It causes release of inflammatory mediators.
    e. It produces hyaline fibrosis of the lung.

43. The following are potential clinical consequences of local invasion of bronchial carcinoma except:
    a. Horner syndrome
    b. Cardiac failure
    c. Pain and numbness in the arm
    d. Hoarseness
    e. Facial oedema

44. Which statement regarding the pathology of lobar pneumonia is incorrect?
    a. It is typically seen in adults between 20 and 50 years.
    b. The common aetiological agent is *Streptococcus pneumoniae*.
    c. Resolution usually begins on days 8–10.
    d. During red hepatization the gross appearance of the lungs is red, solid and dry.
    e. The grey hepatization phase occurs between 2 and 4 days.

45. An 80-year-old male has been exposed to asbestos during his working life as a plumber. Which of these statements regarding asbestos is correct?
    a. Chrysotile is associated with pulmonary mesothelioma.
    b. Amosite is associated with pulmonary mesothelioma.
    c. Amphibole 'blue' fibres penetrate the lungs more deeply than serpentine fibres.
    d. Crocidolite is a flexible, serpentine mineral, composed of long 'woolly' fibres.
    e. Asbestos exposure characteristically leads to adenocarcinoma.

46. Which of the following carcinogens is typically associated with lung carcinoma?
    a. Single chest X-ray
    b. Fallout from nuclear explosions

c. Radium

d. Uranium

e. Thorium dioxide

47. An 80-year-old gentleman presents to the emergency department with abdominal pain localized to the right upper quadrant. You note on examination a right-sided thoracotomy scar through which the patient states a lobectomy for lung cancer was performed 15 years ago. He has a past history of heavy smoking prior to his diagnosis of lung cancer. Which of the following lung cancers is most closely associated with tobacco smoking?

a. Squamous cell carcinoma

b. Small cell carcinoma

c. Large cell carcinoma

d. Adenocarcinoma

e. Mesothelioma

BREAST DISORDERS

48. Which of the following statements is correct with respect to risk factors for carcinoma of the breast?
    a. Menarche at a young age is a known risk factor.
    b. Radiation increases the risk.
    c. Carcinoma of the endometrium is associated with increased risk.
    d. All of the above.
    e. a and c only.

49. A 45-year-old lady presents with a palpable lump in the left breast. Following clinical and radiological assessment in the breast clinic, a core biopsy is performed which reveals the lump to be a sarcoma. Which of the following comments regarding breast sarcoma is correct?
    a. It always follows radiotherapy for previously treated breast cancer.
    b. It develops mainly in the pectoralis major muscle.
    c. Wide local excision is the standard operative procedure.
    d. Formal axillary dissection is mandatory.
    e. Chemotherapy is curative.

50. A 38-year-old woman presents to the breast clinic with a small palpable breast lump. She undergoes triple assessment confirming the presence of a lump. Fine-needle aspiration is inconclusive and the patient requests a formal excision. The histology reveals it to be a phyllodes tumour. Which of the following statements is incorrect?
    a. Phyllodes tumour is a rare form of breast tumour.
    b. Phyllodes tumour is a fibroepithelial neoplasia.
    c. It is best treated with radiotherapy.
    d. About 20% of benign tumours recur, requiring further excision and potential mastectomy.
    e. It has malignant potential.

51. Which of the following is not a recognized risk factor for the development of breast cancer?
    a. Age
    b. Early menarche
    c. Low socioeconomic class
    d. BRCA-2 gene
    e. Nulliparity

52. Breast cancer is the leading cause of cancer-associated death in females in the 15- to 54-year age group. The risk factors for the development include all the following except for which one?
    a. BRCA2
    b. BRCA1
    c. Fibroadenoma
    d. Hormone replacement therapy (HRT)
    e. Early menarche

53. A woman undergoes a right-sided mastectomy for multifocal lobular carcinoma *in situ*; this is accompanied with level 2 axillary lymph node clearance. Up to which level have the nodes been removed?
    a. Medial border of pectoralis minor
    b. Lateral border of pectoralis minor
    c. Level of axillary vein
    d. The border of the first rib
    e. Level of the axillary artery

54. When taking a history from a patient with suspected breast cancer, which of the following criteria is not a recognised risk factor?
    a. Hispanic race
    b. Radiation exposure
    c. Tobacco
    d. Adult weight loss
    e. Menarche starting after 14 years old

55. When examining a breast, in which area are you most likely to palpate a carcinoma?
    a. Subareolar
    b. Upper medial quadrant
    c. Lower medial quadrant
    d. Upper lateral quadrant
    e. Lower lateral quadrant

56. A 55-year-old lady presents with advanced breast cancer. Subsequent investigations are arranged to assess for metastatic spread. Breast cancer metastasizes to which of the following organs?
    a. Bone
    b. Brain
    c. Adrenal gland
    d. All of the above
    e. a and b only

57. Which of the following modes of presentation of breast cancer is the most common?
    a. Breast mass discovered by palpation
    b. Asymptomatic tumour discovered by mammography
    c. Breast pain
    d. Nipple involvement
    e. Distant metastasis

58. A 65-year-old male presents with painless bilateral gynaecomastia. Which of the following medications is associated with gynaecomastia?
    a. Amoxicillin
    b. Thyroxine
    c. Spironolactone
    d. Furosemide
    e. Aspirin

CARDIOVASCULAR SYSTEM

59. A 70-year-old man presents to hospital following a collapse at home 1 h ago. On examination, there is a pulsatile, expansile mass in the abdomen, which is tender. The patient is shocked and hypotensive despite 2 L of crystalloid given by the paramedics. Which of the following statements is true regarding aneurysms and the management in this patient?
    a. The patient should have rapid and fast intravenous (IV) fluids through two large IV cannulae.
    b. The patient should be taken to theatre as soon as possible after discussion with the vascular surgeons.
    c. The patient should be resuscitated and stabilized in the high-dependency area of the emergency department before being taken to theatre.
    d. In this scenario the patient should have a computed tomography scan before any intervention.
    e. In this scenario the patient should have a bedside ultrasound scan (USS) before proceeding to theatre.

60. During a preoperative clinic you examine a patient's heart. While auscultating you hear an ejection systolic murmur, which is loudest in the second intercostal space on the right side. What valvular abnormality is this patient likely to have?
    a. Mitral stenosis
    b. Mitral regurgitation
    c. Aortic stenosis
    d. Aortic regurgitation
    e. Pulmonary stenosis

61. What is considered to be the gold standard investigation for a suspected deep vein thrombosis (DVT)?
    a. Duplex ultrasound Doppler
    b. Magnetic resonance imaging (MRI) of leg
    c. Ascending contrast venography
    d. ^{125}I-fibrogen scanning
    e. Sequential calf measurements

62. A 69-year-old gentleman attends the vascular outpatient clinic following an incidental finding of a pulsatile, expansile mass in his abdomen by his general practitioner (GP). Which of the following is the most common aetiology for an aneurysm?
    a. Infective
    b. Congenital
    c. Atherosclerotic
    d. Inflammatory
    e. Traumatic

63. You are called to see a 67-year-old woman who had a total hip replacement 7 days ago following a hip fracture. She had been mobilizing around the ward earlier that day. On examination you see that her entire right leg is swollen with visible superficial veins. Her calf is noted to be 2.5 cm larger on the right than the left. From the information given what is her Wells score?

    a. 1
    b. 2
    c. 3
    d. 4
    e. 5

ENDOCRINE SYSTEM

64. Which one of the following statements regarding autoimmune thyroid disease is correct?
    a. Antithyroid-stimulating receptor antibodies are seen in Hashimoto disease.
    b. Antithyroid peroxidase antibodies are seen in Hashimoto's (a and b) disease.
    c. There is a high thyroid-stimulating hormone (TSH) in Graves disease.
    d. There is a low free thyroxine (T_4) in Graves disease.
    e. Thyroid acropachy is seen in Plummer disease.

65. Which one of the following statements regarding hyperaldosteronism is correct?
    a. Conn syndrome is an example of secondary hyperaldosteronism.
    b. Secondary hyperaldosteronism is caused by overactivity of the renin–angiotensin system.
    c. Typically, the patient is hypotensive.
    d. Low sodium levels are found in hyperaldosteronism.
    e. Raised potassium levels are found in hyperaldosteronism.

66. Which of the following is not a common cause of secondary diabetes mellitus?
    a. Pancreatitis
    b. Corticosteroids
    c. Down syndrome
    d. Congenital lipodystrophy
    e. Gastrinoma

67. Which of the following is not a recognized cause of Addison disease?
    a. Meningococcal septicaemia
    b. Amyloidosis
    c. Blastomycosis
    d. Tuberculosis
    e. Cytomegalovirus

68. A 57-year-old male attends the preoperative assessment clinic in preparation for his laparoscopic cholecystectomy. He informs you that he has a past history of pheochromocytoma, for which he has undergone treatment. Which of the following statements regarding phaeochromocytoma is correct?
    a. It is characterized by undersecretion of catecholamines.
    b. It originates in the chromaffin cells.
    c. Twenty percent arise from outside the adrenal medulla.
    d. Fifty percent are malignant.
    e. pheochromocytoma is a tumour of multiple endocrine neoplasia (MEN) syndrome type I.

69. A 51-year-old female attends the general surgical clinic with a 3-month history of a palpable neck lump, which appears to be slowly increasing in size. The fine-needle aspiration performed is suspicious of malignancy, and following surgery, the histological report mentions the presence of psammoma bodies in the specimen. Psammoma bodies are seen in which thyroid malignancy?
    a. Follicular carcinoma
    b. Papillary carcinoma
    c. Medullary carcinoma
    d. None of the above
    e. All of the above

70. Which of the following statements is correct regarding gastrointestinal carcinoids?
    a. They rarely produce local symptoms.
    b. Systemic endocrinopathies such as Zollinger–Ellison syndrome, Cushing syndrome and hyperinsulism may occur.
    c. They can manifest with cutaneous flushes, diarrhoea, nausea and vomiting.
    d. All of the above.
    e. a and c only.

71. The following conditions are part of multiple endocrine neoplasia syndrome type I except:
    a. Pituitary adenoma
    b. Parathyroid adenoma
    c. Pheochromocytoma
    d. Pancreatic islet cell tumour
    e. Adrenal cortical adenoma

72. The signs and symptoms of Cushing syndrome include all but which one of the following?
    a. Interscapular fat pad
    b. Hypertension
    c. Thin skin
    d. Weight loss
    e. Impaired glucose tolerance

73. Which one of the following is the most common type of malignant thyroid tumour?
    a. Papillary
    b. Follicular
    c. Lymphoma
    d. Medullary
    e. Anaplastic

74. Which of the following thyroid tumours commonly spreads haematologically?
    a. Papillary
    b. Follicular
    c. Lymphoma
    d. Medullary
    e. Anaplastic

75. Which of the following thyroid tumours is associated with the multiple endocrine neoplasia syndrome?
    a. Papillary
    b. Follicular
    c. Lymphoma
    d. Medullary
    e. Anaplastic

76. Which statement regarding carcinoid tumours and syndrome is incorrect?
    a. Cells are able to reduce silver compounds known as argentaffin cells.
    b. Argentaffin cells express chromogranin.
    c. Carcinoid syndrome is characterized by flushing and diarrhoea.
    d. Excess serotonin production leads to fibrosis.
    e. Thirty percent of carcinoid tumours of the appendix occur at the tip.

77. A 34-year-old male presents with generalized fatigue and neck swelling. Following clinical and biochemical analysis, a diagnosis of Hashimoto thyroiditis is made. Which of these statements regarding Hashimoto's thyroiditis is correct?
    a. It occurs more often in males.
    b. It is an inherited condition.
    c. On microscopy the gland is infiltrated with neutrophils.
    d. It is the most common cause of hyperthyroidism.
    e. It is associated with human leukocyte antigen (HLA) DR5.

78. Concerning hyperparathyroidism, which statement is correct?
    a. Hyperplasia accounts for the majority of cases.
    b. Carcinoma accounts for approximately 5% of cases.
    c. Secondary hyperparathyroidism is characterized by hypercalcaemia and hypophosphataemia.
    d. Tertiary hyperparathyroidism is characterized by hypercalcaemia and hyperphosphataemia.
    e. Multiple adenomas account for 5% of cases.

79. A 48-year-old lady presents to her GP with progressively worsening fatigue, weight loss and occasional diarrhoea. She notes that her skin has become more pigmented despite rarely walking in the sunshine. Blood tests are arranged accordingly. Which of the following best describes the biochemical changes seen in Addison disease?
    a. Hypernatraemia, increased serum adrenocorticotropic hormone (ACTH), decreased cortisol
    b. Increased ACTH, decreased cortisol, hyperkalaemia
    c. Hypokalaemia, hyponatraemia, increased ACTH
    d. Decreased ACTH, increased cortisol, hypernatraemia
    e. Decreased ACTH, increased cortisol, hyperkalaemia

80. Concerning medullary carcinoma of the thyroid, which of the following statements is correct?
    a. It stains with apple-green dichroic birefringence on application of Congo red.
    b. It is associated with multiple endocrine neoplasia type I.

c. It is sporadic in approximately 90% of cases.
d. It is derived from follicular cells.
e. It has a poor prognosis, with a 5-year survival of approximately 10%.

81. A 78-year-old male presents to the surgical clinic with a short history of a rapidly enlarging neck lump and alteration of his voice. On examination, there is evidence of a goitre that is firm and irregular. This clinically appears to be an anaplastic thyroid carcinoma. Which of the following statements regarding this type of thyroid cancer is correct?
   a. It has a 5-year survival rate of 20%.
   b. It is likely to arise from thyroid epithelial cells.
   c. It is associated with multiple endocrine neoplasia type II.
   d. It rarely arises on a background of existing thyroid disease.
   e. It has a prevalence of approximately 15% of thyroid carcinomas.

82. Concerning multiple endocrine neoplasia, which statement is correct?
   a. Type I is characterized by medullary thyroid carcinoma.
   b. Type IIa is characterized by pancreatic adenoma.
   c. Type I is characterized by pituitary adenoma.
   d. Type IIa is characterized by submucosal neurofibromas.
   e. Type I, but not type II, is characterized by parathyroid hyperplasia.

83. Concerning papillary thyroid carcinoma, which statement is correct?
   a. It is the second most common histological variant of thyroid cancer.
   b. It is multifocal in approximately 50% of cases.
   c. It is found incidentally in 25% of postmortem examinations.
   d. It has a 5-year survival rate of 20%.
   e. Its mode of spread is classically haematogenous.

84. A 42-year-old woman has been diagnosed with a lump in her neck. She is referred for fine-needle aspiration cytology (FNAC) of what is identified as a lump in the thyroid gland. An FNAC report reveals Thy5. Which one of the following FNAC reports does this correspond to?
   a. Benign
   b. Insufficient material
   c. Suspicious but not diagnostic of malignancy
   d. Follicular lesion
   e. Definite malignancy

85. Which of the following statements regarding acromegaly is true?
   a. Acromegaly is caused by a decrease in circulating growth hormone (GH).
   b. Acromegaly is associated with excessive sweating.
   c. Acromegaly is associated with a decreased incidence of hernias.
   d. Acromegaly is associated with hypotension.
   e. A drop in circulating GH levels after a glucose load is diagnostic.

86. Which of the following statements about prolactinomas is false?
   a. Prolactinomas account for 10% of hyperfunctioning pituitary adenomas.
   b. Hyperprolactinaemia is only caused by a prolactinoma.
   c. Hyperprolactinaemia causes galactorrhoea.

    d. Prolactinomas do not occur in men.

    e. Prolactinomas are most commonly diagnosed between the ages of 40 and 60 years.

87. Which one of the following statements about Cushing syndrome is true?
    a. Cushing syndrome can be associated with hyperpigmentation.
    b. Cushing syndrome can be caused by a pituitary or adrenal tumour.
    c. Cushing syndrome can be associated with hyperkalaemia.
    d. All of the above.
    e. a and b only.

88. Which of the following are features of hyperthyroidism?
    a. Weight loss
    b. Thyroid acropachy
    c. Heat intolerance
    d. All of the above
    e. None of the above

89. Which of the following are features of hypothyroidism?
    a. Tachycardia
    b. Myxoedema
    c. Weight gain
    d. All of the above
    e. b and c only

GENITOURINARY SYSTEM

90. Which of the following is not a recognized sequela of pelvic inflammatory disease?
    a. Ectopic pregnancy
    b. Dysmenorrhoea
    c. Ovarian tumours
    d. Chronic pain
    e. Infertility

91. The following statements concerning bladder tumours are true except:
    a. Transitional cell carcinoma (TCC) is the most common type.
    b. They may be associated with schistosomiasis infection.
    c. Gonadotrophin-releasing analogues have a role in treatment.
    d. Smoking is a recognised risk factor.
    e. They may spread via the haematogenous route.

92. The following statements regarding testicular tumours are true except:
    a. They are associated with an undescended testis.
    b. Seminoma causes raised α-fetoprotein levels in 90% of cases.
    c. Teratomas are chemosensitive.
    d. Teratomas commonly spread to lungs and liver.
    e. The peak incidence of seminoma occurs in 30- to 40-year-olds.

93. Renal calculi can be formed from a variety of different solutes. Which one of the following most commonly forms renal stones?
    a. Calcium oxalate
    b. Uric acid
    c. Struvite
    d. Cystine
    e. Calcium phosphate

94. A 42-year-old man presents with right-sided loin-to-groin pain with microscopic haematuria. Plain KUB (X-ray showing kidneys, ureter and bladder) shows evidence of renal stone at the level of L3. Of the following potential renal stones, which one is most likely to be causative in his case?
    a. Calcium oxalate
    b. Uric acid
    c. Struvite
    d. Cystine
    e. Calcium phosphate

95. A 65-year-old woman with a history of recurrent urinary tract infection presents with colicky right iliac fossa (RIF) pain radiating to the groin. Her abdomen is tender in the RIF with minimal flank pain. There is no evidence of peritonism. Her urine dip is positive for blood, nitrites and leukocytes. A plain KUB (X-ray showing kidneys, ureter and bladder) does not show any evidence of a stone; however, an intravenous urogram (IVU) shows right-sided

hydronephrosis to the vesicoureteric junction. What is the most likely diagnosis?

a. Calcium oxalate renal stone
b. Appendicitis
c. Struvite renal stone
d. Abdominal aortic aneurysm
e. Calcium phosphate renal stone

96. A 30-year-old man is diagnosed as having testicular teratoma. In which of the following lymph node groups would lymphadenopathy most likely occur?

a. Para-aortic
b. Axillary
c. Superficial inguinal
d. Internal iliac
e. None of the above

97. A 70-year-old man presents with a superficial infection of his scrotal skin. Which of the following lymph node groups is the infection likely to spread to?

a. Para-aortic
b. Axillary
c. Superficial inguinal
d. Internal iliac
e. None of the above

98. A 60-year-old male diabetic attends the accident and emergency department with a 4-day history of progressive discoloration of his scrotum with severe pain and pruritus. On examination he is feverish, tachycardic and the area is erythematous and malodorous. A diagnosis of Fournier gangrene is made by the accident and emergency team. Which one of the following statements regarding his management is correct?

a. The patient can be discharged with oral antibiotics and urology follow-up.
b. Any infected tissue can be debrided on the ward under local anaesthetic.
c. Initiation of intravenous broad-spectrum antibiotics is not necessary.
d. The patient will require gross surgical debridement of the area under general anaesthesia.
e. There is a low risk of systemic infection and multiorgan failure.

99. A young man presents to the Accident and Emergency department with left-sided loin pain radiating to his groin. An intravenous urogram is performed confirming the presence of a urinary tract calculus. Which of the following statements regarding such calculi is incorrect?

a. Urinary calculi occur in 5–10% of the population.
b. Ninety percent of urinary calculi are radio-opaque.
c. Urate stones arise in acidic urine.
d. The most common form is calcium oxalate calculi.
e. Urate stones are radiolucent.

100. A 72-year-old man presents to hospital with painless haematuria and frequency. Cystoscopy confirms the presence of a tumour of the bladder. Which of the following is not a recognized aetiological factor for bladder tumours?
    a. Benzidine
    b. Bladder diverticulae
    c. Ectopia vesicae
    d. Schistosomiasis
    e. Alcohol

101. A 20-year-old man presents to the urology clinic with a painless testicular lump. An ultrasound scan confirms a testicular tumour. Preoperative tumour markers reveal a lactate dehydrogenase (LDH) 1.5 times normal, α-fetoprotein (AFP) levels of 900 ng/mL and human chorionic gonadotrophin (hCG) levels of 4378 mIU/L. Based on these, which one of the following is his serum tumour marker stage?
    a. Sx
    b. S0
    c. S1
    d. S2
    e. S3

102. A 25-year-old man is awaiting retroperitoneal lymph node dissection for a metastatic testicular tumour. Which of the following tumour markers are not routinely used in testicular cancer?
    a. Placental alkaline phosphatase (PLAP)
    b. Lactate dehydrogenase (LDH)
    c. α-Fetoprotein (AFP)
    d. γ-Glutamyltransferase (GGT)
    e. Carcinoembryonic antigen (CEA)

103. A 36-year-old male attends the accident and emergency department with a 4 h history of sudden left testicular pain and vomiting. Clinical examination reveals a very tender cord and swollen left testis. Elevation of the testicles provides some relief. Urine analysis is positive. Which of the following organisms is not known to cause epididymitis?
    a. *Chlamydia trachomatis*
    b. *Streptococcus pyogenes*
    c. *Mycobacterium tuberculosis*
    d. *Amiodarone*
    e. *Escherichia coli*

104. A 65-year-old male presents to the surgical team following a fall from 2 m landing on his right loin. Which of the following statements regarding renal injury is true?
    a. Bruising over the loin is unlikely to indicate renal injury.
    b. If the patient has macroscopic haematuria this may indicate significant renal injury.
    c. Patients with renal injury present with frank bleeding per urethra.
    d. Renal function tests are important in the diagnosis of traumatic renal injury.
    e. A normal ultrasound scan excludes renal injury.

GASTROINTESTINAL SYSTEM

105. All of the following can cause portal hypertension with the exception of which condition?
    a. Congenital atresia
    b. Schistosomiasis
    c. Constrictive pericarditis
    d. Polycythaemia
    e. Gallstones

106. Congenital pyloric stenosis may occur in association with which of the following?
    a. Turner syndrome
    b. Oesophageal atresia
    c. Trisomy 18
    d. All of the above
    e. None of the above

107. Which of the following statements regarding abdominal compartment syndrome is correct?
    a. It is defined as an increased intra-abdominal pressure of >10 mmHg.
    b. Peritoneal dialysis is a recognized cause of secondary abdominal compartment syndrome.
    c. Cardiac effects of abdominal comportment syndrome include a decrease in the central venous pressure.
    d. Pancreatitis is a recognized secondary cause of abdominal compartment syndrome.
    e. Prevention includes tight primary abdominal closure following surgery.

108. Crohn disease is characterized by which of the following pathological features?
    a. Transmural involvement of the bowel with skip lesions
    b. Non-caseating granulomas
    c. Cobblestone appearance of mucosa with crypt abscesses
    d. All of the above
    e. a and b only

109. A 60-year-old lady is referred by the medical team with abdominal pain and distention. An abdominal radiograph shows grossly dilated large bowel. Which of the following is a cause of toxic megacolon?
    a. *Clostridium difficile*
    b. Ulcerative colitis
    c. *Campylobacter*
    d. Ischaemic colitis
    e. All of the above

110. Hamartomatous polyps of the gastrointestinal tract are commonly associated with which one of the following conditions?
    a. Turner syndrome
    b. Kartagener syndrome

   c. Klinefelter syndrome
   d. Peutz–Jeghers syndrome
   e. Di George syndrome

111. What is incarceration of the vermiform appendix within a femoral hernia otherwise known as?
   a. De Garengeot hernia
   b. Amyand hernia
   c. Richter hernia
   d. Spigelian hernia
   e. Littre hernia

112. What is incarceration of the vermiform appendix within an inguinal hernia otherwise known as?
   a. De Garengeot hernia
   b. Amyand hernia
   c. Richter hernia
   d. Spigelian hernia
   e. Littre hernia

113. What is the name given to a hernia occurring between the rectus abdominis and the semilunar line?
   a. De Garengeot hernia
   b. Amyand hernia
   c. Richter hernia
   d. Spigelian hernia
   e. Littre hernia

114. A 20-year-old woman presents to the accident and emergency department with severe central crampy abdominal pain gradually worsening over the past 3 days, associated with absolute constipation and vomiting. She has no relevant past medical or family history. On examination, she is clinically dehydrated, with a heart rate of 120 bpm and blood pressure of 75/50 mmHg. She has circumoral pigmentation. Abdominal X-ray shows an isolated loop of dilated small bowel. At laparotomy she is found to have intestinal intussusception requiring small bowel resection and primary anastomosis. Within this resected segment there are several polyps. Which one of the following is the most likely diagnosis?
   a. Familial adenomatous polyposis
   b. Peutz–Jeghers syndrome
   c. Systemic lupus erythematosus
   d. Crohn disease
   e. Lymphoma

115. Which one of the following is not a cause of pancreatitis?
   a. Gallstones
   b. Hypothermia
   c. Hypocalcaemia
   d. Thiazide diuretics
   e. Corticosteroids

116. A 43-year-old woman is brought by ambulance to the accident and emergency department having been stabbed in the upper abdomen with a kitchen knife. On examination, there is no evidence of active bleeding; however, she has a heart rate of 132 bpm, blood pressure of 94/68 mmHg and is pale. After catheterization, you note that her urine output is 10 mL/h. You start the appropriate trauma management. This woman is suffering from which one of the following?
    a. Stage I haemorrhagic shock
    b. Stage II haemorrhagic shock
    c. Stage III haemorrhagic shock
    d. Stage IV haemorrhagic shock
    e. Cardiogenic shock

117. A 20-year-old woman presents with a 2-day history of right iliac fossa pain, constant in nature. On examination she is haemodynamically stable, with guarding in the right iliac fossa. Her blood tests are unremarkable. A diagnostic laparoscopy is performed to reveal a normal appendix. You perform a thorough investigation of the abdomen and find a Meckel's diverticulum. Which one of the following statements is incorrect regarding Meckel's diverticulum?
    a. It is a remnant of the vitellointestinal duct.
    b. It is more common in males.
    c. It may contain gastric acid–secreting epithelium.
    d. It can present with rectal bleeding.
    e. It always requires surgical removal if found.

118. Complications of Meckel's diverticulum include all of the following. Which one is the least common complication?
    a. Volvulus
    b. Discharging umbilical sinus
    c. Peptic ulceration
    d. Intussusception
    e. Leiomyoma

119. A 25-year-old woman presents with recurrent right iliac fossa pain with increased bowel frequency over the past 5 months. This settles and then returns several days later. She has loss of appetite and significant weight loss. On examination she has swollen lips and oral ulceration. Her abdomen is tender with guarding over the right iliac fossa. Her urine shows low concentration of ketones, with a negative β-Human chorionic gonadotropin (hCG) test. Which one of the following is the most likely diagnosis?
    a. Ulcerative colitis (UC)
    b. Crohn disease
    c. Appendicitis
    d. Ectopic pregnancy
    e. Meckel's diverticulum

120. Which one of the following statements regarding Crohn disease is correct?
    a. Crohn is commonly characterized by continuous lesions.
    b. It is characterized by mucosal non-caseating granulomatous inflammation.
    c. Surgery is curative.

    d. It mainly affects the terminal ileum.

    e. Anal lesions are uncommon.

121. A 40-year-old man presents to the accident and emergency department with a prolonged history of bloody diarrhoea, which has become more frequent. He is occasionally faecally incontinent and has the sudden urge to pass stool. He has no recent history of foreign travel. This is associated with a central crampy abdominal pain. On examination he is pyrexial and tachycardic with a distended abdomen, which is generally tender. Which one of the following is the most likely diagnosis?

    a. Crohn disease

    b. Ulcerative colitis

    c. Infective diarrhoea

    d. Haemorrhoids

    e. Caecal carcinoma

122. Which one of the following statements regarding Ulcerative colitis (UC) is correct?

    a. Fistulae are common in UC.

    b. It is characterized by transmural inflammation.

    c. It rarely involves the rectum.

    d. The risk of colon cancer is similar to that of the general population.

    e. Severe acute UC can lead to toxic megacolon.

123. Which of the following statements regarding cirrhosis is incorrect?

    a. Biliary causes include gallstones and cystic fibrosis.

    b. Methyldopa is a recognized cause of cirrhosis.

    c. Complications of cirrhosis include portal hypertension and hepatocellular carcinoma.

    d. Primary sclerosing cholangitis is associated with ulcerative colitis.

    e. Primary biliary cirrhosis is a chronic disorder which commonly affects women over the age of 70.

124. Which statement concerning gallstones is correct?

    a. The principal constituents of gallstones are cholesterol, phospholipids and peptides.

    b. Carcinoma of the gallbladder is not associated with gallstones.

    c. Cholesterol stones are associated with *Escherichia coli* infection.

    d. Mixed stones make up 80% of gallstones.

    e. Bile pigment stones are usually associated with Crohn disease.

125. What is the name given to the type of hernia where only one sidewall of the bowel is involved, leading to strangulation?

    a. De Garengeot hernia

    b. Amyand hernia

    c. Richter hernia

    d. Spigelian hernia

    e. Littre hernia

126. Which statement regarding tumours of the small intestine is correct?
    a. Peutz–Jeghers syndrome is an autosomal recessive condition.
    b. Approximately 20% of adenocarcinomas occur at the duodenum.
    c. T-cell lymphoma is often seen in patients with a long history of coeliac disease.
    d. Gastrointestinal stromal tumours (GISTs) rarely metastasize to the liver.
    e. A decreased risk of carcinoma is seen with coeliac disease.

127. Which of the following statements about familial adenomatous polyposis (FAP) is correct?
    a. The condition is inherited as autosomal recessive.
    b. Malignancy often develops before the age of 20.
    c. There is male preponderance.
    d. The combination of polyposis, desmoid tumours, osteomas and sebaceous cysts is termed Gardner syndrome.
    e. The gene responsible for the disease is on the long arm of chromosome 6.

128. Concerning diverticulae, which of the following statements is correct?
    a. Meckel's diverticulum is always solitary.
    b. Duodenal diverticula are usually solitary.
    c. A sigmoid diverticulum is a 'true' diverticulum.
    d. A pharyngeal diverticulum occurs at a congenital weakness between the two components of the superior constrictor.
    e. True diverticula are usually acquired.

129. A 42-year-old man presents to the accident and emergency department with severe epigastric pain of sudden onset accompanied by nausea and vomiting. The pain is particularly worse on movement. He has no significant past medical history. Incidentally, he mentions a 4-month history of dyspepsia-like symptoms, which are relieved with over-the-counter antacids, although today the pain is similar in nature but unresolved with medication. Which one of the following is the investigation of choice?
    a. Erect chest X-ray (CXR)
    b. Abdominal X-ray (AXR)
    c. Full blood count (FBC)
    d. Ultrasound (US) abdomen
    e. Oesophagogastroduodenoscopy (OGD)

130. An 8-year-old male presents with a 1-day history of generalized abdominal pain, which has now localized to the right iliac fossa. There is nausea and vomiting and he reports some diarrhoea and passing painless blood per rectum (PR). Which one of the following is the most likely underlying pathology?
    a. Appendicitis
    b. Crohn's colitis
    c. Meckel diverticulum
    d. Diverticulitis
    e. Viral gastroenteritis

131. A 21-year-old female presents with bloody diarrhoea and central abdominal pain. She undergoes a diagnostic colonoscopy, which demonstrates Crohn's colitis. Which of the following histological features supports a diagnosis of Crohn disease over ulcerative colitis?
    a. Granulomas
    b. Mucosal inflammation
    c. Continuous inflammation
    d. Caseating granulomas
    e. Crypt abscesses

132. A 40-year-old man is brought into the accident and emergency department complaining of severe abdominal pain and vomiting. Blood tests show a neutrophil count of 17×10^9/L, lactate dehydrogenase (LDH) of 550 IU/L, glucose of 8 mmol/L and urea of 16.1 mmol/L. Arterial blood gas (ABG) shows pH 7.29, PaO$_2$ 7.6 kPa, PaCO$_2$ 3.1 kPa, BE −6.1 on room air. Which of the following represents his Glasgow prognostic score with the given results?
    a. 3
    b. 4
    c. 5
    d. 6
    e. 7

133. A 45-year-old known alcoholic is brought into hospital with nausea, vomiting and severe epigastric pain that requires large doses of opioid analgesics to control. Which of the following results is associated with an increased risk of severe pancreatitis according to the Glasgow prognostic score?
    a. Albumin 33 g/L
    b. Glucose 9 mmol/L
    c. Age 50 years
    d. Calcium 1.98 mmol/L
    e. Urea 15 mmol/L

134. You are called to see an obese 43-year-old woman who was seen by your colleague in surgical outpatients last week with right upper quadrant pain. She has now presented with worsening pain associated with nausea and vomiting and has been unable to eat or drink anything for 24 h. Which of the following results would classify her as having an increased risk of severe pancreatitis?
    a. Amylase 1000 U/L
    b. Bilirubin 45 μmol/L
    c. Alkaline phosphatase 350 U/L
    d. Urea 19 mmol/L
    e. Amylase 1423 U/L

135. A 39-year-old obese man is referred via his general practitioner for open-access endoscopy after complaining of a 1-year history of dyspepsia. Upper gastrointestinal (GI) endoscopy demonstrates circumferential oesophagitis.

Which of the following stages of endoscopically detectable oesophagitis does this represent?

a. Stage A
b. Stage B
c. Stage C
d. Stage D
e. Stage E

136. A mother notices that her newborn baby boy is drooling excessively. On feeding him, he swallows normally, but moments later starts to cough and appears to choke on the milk, which is brought up through his nose. The diagnosis of oesophageal atresia is confirmed by passing a nasogastric tube, which subsequently coils in the lower oesophagus and is visible on chest X-ray. Which of the following is the most common type of this condition?

a. Type A
b. Type B
c. Type C
d. Type D
e. Type E

137. A newborn presents with profuse bilious vomiting at birth with fullness in the epigastric region. Abdominal X-ray (AXR) shows the 'double bubble' sign. Which of the following genetic conditions is this is associated with?

a. Patau syndrome
b. Edwards syndrome
c. Down syndrome
d. Turner syndrome
e. Fragile X syndrome

138. A 4-week-old baby presents with his mother with a 3-day history of absolute constipation. Examination reveals a diffusely tender abdomen with absent bowel sounds. Plain abdominal X-ray shows a distended colon. Which one of the following pathological findings is consistent with the likely diagnosis?

a. Absence of mural ganglionic cells
b. *KRAS2* gene mutation
c. CFTR gene mutation
d. Small round blue cells
e. *Trypanosoma cruzi* infection

139. An elderly female presents with left iliac fossa pain, a change in bowel habit and a fever. Her abdomen is soft with tenderness and guarding limited to the left iliac fossa. Which of the following management options is best in the initial hour of presentation?

a. IV antibiotics
b. CT scan
c. Mid-stream urine
d. Laparoscopy
e. Laparotomy

DERMATOLOGICAL DISEASES

140. The epidermis is composed of five layers. Which of the following epidermal layers is the most superficial?
    a. Stratum corneum
    b. Stratum lucidum
    c. Stratum granulosum
    d. Stratum spinosum
    e. Stratum basale

141. The epidermis is composed of five layers. Which of the following epidermal layers is the deepest?
    a. Stratum corneum
    b. Stratum lucidum
    c. Stratum granulosum
    d. Stratum spinosum
    e. Stratum basale

142. Which one of the following statements regarding squamous cell carcinoma (SCC) is correct?
    a. It classically has rolled edges.
    b. Immunosuppression is a risk factor.
    c. SCC has no risk of metastasis.
    d. Marjolin's ulcer is an *in situ* SCC.
    e. Bowen disease is defined as a malignant change in a long-standing scar or sinus.

143. A 35-year-old man is brought to the emergency department after being extricated from a vehicle involved in a 60 mph road traffic collision. Following initial assessment, the only injuries of note are burns to his left leg caused by a small fire within the vehicle soon after the impact. Which of the following statements regarding burns is correct?
    a. The zone of coagulation is potentially viable.
    b. A third-degree burn is often exquisitely painful.
    c. The dermis is involved in second-degree burns.
    d. First-degree burns are often characterized by blistering.
    e. The zone of ischaemia is non-viable.

144. Which of the following statements concerning burns is incorrect?
    a. The Advanced Trauma Life Support (ATLS) guideline for fluid resuscitation is 2–4 mL/kg per percent burn.
    b. Coagulopathy can develop due to disseminated intravascular coagulation.
    c. Electrolyte disturbances include hyperkalaemia and hypercalcaemia.
    d. Initial management should include stress ulcer prophylaxis.
    e. Intravenous fluids are recommended if >15% burns in an adult.

145. A 42-year-old female presents to the minor surgical department with an 8-week history of alteration of a small mole on her left arm. The lesion measures 8 mm in diameter and has become more irregular in colour and shape. Which one of the following statements is incorrect regarding malignant melanoma?
    a. Males have a worse prognosis than females.
    b. Nodular melanoma is the most common type.
    c. Malignant melanoma can be mistaken for a subungual haematoma.
    d. Prognosis depends on Breslow thickness.
    e. It can arise from a Hutchinson lentigo.

146. Which type of malignant melanoma usually occurs on the face of elderly patients?
    a. Superficial spreading melanoma
    b. Nodular melanoma
    c. Lentigo maligna
    d. Acral lentiginous melanoma
    e. Amelanotic melanoma

147. A 72-year-old woman presents with a 15 × 12 cm lesion on her left calf, which has gradually been increasing in size over the past 7 years. Her contralateral leg has evidence of varicose veins. The lesion is foul smelling, with raised everted edges. She has a palpable inguinal lymph node. Which of the following is most likely to be the diagnosis of her lesion?
    a. Basal cell carcinoma (BCC)
    b. Nodular melanoma
    c. Squamous cell carcinoma (SCC)
    d. Lymphoma
    e. Bowen disease

148. A 79-year-old farmer presents to your clinic with a 5 mm well-defined lesion over his left temple region with a pearly, rolled edge. Over the lesion you note he has visible small vessels. It has gradually been increasing in size over the past 7 months. What is the most likely diagnosis?
    a. Basal cell carcinoma
    b. Nodular melanoma
    c. Squamous cell carcinoma
    d. Lymphoma
    e. Bowen disease

149. Which layer of the epidermis is important for the production of bipolar lipids to reduce water evaporation?
    a. Stratum corneum
    b. Stratum lucidum
    c. Stratum granulosum
    d. Stratum spinosum
    e. Stratum basale

150. An excised melanoma from a 70-year-old male appears histologically to have invaded the papillary dermis of the skin. Which Clark level does this refer to?
   a. Level I
   b. Level II
   c. Level III
   d. Level IV
   e. Level V

151. Which of the following features is associated with the malignant change in a pre-existing naevus?
   a. Asymmetry
   b. Becoming larger than 3 mm
   c. A rolled edge
   d. None of the above
   e. a and b only

LYMPHORETICULAR SYSTEM

152. Spontaneous rupture of the spleen can occur in which of the following conditions?
    a. Lymphoid neoplasms
    b. Malaria
    c. Infectious mononucleosis
    d. All of the above
    e. None of the above

153. Which of the following cells contribute to the reticuloendothelial system?
    a. Kupffer cells
    b. Histiocytes
    c. Alveolar macrophages
    d. All of the above
    e. b and c only

154. During mobilization of the splenic flexure, a severe laceration in the spleen is made and your consultant opts to perform a splenectomy. Your consultant talks to you about the implications a splenectomy has for the patient. Which of the following statements is true?
    a. An immediate rise in platelets occurs, lasting for 2–3 days.
    b. The risks of overwhelming post-splenectomy infection (OPSI) are highest within the first 2 months.
    c. Patients are particularly susceptible to *Haemophilus influenzae* infections.
    d. Malaria prophylaxis is not essential when in endemic areas.
    e. Children under the age of 15 years have an infection rate of less than 1%.

155. A 22-year-old man has a splenectomy performed after sustaining a splenic rupture following a motorcycle accident. Which one of the following comments is incorrect?
    a. There is increased risk of infection from *Haemophilus influenzae*.
    b. There is increased risk of infection from *Streptococcus pneumoniae*.
    c. There is increased risk of infection from *Neisseria meningitides*.
    d. There is increased risk of infection from fungi.
    e. There is an early thrombocytosis peaking 7 days after the procedure.

156. After a splenectomy is performed, which one of the following statements is true?
    a. There are reduced levels of Howell–Jolly bodies.
    b. There is late thrombocytosis peaking at 1 month post-procedure.
    c. There is increased platelet dysfunction.
    d. There is decreased platelet adhesiveness.
    e. Susceptibility to encapsulated organisms remains unchanged.

157. Which of the following is not an indication for splenectomy in idiopathic thrombocytopenic purpura (ITP)?
    a. Relapse after steroid therapy
    b. Failure to respond to medical management

c. Refractory severe thrombocytopenia

d. Toxic/high-dose steroid used

e. Persistently high platelet count

158. An emergency open splenectomy is performed on a 24-year-old male following a road traffic accident. Which one of the following statements is false?

a. The patient is at risk for meningococcal C infections.

b. Prophylactic antibiotics to protect against encapsulated bacteria should be commenced.

c. The patient is at a low but significant risk of overwhelming post-splenectomy infection.

d. The patient should be vaccinated against influenza yearly.

e. The patient should have vaccinations for meningococcal C within 12 weeks of surgery.

159. Which one of the following statements is incorrect regarding overwhelming post-splenectomy infection?

a. It usually presents within 2 years of splenectomy.

b. It can occur in patients who are hyposplenic.

c. It is more likely in patients with Hodgkin disease than following splenectomy as a result of trauma.

d. It is usually caused by encapsulated bacteria.

e. Treatment must start only after gaining cultures.

160. In the pathogenesis of lymphoma, which one of the following is true?

a. The presence of Reed–Sternberg cells is not important in the diagnosis.

b. Bone marrow biopsy may be warranted.

c. Lymphoma patients are unlikely to manifest intra-abdominal symptoms.

d. Bowel obstruction is never seen.

e. It should be the diagnosis to exclude in all patients with submandibular lymph node enlargement.

161. Which of the following features helps to distinguish Hodgkin from non-Hodgkin lymphoma?

a. Malaise

b. Auer rods on bone marrow biopsy

c. Weight loss

d. Male sex

e. Reed–Sternberg cells

162. Which comment regarding Hodgkin disease is correct?

a. Hodgkin disease accounts for about 50% of lymphomas.

b. Reed–Sternberg cells have large eosinophilic nucleoli within mirror image nuclei.

c. Classical Hodgkin disease is believed to be caused by cytomegalovirus.

d. Ann Arbor Stage II includes disease involving a single node or group of nodes.

e. Ann Arbor Stage IV involves disease on both sides of the diaphragm.

163. Which of the following statements are true for Hodgkin lymphoma?
    a. It usually presents with a painless enlargement of lymph nodes.
    b. It is subclassified into two subtypes.
    c. Identification of Reed–Sternberg cells and their variants is essential for the histological diagnosis.
    d. All of the above.
    e. a and c only.

EAR, NOSE AND THROAT

164. Which of the following statements regarding epistaxis is false?
    a. The most common site of epistaxis is from Little's area.
    b. Anterior bleeds are amenable to direct pressure and cauterization.
    c. Posterior bleeds often need packing.
    d. Foley catheters are often useful for posterior packs.
    e. Sphenopalatine artery ligation is not indicated in severe epistaxis.

165. A 14-year-old boy is discharged from hospital the day after having a tonsillectomy. Once discharged he does not take his analgesia as recommended, and admits to very poor oral hygiene and intake. He returns to the hospital on day 4 with moderate bleeding from the tonsillar fossa. Which type of haemorrhage is this known as?
    a. Primary haemorrhage
    b. Secondary haemorrhage
    c. Tertiary haemorrhage
    d. Reactionary haemorrhage
    e. Delayed haemorrhage

166. A 75-year-old man presents with a 5-month history of an asymptomatic lump in the anterior triangle of the neck. On examination this has a strongly transmitted pulse and investigations yield a positive goblet deformity. Which one of the following is the name given to this lump?
    a. Branchial cyst
    b. Cystic hygroma
    c. Carotid body tumour
    d. Thyroid tumour
    e. Dermoid

167. Which of the following statements regarding acoustic neuromas is correct?
    a. Arise from Schwann cells of cranial nerve VII.
    b. May be a feature of Von Recklinghausen's disease.
    c. Usually occur in the 70- to 80-year age group.
    d. Facial weakness is an early manifestation.
    e. Can lead to bilateral cerebellar signs.

168. Which one of the following comments regarding a lesions of the parotid gland is true?
    a. Adenoid cystic tumours rarely affect the facial nerve.
    b. Monomorphic adenoma is the most common salivary gland tumour.
    c. Warthin tumour is an adenolymphoma.
    d. Warthin tumours are more commonly unilateral.
    e. A small tissue biopsy should be performed in the first instance to gain a histological specimen.

MISCELLANEOUS

169. Which of the following is not a mandatory circumstance for referral to the coroner?
    a. Death within 24 h of an operation or procedure
    b. Death within 72 h of admission to hospital
    c. Death in custody
    d. Death from suicide
    e. Death due to industrial accident

NERVOUS SYSTEM

1. e. The UK brainstem death test includes seven criteria, all of which must be absent for a diagnosis to be made. Also, these tests should be performed by two doctors on two separate occasions. The doctors must not be part of a transplant team, must have more than 5 years experience, must be competent in intensive care treatment or neurology and one of them should be a consultant. The seven tests are:

1. No direct or consensual papillary response to light (cranial nerve [CN] II and CN III)
2. Absent corneal reflex (CN V and CN VI)
3. Absent gag reflex (CN IX and CN X)
4. No motor response to face or limbs after stimuli in any somatic area
5. Absent vestibulo-ocular reflex (CN III, CN VI and CN VIII)
6. Absent cough reflex (CN IX and CN X)
7. No respiratory effort despite a $PaCO_2$ of >6.5 kPa

2. b. Raised intracranial pressure can be caused by space-occupying lesions such as tumours, haematomas, abscesses and cysts. The normal pressure ranges from 0 to 10 mmHg. Systemic effects include Cushing's response, neurogenic pulmonary oedema and Cushing's ulcer. The clinical manifestations include headache, vomiting and papilloedema. Cerebral herniation can cause oculomotor nerve compression, ipsilateral pupil dilatation, contralateral hemiparesis and cortical blindness.

3. e. Cutaneous neurofibromas usually develop in the dermis and subcutaneous fat as a well-delineated but unencapsulated mass. Although they are not invasive, the adnexal structures are sometimes enwrapped by the edges of the lesion. The risk of malignant transformation from these tumours is extremely small. Plexiform neurofibromas occur in patients with neurofibromatosis type 1 as multiple lesions. They have a significant risk for malignant transformation.

4. e. Fat embolus typically occurs between days 3 and 10 following long bone fractures. The source of the embolus is thought to be from the bone marrow. Signs include confusion, fits, dyspnoea, low PO_2 and a petechial rash.

The embolus affects lung and brain microvasculature causing these clinical features. A computed tomography (CT) scan would normally show small subpleural nodular opacities. Early fixation of the fractures is preventative.

5. e.   Brown–Séquard syndrome occurs as a result of hemisection of the spinal cord. Although a rare condition, it may result from trauma to the back or penetrating gunshot or knife injuries. It may also be caused by tumour, ischaemia of the cord from a compromised blood supply, multiple sclerosis or tuberculosis (TB). Typically, it presents with ipsilateral motor paralysis and loss of vibration and proprioception, but contralateral loss of pain and temperature sense. This is because fibres of the spinothalamic tract that conduct pain and temperature cross over to the opposite side before ascending up the spinal cord. Presentation can be progressive and incomplete, with variation from the classic picture not uncommon.

6. b.   Extradural haemorrhage is characterized by a lenticular-shaped haematoma situated between the skull and the dura. It is almost always related to a skull fracture – typically the thin squamous part of the temporal bone near to the middle meningeal artery. It occurs in the younger age group and is characterized by a lucid interval of several hours followed by a rapid increase in intracranial pressure. A subdural haematoma is crescent in shape and occurs between the dura and outer surface of the arachnoid membrane, so the blood is not limited by suture lines. This occurs more commonly in the elderly, owing to brain atrophy, and is caused by rupture of the small bridging veins. Subdural haematomas tend to follow a contrecoup injury.

7. a.   Subarachnoid haemorrhage is characterized by sudden-onset 'thunderclap' headache. It usually results from a spontaneous rather than a traumatic bleed. Most cases are caused by the rupture of an underlying berry aneurysm. It is often difficult to differentiate it from a severe migraine attack or bacterial meningitis. In this case, she has a history of hypertension with sudden onset of symptoms and no preceding visual aura or history of trauma.

8. d.

Affected structure	Clinical manifestations
Oculomotor nerve	Ipsilateral papillary dilatation
Midbrain	Decerebrate rigidity
Reticular formation	Coma
Posterior cerebral artery	Cortical blindness
Cerebral aqueduct	Hydrocephalus
Ipsilateral cerebral peduncle	Contralateral hemiparesis
Contralateral cerebral peduncle	Ipsilateral hemiparesis

9. e.   Extradural haemorrhage is caused by trauma to the skull, commonly fractures of the temporal bone tearing the middle meningeal artery. Clinical features include temporary concussion and recovery. Other features are a falling pulse rate, dilated ipsilateral pupil and contralateral hemiparesis. Subdural haemorrhage is caused by bleeding to the bridging veins. Subarachnoid haemorrhage can be caused by rupture of a berry aneurysm, vascular malformation or intracerebral haematoma. Patients present with headache and signs of meningeal irritation. Ten percent of cases die immediately, and around 50% of patients die within 6 months.

10. c. Paragangliomas derive from neural crest cells. The largest concentration of paraganglionic cells is found in the adrenal medulla. However, paraganglionic tissue is present in the head and neck region, giving rise to paragangliomas such as:

- The carotid bifurcation (most common site for paraganglioma)
- Glomus jugulare (i.e. the jugular bulb – the second most common site)
- Glomus tympanicum (arising from the cochlear promontory of the middle ear)
- Glomus vagale (arising from the vagal nerve)

Lyre's sign refers to splaying of the carotid bifurcation seen on angiography, due to enlargement of an encroaching paraganglioma. The vast majority of paragangliomas are sporadic (90%), but up to 10% are familial. The propensity for malignant spread is low.

11. e. Hyponatraemia occurs post–subarachnoid haemorrhage (SAH) because of cerebral salt wasting where sodium is lost in the urine. It is thought to be caused by rising natriuretic peptides and is associated with hypovolaemia. This is managed with the 'triple H' therapy of SAH consisting of hypervolaemia, hypertension and haemodilution. Aggressive fluid resuscitation with saline is required to prevent hyponatraemia. There is a 3% risk of rebleeding in the first 24 h. Vasospasm is thought to be caused by the breakdown of blood products in the cerebrospinal fluid (CSF), typically occurring after day 3 post-bleed and is treated with calcium channel blockers or triple H therapy with inotropes or vasopressors. Hydrocephalus occurs as a result of the blood in the subarachnoid space interfering with CSF flow. Cardiac abnormalities and electrocardiogram (ECG) changes post-SAH have been reported, particularly abnormalities of the T and U waves and prolongation of the QT interval.

12. c. Vomiting is a less specific sign in children than adults. Vomiting in children may not necessarily indicate any intracranial pathology unless profuse (>3 times). Following the National Institute for Health and Care Excellence (NICE) guidelines for head injury, there is no indication for CT at present. However, he warrants a period of observation in hospital for at least 4 h to assess his progress.

13. d. Meningitis is a potentially life-threatening infection of the subarachnoid space. The symptoms include fever, headache, photophobia and, importantly, neck stiffness. Viral meningitis is the most common cause of meningitis, and this is most frequently caused by echoviruses and coxsackieviruses. Bacterial meningitis is most frequently caused by *Neisseria meningitidis* or *Streptococcus pneumoniae*. *Haemophilus influenzae* was a frequent cause until the introduction of the vaccination programme. Any patient with suspected bacterial meningitis should have immediate empirical antibiotics, with subsequent laboratory cerebrospinal fluid (CSF) and blood culture samples to allow specific antimicrobial targeting. Below is a table of the typical CSF changes in meningitis.

	Normal	Bacterial	Viral	Tuberculosis
Microscopy	Few cells	Neutrophils	Lymphocytes	Lymphocytes
Glucose	50–66% blood level	Low	Normal	Low
Appearance	Clear	Purulent	Turbid	Turbid

14. e. The scenario describes how a classical extradural haematoma presents with devastating consequences. Classically, the pterion (region of the skull formed by the sutures of the frontal, parietal, temporal and sphenoid bones) is fractured resulting in rupture of the middle meningeal artery. The force of the injury knocks the patient unconscious for a few minutes and is followed by a 'lucid interval' before a further deterioration in consciousness. The arterial blood rapidly collects in the extradural space creating a lens-shaped defect due to the attachments of the dura to the cranium. Pressure autoregulation by the brain provides compensation until the expanding haematoma causes a rise in intracranial pressure, deterioration in conscious and subsequent death by 'coning'.

MUSCULOSKELETAL SYSTEM

15. d.   Osteochondromas are also known as exostoses. Multiple osteochondromas develop in multiple hereditary exostoses, which is an autosomal dominant hereditary disease. Solitary osteochondromas are usually first diagnosed in late adolescence and early adulthood, but multiple osteochondromas become apparent during childhood. They are the most common benign bone tumour and usually arise from the metaphysis near the growth plate of long tubular bones, especially about the knee.

16. d.   Osteosarcoma is a malignant mesenchymal tumour more common in men. It is the most common primary malignant tumour of bone. Osteosarcoma occurs in all age groups, but 75% occur in patients younger than age 20 years. Conditions known to be associated with the development of osteosarcoma are Paget's disease, bone infarcts and prior irradiation.

17. b.   Fat embolism occurs after long bone fractures or surgery to correct these types of fractures. Circulating fat emboli are small and multiple, and can cause widespread effects including lodging in the brain microvasculature resulting in agitation and delirium. Other clinical features are hypoxaemia, shortness of breath and a petechial rash. Blood count may show a drop in platelet count. Treatment is conservative. Steroids have been shown to reduce the risk of fat embolism when used prophylactically.

18. a.   Poland syndrome results in underdevelopment or absence of pectoralis muscle, with syndactyly of the ipsilateral hand. It is usually unilateral. It is thought to be caused by interruption of embryonic blood supply to the upper limb toward the end of gestation. Erb's palsy results from an injury to the upper brachial plexus (C5–C7). The most common cause is during a traumatic vaginal delivery. Signs include loss of sensation in the arm and muscular atrophy of deltoid, biceps and brachialis, and forearm pronation and extension, leading to the "waiter's tip" position. Klumpke paralysis results from lower brachial plexus (C8–T1) injury. It involves muscles of the forearm and intrinsic muscles of the hand, with loss of sensation in ulnar nerve distribution. The most common cause is also during a traumatic vaginal delivery, and it may present with Horner syndrome.

19. d.   Poland syndrome results in underdevelopment or absence of pectoralis muscle, with syndactyly of the ipsilateral hand. It is usually unilateral. It is thought to be caused by interruption of embryonic blood supply to the upper limb toward the end of gestation. Erb's palsy results from injury to the upper brachial plexus (C5–C7). The most common cause is during a traumatic vaginal delivery resulting in shoulder dystocia. Signs include loss of sensation in the arm and muscular atrophy of deltoid, biceps and brachialis, and forearm pronation and extension, known as the "waiter's tip" position. Klumpke paralysis results from lower brachial plexus (C8–T1) injury. It involves muscles of forearm and intrinsic muscles of the hand, with loss of sensation in ulnar nerve distribution.

20. c.   Rheumatoid arthritis (RA) is a symmetrical deforming polyarthropathy of the joints that affects the metacarpal phalangeal and proximal interphalangeal joints.

There is wasting of the small muscles of the hand with ulnar deviation at the metacarpal phalangeal joints, swan neck and Boutonniere deformity and Z thumb. Patients with RA can also be anaemic, which can be caused by gastrointestinal bleeding as a result of the use of non-steroidal anti-inflammatory drugs (NSAIDs), bone marrow suppression by indomethacin, anaemia of chronic disease or an associated pernicious anaemia. Felty syndrome is a triad of rheumatoid arthritis, splenomegaly and neutropenia. Extra-articular manifestations of rheumatoid arthritis include episcleritis, pleural effusion, fibrosing alveolitis, rheumatoid nodules, Caplan syndrome (rheumatoid nodules in the lungs associated with a fibrotic reaction), pericarditis, peripheral neuropathy and carpal tunnel syndrome.

21. b.   Poland syndrome is characterized by the underdevelopment or absence of the pectoralis muscle, with syndactyly of the ipsilateral hand. The condition is usually unilateral, and is more common in males. The patient may have an absent or abnormal humerus, radius and ulna, and may have a simian crease in the affected side.

22. d.   The most common cause is an irritable hip (transient synovitis), but this is a diagnosis of exclusion and can be difficult to distinguish from Perthes disease. Perthes disease is an avascular necrosis of the femoral head and is more common in males aged 4–10 years. X-ray features include a mushroom-shaped widened flattened femoral head. In the later stages of the disease it may be painless. Dysplasia of the hip (DDH) results in abnormal development of the hip and would be easily identified on plain radiography in a 9-year-old boy. Slipped upper femoral epiphysis (SUFE) is classically seen in children once they reach puberty (age 10–15 years). A patient with an infected hip joint would be pyrexial, unwell, with a tender, erythematous joint. The history of pain in the groin radiating to the thigh or knee is due to the dual innervation of the hip and knee joint by the femoral nerve.

23. b.   Slipped upper femoral epiphysis (SUFE) is the most common hip disorder in those of pubertal age and is more common in males. The proximal femoral growth plate is unstable, allowing the epiphysis to slide posteriorly. A slip can be classified as chronic or acute, typical or atypical, stable or unstable. Causative factors of SUFE include local trauma, obesity, hormonal imbalances secondary to endocrine pathology or pubertal hormones. Perthes disease is an avascular necrosis of the femoral head, most common in the 4- to 10-year age group.

24. c.   Ewing sarcoma is the second most common primary bone tumour in children. It typically affects the diaphysis of long tubular bones, particularly the femur. Microscopic examination of the tumour reveals small round blue cells of unknown origin. Patients typically present with pain and an enlarging mass. Eighty-five percent have characteristic chromosomal translocation between Ch11 and Ch22. A characteristic periosteal reaction produces reactive bone layer deposition leading to an onion skin appearance on imaging. The tumour involves the diaphysis or metaphysic. Codman's triangle is a characteristic triangular shadow more associated with osteosarcoma. Endosteal scalloping and bony expansion are radiographic signs of bone disease but are not specific to Ewing sarcoma.

25. c. The X-ray findings are suggestive of osteoarthritis (OA). In OA, hyaline joint cartilage initially becomes swollen causing stretching of the matrix collagen network. The cartilage becomes softer and therefore more susceptible to damage. Fibrillations form in superficial layers, gradually deepening perpendicular to the joint surface. The chondrocyte population falls and the matrix diminishes. Subchondral bones are remodelled in response to these metabolic and mechanical changes. Radiological features of both OA and rheumatoid arthritis (RA) include:

- OA (the mnemonic LOSS):
    - **L**oss of joint space
    - **O**steophyte formation
    - **S**ubchondral sclerosis
    - **S**ubarticular bone cysts
- RA:
    - Loss of joint space
    - Periarticular erosions
    - Joint line thickening
    - Juxta-articular osteoporosis
    - No osteophytes

26. d. Calcification may be classified into two main types: orthotopic and heterotopic (which is further divided into dystrophic, metastatic and age related). Orthotopic calcification is the normal process of calcification in tissues such as bones and teeth. Dystrophic calcification is most commonly seen in heart valves, damaged muscle, scars and atheroma in areas of necrosis and parasitic cysts. There are two phases: initiation phase and propagation phase. Metastatic calcification tends to occur in areas where acidic substances are secreted, such as gastric glands and the renal tubules. Dystrophic calcification occurs in damaged tissue, and metastatic calcification occurs in normal tissue in the setting of hypercalcaemia.

27. e. X-ray findings associated with osteoarthritis (OA) include joint space narrowing, osteophyte development, subchondral sclerosis and subchondral cyst formation. Fractures may occur as a result of OA but are not a feature on X-ray of OA. Periosteal osteoporosis, erosions and fractures are all associated with rheumatoid arthritis. Soft tissue swelling is associated with many conditions and is a non-specific X-ray characteristic.

28. c. Open fractures always need reduction in theatre and always require immediate administration of antibiotics. A volar backslab is usually used to immobilize a Smith's fracture. An above-elbow plaster of Paris (POP) is indicated in a proximal ulna/radial fracture. A haematoma block with local anaesthesia is a good analgesic when reducing fractures outside an operating theatre. A Cochrane review has shown all methods including sedation, regional block and general anaesthesia to be effective, with little evidence of sufficient quality to advocate one over the other.

29. d. Neck of femur fractures often occur in elderly patients who may be infirm or confused and often are unable to give a good history. Intracapsular fractures are commonly treated with hemiarthroplasty. A collateral history is usually relied upon to identify perioperative risks. Hip fractures are painful and so parenteral analgesia is often required. Many units now include regular input from care of the elderly physicians to aid preoperative optimization of comorbidities, and to assess and plan for postoperative recovery and discharge.

30. a.   Greenstick fractures involve an incomplete break of the cortex (like breaking a green or young tree branch). These fractures occur in childhood because of the relatively flexible nature of the growing bones and thick periosteum compared to the brittle nature of adult bones and thin periosteum. The usual way of managing fractures is still indicated (i.e. reduce, hold, rehabilitate) due to pain and the possibility of worsening the fracture should repeat injury occur. These fractures are caused by low-energy trauma; therefore vascular compromise is unlikely.

31. c.   Supracondylar fractures usually occur in children and require urgent intervention. The fracture may leave an anterior spike of bone which may lead to injury to the brachial artery or median nerve. The radial nerve is at risk in this injury but due to its anatomical location, injury is not common. They are usually sustained during a fall onto an outstretched arm. The fracture should be immobilized prior to theatre to decrease pain and prevent secondary injury.

32. e.   The anterior humeral line is drawn along the anterior cortex of the distal humerus in the lateral view. This line passes through the anterior third of the capitellum. Following an extension type supracondylar fracture, the capitellum may displace posteriorly allowing the anterior humeral line to erroneously pass anterior to the capitellum, indicating a fracture.

33. b.   This scenario suggests a fat embolism. Symptoms include pulmonary compromise, confusion, anaemia and thrombocytopenia, usually starting within 1–3 days following a fracture of a bone with fatty marrow. However, this presentation rarely occurs following soft tissue trauma or burns. The symptoms are caused by microscopic fat globules entering the circulation after rupture of venules within marrow or adipose tissue. The globules attract platelets and can cause erythrocyte haemolysis. The pulmonary and neurological symptoms are caused by microemboli occluding the pulmonary and cerebral circulations with additional aggregation of platelets and erythrocytes. Interestingly, trauma-related fat embolism occurs in up to 90% of patients with appropriate injuries, but only 10% of those patients actually develop any symptoms.

34. a.   Paget disease is a bone disease of unknown aetiology; however a viral link has been suggested. It is the second most common metabolic bone disease after osteoporosis. It is typified by an increased and chaotic turnover of bone that occurs in localized parts of the skeleton. Any bone or bones can be affected, but Paget disease occurs most frequently in the spine, skull, pelvis, femur and lower legs. Diagnosis is usually made from the clinical picture, characteristic radiological changes (thickened cortex and bone sclerosis) and an elevated serum alkaline phosphatase. Fewer than 5% of patients have symptoms, of which pain is the most common. The affected bones are enlarged, warm and deformed. The main complications of Paget disease include pathological fracture, deafness and rarely (<1%) osteosarcoma.

35. a.   Osteomalacia is a rare disorder which is the result of inadequate mineralization of osteoid. Almost all cases are due to a deficiency in vitamin D. It can be caused by a deficiency in calcium or phosphate, but this is extremely rare. In the UK, those at risk receive little exposure to sunlight such as the elderly who are confined to home and patients who suffer from malabsorption of vitamin D due to coeliac or Crohn disease. The symptoms of osteomalacia are non-specific and include diffuse bony pain and muscle weakness, hence the often delayed diagnosis. Some of the pain is due to microfractures of the weakened bone, known as Looser's zones. Serum alkaline phosphatase levels are raised and serum calcium is either normal or slightly low.

36. d.   Osteosarcomas are malignant mesenchymal tumours where the cancerous cells create new bony matrix. It occurs more commonly in men and usually presents in adolescents. However, there is a smaller, second peak in the elderly. The main symptoms are night pain and localized tenderness. The tumour can occur in any bone but typically arises in the metaphyseal region of the long bones of the limbs. The knee is the most common affected area due to the high level of growth and almost 60% of cases occur here.

37. e.   Osteoarthritis is a very common condition characterized by degenerative joint destruction. Osteoarthritis is usually primary (no identifiable cause), but may be secondary due to pre-existing irregularity (e.g. fracture, meniscal tear). The arthritis develops through recognized stages. First, the articular cartilage softens and becomes fibrillated and fissured. The damaged cartilage is then worn away to expose the subchondral bone. On a radiograph, this thinning and destruction of the cartilage is seen as a loss of joint space. The resultant exposed bone is now under greater stress and becomes thickened and sclerotic, and cysts may form from microfractures. Further along in the disease process the remaining cartilage proliferates and ossifies to form osteophytes. Periarticular erosions are a radiographic feature of rheumatoid arthritis.

38. c.   Pseudogout, also known as chondrocalcinosis, is caused by the deposition of calcium pyrophosphate crystals. The factors leading to intra-articular crystal formation are not completely known but include matrix proteins inappropriately producing and degrading pyrophosphate, leading to build-up and crystallization with calcium. The disorder is usually experienced in old age, with a prevalence rising to 30–60% of those over 85 years of age. There is no increased prevalence across sex- or race-matched individuals. Pseudogout can be hereditary and individuals who develop the disease early in life have associated severe osteoarthritis. Under microscopy the crystals are positively birefringent and are usually 0.5–5 μm long. Joints may have symptoms lasting days to weeks and the attack can either be monoarticular or polyarticular. The most commonly affected joint is the knee, with the wrist, elbow, shoulder and ankle also commonly involved. The first metatarsophalangeal joint is most commonly affected in true gout.

39. a.   Rheumatoid arthritis is a chronic systemic inflammatory condition of unknown aetiology that causes a chronic and symmetric inflammation of joints. The arthritis is characterized by a non-suppurative and proliferative synovitis that leads to the destruction of cartilage and eventually joint ankylosis. The small joints of the wrist and hand are commonly affected. At the wrist one may see ulnar styloid prominence owing to subluxation (the piano key sign). The dorsum of the hand becomes swollen leading to loss of interknuckle valleys and spindling of the proximal joints. The metacarpophalangeal joints are prone to subluxation and ulnar deviation. On the palms, one may see erythema, wasting of the thenar muscles secondary to carpal tunnel syndrome and Z thumb deformity. Boutonniere deformity is flexion of the proximal interphalangeal joint (PIPJ) and hyperextension of the distal interphalangeal joint (DIPJ) caused by rupture of the central slip of the extensor expansion. Swan neck deformity is hyperextension of the PIPJ and flexion of the DIPJ because of rupture of the lateral slip of the extensor expansion. Heberden's nodes are nodular swellings of the DIPJ caused by osteophytes in osteoarthritis. Bouchard's nodes are swellings seen at the PIPJ. They are less common than Heberden's nodes and may also be found in rheumatoid arthritis.

40. b.   Rheumatoid arthritis is a chronic autoimmune systemic inflammatory condition, the exact cause of which is unknown. It is thought that an unknown arthritogenic antigen activates CD4$^+$ helper T-cells and other lymphocytes via genetic susceptibility (human leukocyte antigen DR4) to secrete proinflammatory cytokines (tumour necrosis factor and interleukin-1 are important). These cytokines have a range of activating functions, of which the formation of rheumatoid factor is one (immunoglobulin M [IgM] is sensitized against the Fc portion of IgG). Rheumatoid factor is present in many people without rheumatoid arthritis and many patients with classic rheumatoid do not have it. Therefore, the presence of rheumatoid factor is not diagnostic. However, high titres≈indicate progressive disease and can be used as a prognostic indicator. Usually the small joints of the hand are involved first.

RESPIRATORY SYSTEM

41. d.   The causes of acute respiratory distress syndrome (ARDS) can be divided into direct pulmonary and indirect causes. Direct causes include pneumonia, smoke inhalation and gastric content aspiration. Indirect causes include sepsis, trauma, acute pancreatitis and massive blood transfusion. Acute renal failure can result from ARDS but does not cause it.

42. c.   Acute respiratory distress syndrome (ARDS) is an acute severe lung disease characterized by inflammation of the lung parenchyma leading to impaired gas exchange and systemic release of inflammatory mediators. Diagnosis requires a recognized cause, hypoxia that is refractory to O_2 (PO_2:FiO_2 ratio of <200 mmHg), bilateral pulmonary infiltrates on chest films and no evidence of cardiac failure (pulmonary artery wedge pressure <18 mmHg). There is increased vascular permeability causing protein-rich exudates to fill the alveoli and form hyaline membranes. This leads to lung fibrosis and reduced compliance. ARDS is commonly managed in a high-dependency unit setting as the patient usually requires respiratory and circulatory support.

43. b.   Local invasion of bronchial carcinoma into adjacent structures can cause a multitude of symptoms. It can invade into the cervical sympathetic chain (Horner syndrome), brachial plexus, recurrent laryngeal nerve as well as superior vena cava, causing obstruction and facial oedema.

44. e.   Lobar pneumonia is commonly seen in adults between the age of 20 and 50 years, more in males. The most common aetiological agent is *Streptococcus pneumoniae* with occasionally *Klebsiella pneumoniae* a causative agent in the elderly or alcoholics. Symptoms include fever/rigors and a cough with rusty sputum production.

Phase 1: Congestion – 1–2 days. The lungs are dark red and wet on gross appearance.
Phase 2: Red hepatization – 2–4 days. The lungs are solid, red and dry on gross appearance.
Phase 3: Grey hepatization – 4–8 days. The lungs are solid and grey on gross appearance.
Phase 4: Resolution – 8–10 days.

45. c.   Asbestos is a fibrous silicate, of which there are more than 50 types. The three types that are pathological to humans may be summarized as follows:

- *Chrysotile:* A curled 'white' asbestos. Fibres are long and woolly, and thus do not penetrate lung tissue deeply. It is associated with pulmonary fibrosis. Most of the asbestos used in industry is of this subtype.
- *Amosite:* An amphibole 'brown' asbestos. Fibres are long, straight and brittle. Associated with pulmonary fibrosis.
- *Crocidolite:* An amphibole 'blue' asbestos. Fibres are short, straight and brittle – penetration into lung tissue is deeper and thus fibres are more pathogenic; associated with pulmonary fibrosis and malignant mesothelioma.

46. d. Radiant energy can be a potent carcinogen, whether in the form of ultraviolet light or ionizing electromagnetic and particulate radiation. Inhalation of dust by uranium miners predisposes them to lung cancer. X-rays are associated with skin cancers and leukaemia. Radiologists, among others, are at increased risk, especially if unshielded during work. Nuclear fallout causes an increase in leukaemia, breast and thyroid cancers. In the past, ingestion of radium occurred when painters of luminescent watches licked their paint brushes, and these activities put them at risk of developing osteosarcoma. Radionuclide imaging exposes people to Thorotrast, which is composed of thorium dioxide and can cause angiosarcoma of the liver.

47. a. About 87% of lung cancers occur in active smokers and those who have recently stopped. There is an invariable statistical association between the incidence of lung cancer and the volume of daily smoking, inhalation and length of habit. Observations of the epithelial lining of the respiratory tract in smokers show that there are sequential histological changes from metaplasia to invasive carcinoma. These changes have been best seen in squamous cell carcinoma and begin with squamous metaplasia, followed by squamous dysplasia, carcinoma *in situ* and finally invasive carcinoma.

BREAST DISORDERS

48. d.   Women who reach menarche when younger than 11 years of age have a 20% increased risk compared with women who reach menarche when more than 14 years of age. Women who have been exposed to therapeutic or non-therapeutic radiation have a higher rate of breast cancer. Carcinoma of the endometrium and contralateral breast are also associated with increased risk.

49. c.   Sarcoma of the breast is a rare tumour arising from the mesenchymal tissue. They can develop *de novo* or may follow chest wall radiotherapy for previously treated breast cancer. The tumour usually develops in breast tissue and overlying skin. Treatment can range from wide local excision to radical mastectomy. Metastatic spread is uncommon, so axillary sampling or sentinel node biopsy is regarded as adequate. Radiotherapy can be used if not done so previously; however, chemotherapy has little adjuvant benefit.

50. c.   Phyllodes tumour is a rare fibroepithelial neoplasia, the majority of which are benign. Approximately 20% of benign phyllodes recur, needing further excision and potential mastectomy. It has malignant potential. In malignant conditions the sarcomatous element is known to recur, with potential for metastatic spread.

51. c.   Risk factors for the pathogenesis of breast cancer can be summarized as follows:

- Age, female sex
- Early menarche, late menopause
- Oral contraceptive pill (OCP) (controversial)
- Nulliparous
- Western prevalence
- High socioeconomic class
- Unmarried
- Obesity (if >55 years old)
- Genetic factors (family history, BRCA 1 and 2 gene)

52. c.   Benign breast disorders such as fibroadenomas are not risk factors for breast cancer. About 5% of diagnoses are attributed to a genetic cause. Carriers of the *BRCA1* (chromosome 17) and *BRCA2* (chromosome 13) genes are at 30–40% increased risk of developing breast and ovarian cancer. An individual has double the normal risk of developing breast cancer if a first-degree relative had the condition. The greater the number of menstrual cycles, the greater the risk. Hormone replacement therapy (HRT) has also increased the incidence of breast cancer.

53. a.   Axillary lymph node clearance is established practice for treatment of invasive breast cancer. It clears local disease and yields prognostic information, helping to stage disease as well as influence postoperative therapy:

Level 1 – border of axillary vein; up to the lateral border of pectoralis minor
Level 2 – medial border of pectoralis minor
Level 3 – beyond the medial border of pectoralis minor up to the outer border of first rib

Axillary sampling involves removing four nodes from the axillary fat pad to stage the disease. Novel sampling techniques in current practice involve sentinel node biopsy. An important randomized multicentre trial (ALMANAC trial) comparing sentinel node biopsy with standard axillary therapy demonstrated that sentinel node biopsy is an accurate procedure with significantly less morbidity than standard axillary node clearance.

54. c. The major risk factors for breast cancer are hormonal and genetic. Caucasian women have a higher rate, on average, of developing invasive carcinoma than African, Asian or Hispanic women. Women who have had any significant radiation exposure have an increased risk. Hormone replacement also increases breast cancer risk, and when oestrogen and progesterone are combined, the risk is greater than with oestrogen alone. The risks of hormone replacement tie in with the risks of an overall long oestrogen exposure as women with an early menarche and late menopause are at higher risk. Smoking tobacco does not increase the risk of breast cancer but it does increase the risk of periductal mastitis or a subareolar abscess. Adult weight gain is a strong and consistent predictor of postmenopausal breast cancer risk.

55. d. The upper lateral quadrant is the most common site of carcinomas at 45%. Subareolar tumours are second with 25%. Upper medial (15%), lower lateral (10%) and lower medial (5%) tumours are less common.

56. d. Invasive breast cancer is able to spread via the lymphatic and vascular systems. Metastatic spread can affect anywhere in the body; however, the most common organs affected are the lungs, liver, brain, bones and adrenal glands. The ipsilateral lower axillary nodes are the most commonly affected lymph nodes. From there, the tumour cells spread to the apical lymph nodes and the supraclavicular lymph nodes. In addition, tumours from each area of the breast are able to spread to the internal thoracic chain of lymph nodes. Involvement of this chain is generally a poor prognostic sign as it indicates potential spread to the mediastinal lymph nodes and pleural cavities.

57. a. Carcinoma of the breast typically presents as a breast lump with direct palpation of the lesion by the patient herself or by a doctor. The second most common method is by mammography. These two modes account for 80–90% of all cases discovered. Breast pain is the most common breast symptom but is actually an uncommon presenting feature of breast carcinoma. Nipple discharge is an uncommon presenting symptom but is more concerning when it is either unilateral or spontaneous. The presence of metastatic spread as the method of diagnosis is uncommon.

58. c. Gynaecomastia is defined as the proliferation of male breast tissue. It is a benign condition that may be secondary to physiological or pathological processes. Spironolactone is well known to cause gynaecomastia.

CARDIOVASCULAR SYSTEM

59. b.   The patient has a clinically ruptured abdominal aortic aneurysm. He is currently shocked and too unstable for a computed tomography scan. He should not receive fast intravenous fluids despite the hypotension, as evidence suggests that increasing the blood pressure above 100 mmHg systolic will cause further bleeding. Performing an ultrasound scan will not provide any further information as the diagnosis has already been made clinically. Therefore, a vascular opinion needs to be obtained and theatres mobilized.

60. c.   Accurate diagnosis of valvular pathology is an important skill. The findings above are indicative of aortic stenosis. Other features may include a low-volume, slow-rising carotid pulse and a prominent, but not displaced, apex beat. On auscultation, the murmur is typically rough in quality and has a crescendo and decrescendo nature. It is best heard in the aortic area (right second intercostal space, as opposed to left for pulmonary valve pathology) and the murmur can radiate up to the carotid arteries and throughout the precordium. The surgical implications are twofold: first, the valve can be surgically replaced, whether open or endovascularly, and second, it increases a patient's anaesthetic risk. The stenosed value limits the stroke volume and therefore prevents the compensatory rise in cardiac output needed for when the anaesthetic agents cause vasodilation.

61. c.   There are a number of methods for detecting a lower-limb deep vein thrombosis with ascending contrast, venography being technically the definitive test of choice. However, the most commonly performed and easily accessible investigation is the duplex ultrasound Doppler, and it is non-invasive when compared to venography.

62. c.   An aneurysm is defined as an abnormal localized blood-filled dilatation of a blood or lymphatic vessel caused by disease or weakening of the vessel's wall. The most common location is the abdominal aorta, but any vessel in the body can be affected. A 'true' aneurysm involves all three layers of the arterial wall. Conversely, a 'false' aneurysm is created when the wall of the vessel has been ruptured and the extravasated blood is contained in a sac, which consists of compressed connective tissues. The most common cause is atherosclerosis. The pathogenesis is not fully understood, but ultimately there is weakening of the components of the arterial wall. Infective causes include syphilis, tuberculosis and osteomyelitis. Congenital aneurysms within the circle of Willis are called berry aneurysms. Inflammatory aneurysms make up 5–10% of abdominal aortic aneurysms and are associated with retroperitoneal fibrosis as well as Behçet disease, Takayasu disease and polyarteritis nodosa.

63. c.   The Well's score (2006) is used to determine the probability of a spontaneous deep vein thrombosis (DVT). One point is awarded for each of the following factors:

- Active cancer, or treated cancer within the last 6 months
- Recently bedridden for >3 days or major surgery within the last month
- Immobile, paralysed or recent lower-limb POP cast
- Entire leg swelling

- Calf >3 cm bigger than adjacent patient's leg
- Localized calf tenderness
- Pitting oedema more than patient's other leg
- Collateral superficial veins which are not varicose in nature
- Previous documented deep vein thrombosis
- Alternative diagnosis at least as likely (–2 points)

Score of 2 or higher — DVT likely. Consider imaging the leg veins.
Score of less than 2 — DVT unlikely.

ENDOCRINE SYSTEM

64. b. Antithyroid-stimulating hormone receptor antibodies are detected in Graves disease, whereas antithyroid peroxidase antibodies are detected in Hashimoto thyroiditis. The biochemistry of Graves disease is of a low thyroid-stimulating hormone, raised free thyroxine (T_4) and triiodothyronine (T_3), thyroid receptor antibodies and hot nodules on radioisotope scan. Thyroid acropachy, pretibial myxoedema and exophthalmus are only seen in Graves disease. Plummer disease is hyperthyroidism caused by a toxic solitary adenoma.

65. b. Hyperaldosteronism is caused by excessive aldosterone production by the zona glomerulosa. It can be primary, where there is autonomous hypersecretion of aldosterone, such as in Conn syndrome characterized by an adrenal cortical adenoma, or secondary, caused by increased production of angiotensin II followed by activation of the renin–angiotensin system. Secondary hyperaldosteronism may be precipitated by congestive cardiac failure, hepatic failure and cirrhosis. The biochemistry seen in hyperaldosteronism shows raised sodium and low potassium. The plasma renin is reduced in Conn syndrome but raised in secondary hyperaldosteronism. They typically suffer from hypertension.

66. e. Secondary causes of diabetes mellitus include:

- *Pancreatic causes* – pancreatitis, pancreatic cancer
- *Insulin antagonists* – acromegaly, glucagonoma, phaeochromocytoma
- *Drugs* – corticosteroids, thiazide diuretics
- *Genetic syndromes* – Down syndrome
- *Insulin receptor abnormality* – congenital lipodystrophy

Gastrinomas are small tumours seen in the pancreas or small intestine producing high levels of gastrin. Between 50% and 66% of tumours are malignant, which can spread to local lymph nodes or the liver. Symptoms include abdominal pain and vomiting. Gastrinomas can be found as part of multiple endocrine neoplasia (MEN) type I.

67. e. Addison disease is adrenocortical insufficiency due to bilateral adrenal cortex dysfunction. The lack of cortisol and aldosterone leads to a decreased mineralocorticoid release with hyponatraemia and hyperkalaemia. Increased levels of adrenocoricotropic hormone (ACTH) are produced by the anterior pituitary gland due to the negative feedback loop. Patients present with malaise, weight loss and excess skin pigmentation. Common causes include autoimmune disease, amyloidosis, sarcoidosis, meningococcal septicaemia (Waterhouse–Friderichsen syndrome), metastatic disease and fungal infections such as blastomycosis.

68. b. A pheochromocytoma is a neuroendocrine tumour of the adrenal medulla originating in the chromaffin cells. They cause excess secretion of catecholamines, adrenaline and noradrenaline. Ten percent are malignant, 10% multiple and 10% arise outside the adrenal medulla. Pheochromocytoma is a tumour of the multiple endocrine neoplasia syndrome types IIa and IIB. The signs and symptoms of the tumour are those of sympathetic overactivity, elevated heart rate and blood pressure, palpitations and anxiety and headaches.

69. b. Psammoma bodies are concentric calcified structures that are a pathognomic feature of papillary carcinoma of thyroid. They are usually present in the cores of the papillae but may also be noted in draining lymph nodes and adjacent tissues.

70. d. The term *carcinoid* was formulated by S. Oberndorfer to describe a carcinoma-like lesion but with a much more indolent clinical course. The common sites of occurrence are the gastrointestinal tract and lung and are derived from resident endocrine cells. Depending on their anatomic site disease manifestation can vary (gastric: Zollinger–Ellison syndrome related to excess elaboration of gastrin; peripancreatic: Cushing syndrome associated with corticotropin secretion; pancreatic: hyperinsulinism). Intestinal hypermotility can result in diarrhoea, cramps, nausea and vomiting.

71. c. Multiple endocrine neoplasia (MEN) syndromes are a rare autosomal dominant condition in which a single gene defect causes multiple endocrine tumours within a patient. Tumours are either benign or malignant. They can be divided into several subgroups according to the types of tumour:

- MEN I – parathyroid adenoma, pituitary adenoma, pancreatic islet cell tumour (gastrinoma and insulinoma), adrenal cortical adenoma, thymic carcinoid tumour, thyroid adenoma
- MEN IIa – medullary thyroid cancer (MTC), phaeochromocytoma, primary parathyroid hyperplasia
- MEN IIb – MTC, multiple endocrine neoplasia, mucosal neuromas
- MEN IIb is similar to MEN IIa but has neurocutaneous signs and marfanoid habitus. It does not, however, include parathyroid hyperplasia.

72. d. The biological actions of cortisol can lead to impaired glucose tolerance resulting in diabetes. Cortisol can cause an increase in body fat, with fat redistribution leading to a moon face and interscapular fat pad, thin skin and easy bruising, striae, hypertension and proximal myopathy. Patients are likely to gain rather than lose weight.

73. a. Papillary carcinoma is the most common tumour. It is slow growing with an excellent prognosis and spreads lymphatically. Follicular carcinoma is histologically similar to follicular adenoma but can be differentiated by its invasion of the capsule. It spreads haematologically. Medullary carcinoma is a tumour arising from the parafollicular C-cells, which synthesize and secrete calcitonin. It can be associated with carcinoid syndrome and commonly occurs in the elderly. Medullary carcinoma can form part of multiple endocrine neoplasia type II, which is a group of medical disorders associated with tumours of the endocrine system. Anaplastic carcinoma is highly malignant and poorly differentiated with rapid local invasion of structures, especially to the trachea. Lymphoma can also affect the thyroid gland.

74. b. Follicular thyroid cancer spreads haematologically whereas papillary thyroid carcinoma, the most common thyroid cancer, metastasizes via the lymphatics. Anaplastic thyroid cancer is very aggressive and invasive locally and is at high risk of encroaching on the airway. Medullary carcinoma and primary lymphoma of the thyroid also spread via the lymphatics.

75. d. Papillary adenocarcinoma is the most common tumour. It is slow growing with an excellent prognosis and spreads lymphatically. Follicular carcinoma is histologically similar to follicular adenoma, but can be differentiated by its invasion of the capsule. It spreads haematologically. Medullary carcinoma is a tumour arising from the parafollicular C-cells, which synthesize and secrete calcitonin. It can be associated with carcinoid syndrome and commonly occurs in the elderly. Medullary carcinoma can form part of multiple endocrine neoplasia type II, which is a group of medical disorders associated with tumours of the endocrine system. Anaplastic carcinoma is highly malignant and is poorly differentiated with rapid local invasion of structures, especially to the trachea.

76. e. Carcinoid tumours can occur in the gut and the lung. The most common sites in the gut are the small intestine and appendix. Seventy percent of tumours in the appendix occur at the tip, with 10% at the base. Argentaffin cells reduce silver compounds and contain neurosecretory granules and express chromogranin. Carcinoid syndrome by excess serotonin causes flushing and diarrhoea. Serotonin also causes fibrin formation and deposition on the cardiac valves leading to fibrosis and stenosis.

77. e. Hashimoto thyroiditis is an autoimmune disease, believed to be one of the most common causes of primary hypothyroidism. It occurs more often in women than men (10–20:1) with a prevalence during middle age. It is associated with human leukocyte antigen (HLA) DR5. Progression of the disease leads to atrophy and fibrosis of the gland. Microscopically the gland is infiltrated with lymphocytes and plasma cells.

78. e. Hyperplasia accounts for approximately 10% of cases of hyperparathyroidism, carcinoma accounts for <1% of cases, multiple adenomas account for 5% of cases, whereas single adenomas account for approximately 85% of cases. Secondary hyperparathyroidism refers to the parathyroid glands' response to chronic hypocalcaemia. Serum calcium is low (or normal), the phosphate is high (or normal) and parathyroid hormone (PTH) is high. Tertiary hyperparathyroidism refers to autonomous secretion of PTH following chronic stimulation of the parathyroid glands following prolonged secondary hyperparathyroidism. This results in parathyroid hyperplasia and a loss of response to serum calcium change levels. Therefore, biochemically, there is hypercalcaemia and hypophosphataemia.

79. b. Addison disease refers to bilateral destruction of the adrenal cortices, resulting in adrenocortical insufficiency. Causes include tuberculosis, Waterhouse–Friderichsen syndrome (following meningococcal sepsis), malignancy, amyloidosis, haemochromatosis, various drugs (i.e. ketoconazole) and sudden withdrawal of chronic corticosteroid therapy. The biochemical changes are hyponatraemia, hyperkalaemia, decreased aldosterone, decreased cortisol and increased adrenocorticotropic hormone.

80. a. Medullary carcinoma of the thyroid has an overall prevalence of approximately 5% of thyroid carcinomas and is derived from thyroid parafollicular C-cells, which are responsible for the synthesis and secretion of parathyroid hormone. Medullary carcinoma of the thyroid can usually be demonstrated with histological staining of biopsy tissue with Congo red. This shows apple-green dichroic birefringence suggesting the presence of amyloid. It is associated with multiple endocrine nei type II. Hereditary medullary thyroid cancer accounts for approximately 30% of cases. Overall 5-year survival is approximately 80%.

81. b.   Anaplastic thyroid carcinoma is a locally aggressive neoplasm, which metastasizes early via lymphatic and haematogenous spread. It accounts for approximately 2–5% of thyroid carcinomas, and almost certainly arises from thyroid epithelial cells, most commonly on a background of thyroid disease (such as pre-existing carcinoma and goitre). Five-year survival rates are incredibly poor (<5%) despite combined treatments of surgery, chemotherapy and radiotherapy.

82. c.   Multiple endocrine neoplasia/adenopathy can be classified as follows:

Type I
- Pancreas → adenoma/carcinoma islet cells
- Pituitary → adenoma (rarely carcinoma)
- Parathyroids → hyperplasia

Type IIa
- Thyroid → medullary carcinoma
- Adrenal → pheochromocytoma
- Parathyroids → hyperplasia

Type IIb
- Thyroid → medullary carcinoma
- Adrenal → pheochromocytoma
- Parathyroids → hyperplasia

Palatal submucosal neurofibromas

83. b.   Papillary thyroid cancer is the most common histological variant, accounting for approximately 80% of cases. It is multifocal in approximately 50% of cases. It is found incidentally in approximately 1–5% of postmortem examinations. The prognosis is excellent, with 5-year survival rates of approximately 90%. Its mode of spread is classically via lymphatics.

84. e.   Thyroid fine-needle aspiration cytology (FNAC) is reported as:

- *Thy1* – insufficient material
- *Thy2* – benign
- *Thy3* – follicular lesion
- *Thy4* – suspicious but not diagnostic of malignancy
- *Thy5* – definite malignancy

A follicular lesion could be either an adenoma or cancer and requires excision biopsy and histological analysis to distinguish the two.

85. b.   Acromegaly is caused by an increase in growth hormone (GH) production. This is normally caused by a GH-secreting pituitary adenoma. However, very rarely, ectopic secretion from a carcinoma of the lung, pancreas or small bowel can occur. The most prominent clinical findings are excessive sweating and an enlargement of the hands, feet, nose and jaw (prognathism). Additional features are bitemporal hemianopia, organomegaly, hyperostosis and metabolic disorders such as hyperglycaemia and hypertension. Diagnosis of pituitary GH excess requires elevated serum GH and insulin-like growth factor-1 (IGF-1) levels. In addition, failure to suppress GH production significantly after a glucose load is a sensitive test.

86. c. Prolactinomas are the most common type of hyperfunctioning pituitary adenoma accounting for approximately 30% of all recognized pituitary adenomas and occur most commonly under the age of 40. Hyperprolactinaemia may be caused by physiological events such as pregnancy and nipple stimulation. The main clinical features in women of reproductive age are amenorrhoea and galactorrhoea. In men, the clinical symptoms may be subtle, such as loss of libido and infertility. Prolactin induces lactation but inhibits both hypothalamic gonadotrophin-releasing hormone (GnRH) secretion and the actions of luteinizing hormone (LH) on the gonads.

87. e. Cushing syndrome is an eponymous term used for the physiological state of increased serum glucocorticoid. It most frequently occurs with the administration of long-term exogenous steroids. Endogenous causes of Cushing syndrome are either an adrenocorticotrophin (ACTH)-releasing pituitary or non-pituitary tumour, a primary excess of cortisol secretion by nodular hyperplasia or an adrenal tumour with subsequent ACTH suppression. The main clinical features of glucocorticoid excess include pigmentation in only ACTH-dependent causes, a Cushingoid appearance (characteristic features include a moon face, thin skin, bruising, hypertension, proximal myopathy and striae), impaired glucose tolerance and hypokalaemia, which is caused by the relative increase in the mineralocorticoid action of cortisol.

88. d. The basal metabolic rate of most nucleated cells and the sensitivity of β-adrenergic receptors are controlled by the thyroid hormones L-thyroxine (T_4) and triiodothyronine (T_3). T_3 is the main hormone acting at the cellular level, while T_4 is the prohormone converted to T_3 in peripheral tissues such as the liver and kidney. Hyperthyroidism is a common condition affecting 2–5% of all females; the peak incidence is between 20 and 40 years of age. The diverse clinical features result from the wide physiological effects, disease aetiology and age of the patient. The symptoms focus on increased metabolic activity leading to weight loss despite an increased appetite. Tremor, hyperkinesis and heat intolerance are common. In the elderly, atrial fibrillation and tachycardia are frequently found. The recognized eye signs (exophthalmus, ophthalmoplegia, chemosis and lid retraction), pretibial myxoedema and thyroid acropachy are only seen in Graves disease.

89. e. The basal metabolic rate of most nucleated cells and the sensitivity of β-adrenergic receptors are controlled by the thyroid hormones L-thyroxine (T_4) and triiodothyronine (T_3). T_3 is the main hormone acting at the cellular level, while T_4 is the prohormone converted to T_3 in peripheral tissues such as the liver and kidney. Hypothyroidism is one of the most common endocrine conditions and carries a lifetime prevalence of almost 9% in females and 1% in males. It is most commonly caused by antithyroid antibodies leading to lymphoid infiltration, but other causes include Hashimoto thyroiditis and dietary iodine deficiency. Myxoedema (an alternative term for hypothyroidism) refers to the build-up of mucopolysaccharides in the subcutaneous tissues. The clinical features of hypothyroidism commonly result in dry-haired, thick-skinned, slow patients who put on weight despite eating less. Patients are cold intolerant and can suffer from constipation.

GENITOURINARY SYSTEM

90. c. Pelvic inflammatory disease is a combined infection often involving the fallopian tubes, the ovaries and the peritoneum. It often results from an ascending infection from the vagina or cervix. Common organisms include chlamydia or gonorrhoea. Acute pelvic inflammatory disease can cause salpingitis, pyosalpinx, hydrosalpinx pelvic peritonitis, tubo-ovarian abscesses and adhesions. Sequelae of the disease include chronic pain, subfertility/infertility, ectopic pregnancy, dysmenorrhoea and dyspareunia.

91. c. The most common type of bladder cancer is transitional cell carcinoma (TCC). Other types include adenocarcinoma and squamous cell carcinoma (SCC). Schistosomiasis infection can predispose to SCC of the bladder. It has a higher male preponderance. Other risk factors include smoking, industrial dye and drugs (cyclophosphamide and phenacetin). It may present with painless haematuria, recurrent urinary tract infections (UTIs) as well as voiding irritability. Bladder cancer can spread locally or via lymphatics (iliac and para-aortic nodes) or haematogenous spread to liver and lungs. Treatment is dependent on stage and grade of disease. Options of treatment are cystectomy, chemotherapy and radiotherapy. Gonadotrophin releasing hormone agonists are used to treat prostate cancer.

92. b. Testicular tumours are the most common malignancy in younger men between 18 and 40 years. It is associated with undescended testis as well as higher levels of exogenous oestrogen exposure prenatally or in childhood. The two most common forms of testicular cancer are seminoma and teratoma (non-seminomatous germ cell tumour [NSGCT]). Seminomas are radiosensitive and very rarely have raised tumour markers (α-fetoprotein or β-human chorionic gonadotrophin [hCG]). The peak incidence of seminoma is in 30- to 40-year-olds. Seminomas commonly spread via lymphatics to iliac and para-aortic nodes. Teratomas are chemosensitive and raised tumour markers can be detected in 60–70% of cases. Peak incidence is in 20- to 30-year-olds. Teratomas commonly spread via haematogenous route to lungs and liver.

93. a. The most common form of renal stone is from calcium oxalate, occurring in 80% of cases. Uric acid forms 10% of cases and produces radiolucent stones. Struvite stones are associated with urea-splitting bacteria and form in an alkaline urine. They account for 10% of urinary calculi. Calcium phosphate stones are generally associated with primary hyperparathyroidism. Cystine stones are associated with patients suffering from cystinuria, a condition where patients accumulate cystine in their urine because of inadequate reabsorption of cystine in the proximal convoluted tubule.

94. a. The most common form of renal stone is from calcium oxalate, occurring in 80% of cases. These stones can sometimes be seen on plain KUB X-ray films. Uric acid forms 10% of cases and produces radiolucent stones. Struvite stones are associated with urea-splitting bacteria and form in an alkaline urine; they account for 10% of urinary calculi. Calcium phosphate stones are generally associated with primary hyperparathyroidism. Cystine stones are associated with patients suffering from cystinuria, a condition where patients accumulate cystine in their urine because of inadequate reabsorption of cystine in the proximal convoluted tubule.

95. c.   The history and intravenous urogram are suggestive of renal stones. The most common form of renal stone is from calcium oxalate, occurring in 80% of cases. These stones can sometimes be seen on plain KUB X-ray films. Uric acid forms 10% of cases and produces radiolucent stones. Struvite stones are associated with urea-splitting bacteria and form in alkaline urine; they account for 10% of urinary calculi. Calcium phosphate stones are generally associated with primary hyperparathyroidism. Cystine stones are associated with patients suffering from cystinuria, a condition where patients accumulate cystine in their urine because of inadequate reabsorption of cystine in the proximal convoluted tubule.

96. a.   Lymphatics from the testicles follow the arterial supply and drain into the para-aortic lymph nodes. The superficial inguinal nodes drain lymph from the lower part of the anal canal, scrotum and abdominal wall below the umbilicus. The internal iliac nodes surround the internal iliac artery and receive supply from the deep perineum and parts of the urethra. The axillary nodes drain the breast and are important in breast cancer.

97. c.   Lymphatics from the testicles follow the arterial supply and drain into the para-aortic lymph nodes. The superficial inguinal nodes drain lymph from the lower part of the anal canal, scrotum and abdominal wall below the umbilicus. The internal iliac nodes surround the internal iliac artery and receive supply from the deep perineum and parts of the urethra. The axillary nodes drain the breast and are important in breast cancer.

98. d.   Fournier gangrene is a rare condition, which is a surgical/urological emergency. It is characterized by a necrotizing fasciitis of the scrotum and perineum, requiring gross surgical debridement with intravenous broad-spectrum antibiotic treatment with aggressive fluid resuscitation prior to theatre. Diabetes is present in up to 60% of cases. The exact mortality rate is unknown but can be around 20%. Death usually results from systemic sepsis leading to multiorgan failure and many patients require critical care support.

99. a.   Urinary calculi occur in 1–5% of the population. Ninety percent of these calculi are radio-opaque. There are various types of calculi according to their composition. Calcium oxalate make up 75% of all calculi occurring in alkaline urine. Struvite stones (15%) enlarge rapidly and can fill the calyces forming staghorn calculi. Both urate and cysteine calculi occur in acidic urine. Urate stones are radiolucent. The rarest forms of calculi are xanthine and pyruvate stones caused by inborn errors of metabolism.

100. e.   Epithelial tumours of the bladder are common, with the majority being transitional cell carcinoma. A small proportion are squamous cell carcinomas, with adenocarcinomas being rare. Chemical substances such as β-naphthylamine and benzidine have been recognized as aetiological agents. Smoking and schistosomiasis are also causative. Tumours complicate approximately 2% of bladder diverticulae. Leucoplakia has been associated with squamous cell carcinoma, with adenocarcinoma a recognized complication of ectopia vesicae. There is no evidence to suggest that alcohol is an aetiological factor.

101. c. Testicular tumours are staged using the Union Internationale Contre le Cancer (UICC) 2002 system which, in addition to TNM (Tumour, node, metastasis) categories, uses an S category for serum tumour markers. Serum markers used include lactate dehydrogenase (LDH), which is secreted by seminomas and is seen in non-seminomatous disease, and appears to be a marker of tumour bulk; human chorionic gonadotrophin (hCG), which is produced by all non-seminomatous tumours containing choriocarcinoma elements; and α-fetoprotein (AFP), which is raised in non-seminomatous tumours only. Serum marker stages are:

- Sx: Serum markers not available
- S0: Serum markers within normal limits
- S1: LDH 1.5× normal, hCG < 5000 mIU/L and AFP < 1000 ng/mL
- S2: LDH 1.5–10× normal or hCG 5000–50,000 mIU/L or AFP 1000–10,000 ng/mL
- S3: LDH >10× normal or hCG > 50,000 or AFP > 10,000

102. e. Carcinoembryonic antigen is not a testicular tumour marker but is a non-specific marker for many cancers, particularly colorectal carcinoma. Placental alkaline phosphatase (PLAP) can be detected in up to 65% of seminomas and is a sensitive marker for metastatic seminomatous disease. Lactate dehydrogenase is not specific for testicular cancer but appears to be a good marker of tumour bulk. It is secreted by seminomas and non-seminomatous cancers. γ-Glutamyltransferase (GGT) is a tumour marker for seminoma and non-seminomatous germ cell tumours.

103. b. Elevation of the testicles in the supine position providing relief may point toward a diagnosis of epididymitis – a positive Prehn sign. However, this is not very reliable and any clinical suspicion of torsion should mandate scrotal exploration. Amiodarone is a rare non-infective cause of epididymitis; it accumulates in high concentrations in the epididymis causing inflammation. *Mycobacterium* is also a rare cause where the epididymis feels like a beaded cord. In men <35 years old, the infective organism is usually *Neisseria gonorrhoeae*, *Chlamydia trachomatis* or coliform bacteria. *Streptococcus pyogenes* is responsible for a range of pathologies from superficial skin infections to life-threatening nectrotizing fasciitis.

104. b. Signs of renal injury include bruising and macroscopic and microscopic haematuria. Frank haematuria is very rare. Renal function blood results may be normal at the time of presentation. A normal ultrasound scan does not exclude any renal injury, whereas computed tomography scanning allows thorough anatomical assessment of the kidneys and urinary tract. This modality can assess the injury together with aiding the diagnosis of concurrent injuries.

GASTROINTESTINAL SYSTEM

105. e.   Portal hypertension refers to abnormally high pressures in the hepatic portal vein, usually defined as pressure >12 mmHg (normal range 5–10 mmHg). It has several causes categorized as pre-hepatic, hepatic and post-hepatic. Pre-hepatic causes include obstruction of the portal vein, portal vein thrombosis, congenital atresia of the vein and extrinsic compression from a tumour. Hepatic causes relate to obstruction of portal flow within the liver, for example chronic liver disease with cirrhosis, sarcoidosis and schistosomiasis infection. Post-hepatic causes arise from outflow obstruction and can occur at any level from the liver to the right side of the heart, for example hepatic vein thrombosis (Budd–Chiari syndrome, polycythaemia) and constrictive pericarditis. In the United Kingdom the most common cause of portal hypertension is cirrhosis, whereas worldwide it is schistosomiasis.

106. d.   Congenital hypertrophic pyloric stenosis is encountered in infants, particularly males. It presents with regurgitation and persistent, projectile, non-bilious vomiting, usually appearing in the second or third week of life. Examination reveals visible peristalsis and a firm, ovoid palpable mass in the region of the pylorus or distal stomach. It is caused by hypertrophy and hyperplasia of the muscularis propria of the pylorus. Surgical correction of stenosis is usually indicated.

107. b.   Abdominal compartment syndrome is a combination of adverse physiological effects of a raised intra-abdominal pressure (>20 mmHg). Primary causes (acute with abdominal pathology) include intra-abdominal haemorrhage, pancreatitis and penetrating trauma. Secondary causes occur without an intra-abdominal injury due to fluid accumulation. These include sepsis, peritoneal dialysis and cirrhosis. Direct effects include compression of vasculature of the gastrointestinal tract (GIT) leading to mucosal oedema and thrombosis, portal vein collapse, ventilator difficulties and an increase in the central venous pressure.

108. d.   Crohn disease is an inflammatory bowel disease that affects a wide spectrum of age groups with a particular peak noted in the second and third decades of life. It is characterized pathologically by (1) sharply delimited transmural involvement of the bowel by inflammatory processes with mucosal damage, (2) the presence of non-caseating granulomas and (3) fissuring with formation of fistulae. Intestinal symptoms are a result of malabsorption because of inflammation.

109. e.   Toxic megacolon is the term used to describe an acute toxic colitis with colonic dilatation. It is a potentially life-threatening condition, requiring prompt medical and sometimes surgical management. All of the above are known to cause toxic megacolon. The classic causes are ulcerative colitis, Crohn disease and pseudomembranous colitis.

110. d.   Peutz–Jeghers syndrome, also known as hereditary intestinal polyposis syndrome, is an autosomal dominant genetic disease characterized by the development of benign hamartomatous polyps in the gastrointestinal tract and hyperpigmented macules on the lips and oral mucosa.

111. a. De Garengeot hernia is incarceration of the vermiform appendix within a femoral hernia. Amyand hernia is incarceration of the vermiform appendix within an inguinal hernia. Richter hernia is a hernia involving only one sidewall of the bowel, which may result in bowel strangulation without the signs of bowel obstruction. Spigelian hernia is a hernia occurring between the rectus abdominis muscle medially and the semilunar line laterally. This most commonly occurs below the arcuate line. Littre hernia is incarceration of a Meckel's diverticulum within a hernial sac.

112. b. Amyand hernia is incarceration of the vermiform appendix within an inguinal hernia. De Garengeot hernia is incarceration of the vermiform appendix within a femoral hernia. Richter hernia is a hernia involving only one sidewall of the bowel, which may result in bowel strangulation without the signs of bowel obstruction. Spigelian hernia is a hernia occurring between the rectus abdominis muscle medially and the semilunar line laterally. This most commonly occurs below the arcuate line. Littre hernia is incarceration of a Meckel's diverticulum within a hernial sac.

113. d. Spigelian hernia is a hernia occurring between the rectus abdominis muscle medially and the semilunar line laterally. This most commonly occurs below the arcuate line. De Garengeot hernia is incarceration of the vermiform appendix within a femoral hernia. Amyand hernia is incarceration of the vermiform appendix within an inguinal hernia. Richter hernia is a hernia involving only one sidewall of the bowel, which may result in bowel strangulation without the signs of bowel obstruction. Littre hernia is incarceration of a Meckel diverticulum within a hernial sac.

114. b. Peutz–Jegers syndrome is an autosomal dominant inherited syndrome characterized by intestinal hamartomatous polyposis and pigmentation around the lips. A patient with Peutz–Jegers syndrome can present in many ways such as with intestinal obstruction, or with intussusception causing recurrent colicky abdominal pain. There can also be rectal bleeding either causing a frank bleed or leading to iron deficiency anaemia. Malignant transformation is rare.

115. c. Causes of acute pancreatitis include gallstones, ethanol, trauma, shock, mumps, polyarteritis nodosa, autoimmune disease, hypercalcaemia, hyperlipidaemia, hypothermia, endoscopic retrograde cholangiopancreatography (ERCP) and drugs such as thiazide diuretics, corticosteroids and azathioprine. The mnemonic GET SMASHED is the most commonly used to remember these. Hypocalcaemia is used as part of a score to mark the severity of the condition.

116. c. With a heart rate above 120 bpm, hypotension and low urine output, she is likely to be in stage III haemorrhagic shock. In this stage she has lost approximately 30–40% of her blood volume, equating to 1500–2000 mL. Stage I occurs with blood loss of less than 750 mL. The patient may be haemodynamically stable, but slightly anxious. Stage II shock has a reduced pulse pressure, slight tachycardia and occurs with blood loss up to 1500 mL. Stage IV shock patients have lost more than 2000 mL and are tachycardic, hypotensive and anuric with severely reduced consciousness.

117. e. Meckel's diverticulum occurs as a result of incomplete regression of the vitellointestinal duct during the embryonic period. There is a 'rule of twos' for Meckel's diverticulum: it affects 2% of the population, it is 2 in. (2.5 cm) in length and it is 2 ft (61 cm) from the ileocaecal valve. The lining is similar in nature to the small bowel epithelium and is often mixed with the gastric acid–secreting epithelium or heterotopic pancreatic tissue. It occurs in 2% of the population and is found more frequently in males than females, with a ratio of about 3:1. Complications include volvulus, inflammation, peptic ulceration and intussusception. If found incidentally with none of the above complications it does not require excision.

118. e. Common complications include volvulus, haemorrhage, peptic ulceration and intussusception. There is a small risk of malignant change in complicated cases (4–5%), and in this situation, the most common tumour type is a leiomyoma. Umbilical anomalies occur in 10% of cases, and patients may present with a chronically discharging umbilical sinus.

119. b. Crohn disease affects any part of the gastrointestinal system from mouth to anus, in particular the terminal ileum. Ulcerative colitis (UC) affects the rectum and spreads proximally. In Crohn disease, there are skip lesions with bowel wall thickening, strictures and adhesions. Microscopically there is transmural non-caseating granulomatous inflammation, whereas in UC the inflammation is diffuse, affecting the mucosa and submucosal region. Anal lesions are present in 75% of Crohn disease patients with anal fistulae and fissures. Fistulae are more common in Crohn disease than UC. The risk of colonic carcinoma is raised in UC. Surgery is not curative in Crohn disease and is usually avoided unless absolutely necessary.

120. d. Crohn disease affects any part of the gastrointestinal system from mouth to anus, in particular the terminal ileum. Ulcerative colitis (UC) affects the rectum and spreads proximally. In Crohn's disease, there are skip lesions with bowel wall thickening, strictures and adhesions. Microscopically there is transmural non-caseating granulomatous inflammation, whereas in UC the inflammation is diffuse, affecting the mucosa and submucosal region. Anal lesions are present in 75% of Crohn disease patients with anal fistulae and fissures. Fistulae are more common in Crohn disease than UC. The risk of colonic carcinoma is raised in UC. Surgery is not curative in Crohn disease and is usually avoided unless absolutely necessary.

121. b. Ulcerative colitis (UC) affects the rectum and spreads proximally. Crohn disease affects any part of the gastrointestinal system from mouth to anus, in particular the terminal ileum. In Crohn disease, there are skip lesions with bowel wall thickening, strictures and adhesions. Microscopically there is transmural non-caseating granulomatous inflammation, whereas in UC the inflammation is diffuse, affecting the mucosa and submucosal region. Anal lesions are present in 75% of Crohn disease patients with anal fistulae and fissures. Fistulae are more common in Crohn disease than UC. The risk of colonic carcinoma is raised in UC.

122. e. Ulcerative colitis (UC) affects the rectum and spreads proximally. In Crohn disease, there are skip lesions with bowel wall thickening, strictures and adhesions. Microscopically there is transmural non-caseating granulomatous inflammation, whereas in UC the inflammation is diffuse, affecting the mucosa and submucosal region. Fistulae are more common in Crohn disease than UC. The risk of colonic carcinoma is raised in UC. Toxic megacolon is a surgical emergency.

123. e. Cirrhosis is a diffuse process characterized by fibrosis and formation of abnormal nodules. The aetiology includes drugs such as methotrexate and methyldopa, hepatitis B and C infections, autoimmune diseases, metabolic conditions such as haemochromatosis and biliary obstruction including gallstones. The major complications include portal hypertension, hepatocellular failure and hepatocellular carcinoma. Primary biliary cirrhosis is a chronic disorder affecting women between 40 and 70 years of age leading to destruction of the intrahepatic ducts, leading to cirrhosis. Primary sclerosing cholangitis usually affects men, attacking both intra- and extrahepatic ducts. There is a strong association with ulcerative colitis.

124. d. Gallstones are found in 10–20% of the population. The principal constituents are cholesterol, phospholipids and bile acids. Mixed stones account for 80% of gallstones. Bile pigment stones are usually due to chronic haemolysis or infection with *Escherichia coli*. Carcinoma of the gallbladder is usually associated with gallstones.

125. c. Richter hernia is a hernia involving only one sidewall of the bowel, which may result in bowel strangulation without the signs of bowel obstruction. De Garengeot hernia is incarceration of the vermiform appendix within a femoral hernia. Amyand hernia is incarceration of the vermiform appendix within an inguinal hernia. Spigelian hernia is a hernia occurring between the rectus abdominis muscle medially and the semilunar line laterally. This most commonly occurs below the arcuate line. Littre hernia is incarceration of a Meckel's diverticulum within a hernial sac.

126. c. Benign tumours of the small intestine include adenomas and leimyomas. Peutz–Jeghers syndrome is an autosomal dominant condition characterized by hamartomatous polyps and melanotic pigmentation of the lips and mouth. Adenocarcinoma is 50 times rarer in the small intestine than the colon. T-cell lymphoma is seen in middle-aged patients with a history of coeliac disease. B-cell lymphoma is usually of the mucosa-associated lymphoid tissue (MALT) type. Gastrointestinal stromal tumours (GISTs) may present with bleeding or obstruction and often metastasize to the liver.

127. d. Familial adenomatous polyposis (FAP) is a rare condition inherited as autosomal dominant. It involves the development of hundreds of polyps within the colon and rectum from adolescence which can bleed or develop malignancy. The condition has an equal sex incidence. The gene responsible for the disease is found on chromosome 5. Gardner syndrome refers to the combination of desmoid tumours, osteomas of the mandible, polyposis and sebaceous cysts.

128. a. Meckel's diverticulum is always solitary, occurring in the ileum 2 ft from the ileocaecal valve in 2% of the population and is usually 2 in. long. Duodenal diverticula are congenital, and usually multiple. False diverticula have only part of their wall outpouching from a hollow viscus into the surrounding tissues – examples include sigmoid diverticula and pharyngeal diverticulum (herniation of pharyngeal mucosa between the two components of the inferior constrictor muscle: thyropharyngeus and cricopharyngeus). True diverticula contain all layers of the viscus wall and are usually congenital. False diverticula are usually acquired.

129. a. This scenario describes a case of upper gastrointestinal perforation. The main investigation is an erect chest X-ray (CXR), which in approximately 70% of cases of perforation will show air under the diaphragms. Depending on the clinical state of the patient and hospital resources, a computed tomography scan may be more appropriate for diagnostic and management purposes. An abdominal X-ray (AXR) is of limited value as Rigler's sign may be subtle in many cases.

130. c. Meckel's diverticulum is the most common congenital defect of the gastrointestinal tract. It is a vestigial remnant of the vitellointestinal duct and is present in 2% of the population. It is found approximately 60 cm proximally from the ileocaecal valve on the antimesenteric border and has its own blood supply. There are two types of common ectopic tissue present in Meckel diverticulum: gastric or pancreatic. In most individuals affected it normally presents before the age of 2 years. It is symptomatic in 2% of individuals and can present with painless haematochezia, obstructive symptoms, a volvulus or intussusception. It can present in a fashion similar to acute appendicitis.

131. a. Crohn disease affects the full thickness of the bowel wall. It appears in skip lesions, whereas ulcerative colitis involves only the mucosa and normally starts in the rectum spreading proximally in a continuous fashion. Fistulae are more commonly associated with Crohn's. Histological findings on biopsy often demonstrate non-caseating granulomas. Crypt abscesses are typically seen in UC.

132. a. The Glasgow scoring system is used to predict severe pancreatitis outcome within the first 48 h of admission with pancreatitis, although other scoring systems may be used by certain institutions. Score for age >55 years, white cell count (WCC) >15 × 10^9, urea >16 mmol/L, albumin >32 g/L, aspartate aminotransferase (AST) >200 IU/L, lactate dehydrogenase (LDH) >600 IU/L, calcium <2 mmol/L, glucose >10 mmol/L, PaO$_2$ <8 kPa. A score of 3 or more constitutes a severe attack and consideration should be made for management on a level 2 or 3 ward.

133. d. The Glasgow scoring system is used to predict severe pancreatitis outcome within the first 48 h of admission with pancreatitis. Score for age >55 years, white cell count >15 × 10^9, urea >16 mmol/L, albumin >32 g/L, aspartate aminotransferase >200 IU/L, lactate dehydrogenase >600 IU/L, calcium <2 mmol/L, glucose >10 mmol/L, PaO$_2$ <8 kPa.

134. d. The Glasgow criteria are used to predict severe pancreatitis outcome within the first 48 h of admission with pancreatitis. Score for age >55 years, white cell count >15 × 10⁹, urea >16 mmol/L, albumin >32 g/L, aspartate aminotransferase >200 IU/L, lactate dehydrogenase >600 IU/L, calcium <2 mmol/L, glucose >10 mmol/L, PaO_2 <8 kPa.

135. d.   Gastro-oesophageal reflux (GOR) is the most common upper gastrointestinal diagnosis made. Patients over the age of 55 years with new symptoms of GOR should be investigated; those younger than 55 years with no worrying symptoms justify a trial of medical therapy alone with no further investigation. Worrying symptoms include weight loss, anaemia, anorexia, family history or Barrett's oesophagus. It is important to remember that 30% of patients with significant reflux may have a normal endoscopy. The stages are defined according to the Los Angeles classification:

Stage A: One or more mucosal breaks <5 mm
Stage B: One or more mucosal breaks >5 mm
Stage C: Mucosal breaks extending above >2 mucosal folds but <75% oesophageal circumference
Stage D: >75% oesophageal circumference
Stage E: There is no stage E.

136. c.   Oesophageal atresia is a congenital condition affecting 1 in 3000–4500 births. It is a developmental disorder resulting in the oesophagus ending as a blind-ended pit. Only 10% of those born with this congenital condition have this in isolation, with the remainder having some other form of congenital abnormality. Two-thirds of those born with this condition also have a tracheo-oesophageal fistula (TOF) present. Other associated abnormalities include vertebral anomalies, anorectal anomalies, and cardiac, renal and limb malformations – the so-called VACTERL association. Diagnosis is confirmed by passing a nasogastric tube, which subsequently coils in the lower oesophagus and is visible on chest X-ray. It is considered a surgical emergency. There are five major anatomical variations of oesophageal atresia. The most common is type C (oesophageal atresia with distal TOF), occurring in 75–85% of cases, followed by type A (pure oesophageal atresia alone in 10%). Type B is oesophageal atresia with TOF between the proximal oesophageal segments and trachea. Type D is oesophageal atresia with TOF between both the proximal and distal ends of the oesophagus and trachea, and type E has TOF but not oesophageal atresia.

137. c.   The incidence of duodenal atresia is 1 in 5000 births in the UK. The 'double bubble' sign indicates gas in the stomach and proximal duodenum. If not treated it becomes fatal as a result of fluid shifts and electrolyte imbalances. Fullness in the epigastric region is a result of a distended stomach. With oesophageal atresia, the baby typically presents with choking rather than vomiting. In gastric outlet obstruction there is no bile in the vomit, and most importantly, it presents later at about 4 weeks, whereas duodenal atresia presents at birth. In congenital intestinal obstruction a plain film will show more pathognomonic features of obstruction. No predisposing maternal risk factors are known. Although up to one-third of patients with duodenal atresia have Down syndrome (trisomy 21), it is not an independent risk factor for developing duodenal atresia.

138. a. Hirschsprung disease is a congenital disease where the affected individuals lack mural ganglionic cells in the colon leading to constipation and abdominal distension. Rectal biopsy is the diagnostic tool of choice to demonstrate the deficiency. Genes involved in the pathogenesis of Hirschsprung disease include *RET* (c10), *EDNRB* (c13), *GDNF* (c5), *EDN3* (c20), *SOX10* (c22), *ECE1* (c1), *NTN* (c19) and *SIP1* (c2).

139. a. Diverticulitis is the most likely diagnosis in this case. A CT scan and urine dip are useful investigative tools, but they can wait. Intravenous antibiotics should be started immediately as recommended by the Surviving Sepsis Campaign. Operative intervention may be required should the patient's condition worsen, but it is not the initial management option.

DERMATOLOGICAL DISEASES

140. a. The epidermis is the outer layer of skin acting as a barrier. It is composed of the stratified squamous epithelium and is aneural and avascular. The epidermis can be divided into five layers. These layers, from superficial to deep, are stratum corneum, stratum lucidum, stratum granulosum, stratum spinosum and stratum basale.

141. e. The epidermis can be divided into five layers. These layers, from superficial to deep, are stratum corneum, stratum lucidum, stratum granulosum, stratum spinosum and stratum basale.

142. b. Squamous cell carcinoma (SCC) is a common invasive malignant epidermal tumour with low but recordable risk of metastasis. Risk factors include sunlight exposure and immunosuppression. It can develop in long-standing scars or sinuses – Marjolin's ulcer. SCC has raised averted edges with a central scab. *In situ* SCC is where the lesion has not invaded through the basement membrane of the dermoepidermal junction. Bowen disease is an *in situ* SCC. Lesions are red and scaly plaques.

143. c. There are three components to a burn:

- *Zone of hyperaemia:* Inflammatory mediators induce vasodilation at the periphery of a burn.
- *Zone of ischaemia:* Microvascular injury resulting in stasis of blood and devitalization of tissues – potentially salvageable.
- *Zone of coagulation:* Non-viable coagulative necrosis at the centre of a burn.

First-degree burns involve the epidermis and do not typically blister; they are often exquisitely painful but heal without scarring. Second-degree burns involve the epidermis and dermis, typically blister and are painful – such burns take longer to heal and may do so with scarring. Third-degree burns are full thickness, including the subcutaneous nerves – as a result such burns are typically insensate. They have a white, leathery characteristic appearance, with healing always resulting in scarring.

144. c. Systemic complications of burns include:

- Burn shock
- Electrolyte disturbances – hyperkalaemia, hypocalaemia
- Hypothermia
- Systemic inflammatory response syndrome (SIRS)/sepsis
- Gastric ulceration
- Coagulopathy
- Haemolysis

Resuscitation includes intravenous fluids, analgesia, prevention of hypothermia, stress ulcer prophylaxis and nutritional support. Intravenous fluids are recommended in >15% burns in adults and >10% in children. The Advanced Trauma Life Support (ATLS) guideline for fluid resuscitation is 2–4 mL/kg per percent burn over the first 24 h.

145. b. Malignant melanomas are epidermal tumours of melanocytes with significant metastatic potential. They can be classified into various forms. Superficial spreading melanoma, which is the most common type, occurs anywhere on the body. Nodular melanoma has a thick irregular outline that may ulcerate. Hutchinson lentigo is also known as lentigo maligna. Acral lentiginous melanoma including subungual melanoma is rare but can present as a subungual haematoma. The prognosis of melanomas depends on Breslow thickness, nodal involvement and metastasis. Melanoma *in situ* must be excised with a 5 mm margin with a greater margin (1–3 cm) for deeper lesions.

146. c. Lentigo maligna is also known as a Hutchinson lentigo and is most commonly found on the face. Acral lentiginous melanoma usually arises from thick epidermal regions such as the sole of the foot. Superficial spreading melanoma is the most common malignant melanoma and is found usually on the legs commonly in women and the upper back in men.

147. c. Squamous cell carcinoma (SCC) is a common invasive malignant epidermal tumour with low but recordable risk of metastasis. A Marjolin's ulcer is a SCC developing in a long-standing scar or sinus. It has raised averted edges with a central scab. Bowen disease is an *in situ* SCC. Lesions are red and scaly plaques.

148. a. Basal cell carcinoma (BCC) is a common slow-growing malignant epidermal tumour that rarely metastasizes. It is the most common skin cancer, characterized by raised, rolled edges, with pearly nodules and visible fine blood vessels. BCCs are slow-growing, have central ulceration and scabbing. Unlike squamous cell carcinomas (SCC), they are not characterized by prickle cells. Approximately 90% of BCCs occur on the face.

149. d. The stratum spinosum is also known as the prickle layer of the epidermis because of its desmosomal connections with adjacent cells. It is important in bipolar lipid production to reduce water evaporation. The stratum corneum is the outermost layer of the epidermis and consists of keratin-filled anuclear cells. The thickness of this layer is determined by what it is exposed to. For example, on the plantar surface of the feet the skin is subject to greater insult than that on the dorsal surface, and so will have a thicker protective stratum corneum. Melanocytes are found in the stratum basale.

150. b. Clarke's levels are an anatomical classification of melanoma thickness. These are:

Level I – an epidermal melanoma that has not penetrated the basement membrane and therefore does not metastasize (100% 5-year survival)
Level II – a melanoma that has breached the basement membrane to reach the papillary dermis (90–100% 5-year survival)
Level III – a melanoma that fills the papillary dermis and has begun to encroach into the reticular dermis (80–90% 5-year survival)
Level IV – a melanoma that has invaded the reticular dermis (60–70% 5-year survival)
Level V – a melanoma that has invaded the subcutaneous fat (15–30% survival)

Owing to the varying thickness of the skin over the body, Clarke's levels have less significance in modern clinical practice than the Breslow thickness, which serves as a more reliable prognostic indicator.

151. a. Malignant melanoma may arise from the melanocytes of pre-existing naevi (>50% arise *de novo*). Some of the features that raise concern in a pre-existing naevus are asymmetry, border irregularity, colour variegation and having a dimension >6 mm (these four features can be remembered with the aide-memoire ABCD). Other worrying features include itching or pain, bleeding, ulceration, satellite lesions and the development of regional lymph nodes. A rolled edge is associated with a basal cell carcinoma.

LYMPHORETICULAR SYSTEM

152. d.   Splenic rupture is usually precipitated by a crushing injury or severe blow. However, it can also occur in non-traumatic conditions such as infectious mononucleosis, malaria, typhoid fever and lymphoid neoplasms. It is caused by rapid splenic enlargement, producing a thin, tense splenic capsule that is susceptible to rupture.

153. d.   The total combination of monocytes, mobile macrophages, fixed tissue macrophages and a few specialized endothelial cells in the bone marrow, spleen and lymph nodes is called the reticuloendothelial system. Sinusoids of the liver are lined with tissue macrophages called Kupffer cells, which form an effective particulate filtration system for bacteria entering from the gastrointestinal tract. Tissue macrophages in the skin and subcutaneous tissues constitute histiocytes, which play a useful role in subcutaneous tissue infection. Large numbers of tissue macrophages are present as integral components of the alveolar walls. These can phagocytose particles that become entrapped in the alveoli.

154. c.   Splenectomy is mainly performed for trauma, autoimmune thrombocytopenic purpura, haemolytic anaemias and hypersplenism. Problems post-splenectomy include a rise in platelets (600–1000×10^9) for 2–3 weeks. During this time the patient is at an increased risk of thromboembolic phenomena. In the longer term, the patient is particularly at risk for overwhelming sepsis by encapsulated bacteria (pneumococcus, *H. influenzae* and meningococcus), but problems from infections by *E. coli*, malaria and babesiosis (from tick bites) can occur. The greatest risk is within the first 2 years, and an increased risk is probably present for life. Children aged 5 years or less have an infection rate of more than 10%, which is more than 10 times the adult rate. All patients who have had a splenectomy should have pneumococcal, *Haemophilus* and meningococcal group C vaccinations and have prophylactic penicillin.

155. d.   Post-splenectomy there is an early thrombocytosis peaking at 7–10 days postoperatively with increasing levels of circulating target cells, Howell–Jolly bodies and sideroblasts (red blood cells containing granules of free iron). There is increased platelet adhesiveness and platelet dysfunction. There is also an increased susceptibility to sepsis caused by encapsulated organisms such as *Haemophilus influenzae*, *Streptococcus pneumoniae* and *Neisseria meningitidis*.

156. c.   Post-splenectomy there is an early thrombocytosis peaking at 7–10 days postoperatively with increasing levels of circulating target cells, Howell–Jolly bodies and sideroblasts (red blood cells containing granules of free iron). There is increased platelet adhesiveness and platelet dysfunction. There is also an increased susceptibility to sepsis caused by encapsulated organisms such as *Haemophilus influenzae*, *Streptococcus pneumoniae* and *Neisseria meningitidis*.

157. e.   Indications for splenectomy in idiopathic thrombocytopenic purpura (ITP) include refractory severe thrombocytopenia, failure to respond to medical therapy, relapse after steroids, or if the steroid concentration required to increase the platelet count is very high or at toxic doses. A persistently high platelet count is not an indication for splenectomy.

158. e.   Emergency splenectomy is usually performed as an open procedure. Post-splenectomy infection is a significant but low risk of splenectomy after trauma when compared with haematological conditions. Ideally, the patient should receive vaccinations for meningococcal C, *Haemophilus influenzae* and pneumococcus within 2 weeks of emergency splenectomy.

159. e.   Overwhelming post-splenectomy infection is usually caused by encapsulated bacteria and presents mainly within the first 2 years after splenectomy, or in patients with hyposplenism. It is usually fatal without treatment. Its incidence can be reduced by vaccinations (meningococcal C, *Haemophilus influenzae* and pneumococcal vaccine) and prophylactic antibiotics. Urgent cultures and treatment with antibiotics are recommended at the first sign of infection. Risk factors that increase the likelihood of post-splenectomy infection include Hodgkin disease, young age, lymphoma and trauma. Trauma has a low but significant risk of overwhelming post-splenectomy infection.

160. b.   Lymphoma is a group of cancers affecting cells of the lymphatic system. Lymphomas can be classified according to the World Health Organization or Revised European-American Lymphoma system. Reed–Sternberg cells are giant cells identified on biopsies, which are essential for the diagnosis of Hodgkin lymphoma. They are derived from B-lymphocytes. Diagnosis can be made by biopsy of any masses or bone marrow biopsy, which can also be used for assessing treatment response.

161. e.   Reed–Sternberg cells are pathognomonic for Hodgkin lymphoma and help to differentiate it from non-Hodgkin lymphoma. Both may have similar presentations with malaise, weight loss and lymph node masses being features. Auer rods are commonly seen in the diagnosis of acute myeloid leukaemia.

162. b.   Hodgkin disease accounts for about 20% of lymphomas. Most patients present with painless enlargement of lymph nodes with one-quarter complaining of systemic symptoms. Classical Hodgkin disease is probably caused by Epstein–Barr virus. Reed–Sternberg cells are distinctive tumour cells containing mirror-image nuclei with large eosinophilic nucleoli.

Ann Arbor:

Stage I – disease involving single node or group of nodes
Stage II – disease in more than one site, all either above or below the diaphragm
Stage III – disease on both sides of the diaphragm
Stage IV – widespread involvement of extralymphoid sites

163. e.   Hodgkin lymphoma is a common form of lymphoid malignancy in young adults. It arises in a single node or chain of nodes and spreads first to the anatomically contiguous nodes. It is characterized morphologically by the presence of distinctive neoplastic giant cells, called Reed–Sternberg cells, which induce the accumulation of reactive lymphocytes, histiocytes (macrophages) and granulocytes. The World Health Organization (WHO) classification recognizes five subtypes of Hodgkin lymphoma: nodular sclerosis, mixed cellularity, lymphocyte rich, lymphocyte depletion and lymphocyte predominance.

EAR, NOSE AND THROAT

164. e. A vast majority of epistaxis occur anteriorly in Little's area, which can often be controlled with pressure. Posterior bleeds are often more prolonged and difficult to control. Sphenopalatine, maxillary and external carotids are all ligation targets in uncontrollable epistaxis.

165. b. This is known as secondary haemorrhage occurring days after the primary procedure, and is usually secondary to infection. Reactionary haemorrhage occurs in the period immediately after the procedure once the individual has recovered from the anaesthetic and the physiological parameters are restored to normal levels (24–48 h). Primary haemorrhage occurs during the operative procedure, caused by transecting a blood vessel. Tertiary heamorrhage does not exist.

166. c. Carotid body tumours, also known as chemodectomas or paragangliomas, arise from chemoreceptors of the carotid body found at the bifurcation of the carotid artery. They are benign, slow-growing lumps and can be bilateral. However, in 10% of cases they can be malignant. On examination, a pulsation will be felt on palpation and a bruit may be heard on auscultation. Investigations will include computed tomography, carotid angiography (illustrating the goblet sign – splaying apart of the carotid bifurcation), Doppler study and magnetic resonance imaging (MRI). Surgical excision is recommended as the infiltrate locally.

167. b. Acoustic neuromas arise from Schwann cells of the nerve sheath of cranial nerve VIII. On expanding it extends into the cerebellopontine angle compressing the pons and cerebellum. It can be a feature of Von Recklinghausen's disease and commonly occurs in the 30- to 60-year age group. The most common presentation is unilateral sensorineural deafness with tinnitus. Facial weakness is usually a late manifestation as are unilateral cerebellar signs.

168. c. Parotid gland tumours account for approximately 80% of all salivary gland tumours, of which two-thirds are pleiomorphic adenomas. Monomorphic adenomas account for the remaining third, the most common of which is Warthin tumour, which is an adenolymphoma. These are more commonly bilateral. Weakness of the facial nerve suggests malignant infiltration. Adenoid cystic carcinomas are highly malignant tumours of the parotid gland, often causing facial nerve palsy. They are hard and fixed on examination. A parotid lump should not be cut into because of the risk of implantation and recurrence. A fine-needle aspiration (FNA) can be performed followed by wide local excision if needed.

MISCELLANEOUS

169. b. The following circumstances require mandatory referral to the coroner:

- Cause of death unknown
- Patient's normal medical practitioner did not attend within 14 days of the death
- Within 24 h of an operation
- Within 24 h of admission to hospital
- Industrial accident/road traffic accident/domestic accident
- Poisoning/suicide/neglect
- Death in custody
- Death surrounding negligence

PART V

PRACTICE PAPER

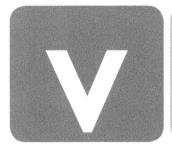

CHAPTER 9
PRACTICE PAPER

Questions

1. At which vertebral level does the oesophagus cross the diaphragm?
   a. T8
   b. T9
   c. T10
   d. T11
   e. T12

2. A 47-year-old male presents with a 3 × 4 cm superficial abdominal wall abscess. Which of the following statements regarding the pathology of abscesses is correct?
   a. They are enclosed in a pyogenic membrane composed of fibrotic connective tissue.
   b. *Staphylococcus aureus* is always the cause of a pilonidal abscess.
   c. Coliforms are most often the cause of a psoas abscess.
   d. A sterile abscess may contain bacteria.
   e. Pus contains a mixture of dead and live neutrophils.

3. Which of the following viruses is correctly paired with the tumours they may cause?
   a. Human herpes virus 8 – hepatocellular carcinoma
   b. Human papilloma virus – anal carcinoma
   c. Epstein–Barr virus – Kaposi's sarcoma
   d. Hepatitis B virus – cervical carcinoma
   e. Human T-cell leukaemia virus – nasopharyngeal cancer

4. A 45-year-old has had several units of blood following a significant road traffic collision. He feels unwell and you perform an electrocardiogram (ECG) to look for evidence of hyperkalaemia. Which of the following ECG changes would you expect to find?
   a. Peaked T waves
   b. Prolonged PR interval
   c. Prolonged QT interval
   d. All of the above
   e. a and b only

5. Which of the following is not a site for communication between the portal and systemic venous systems?
   a. Between the oesophageal branch of the left gastric vein and the azygous system
   b. Between the portal tributaries in the mesentery and retroperitoneal veins communicating with the renal, lumbar and phrenic veins
   c. Between portal branches in the liver and the veins of the abdominal wall
   d. Between the superior rectal branch of the inferior mesenteric vein and the inferior rectal veins
   e. Between the superior and inferior pancreaticoduodenal veins

6. Which of the following statements regarding the inferior epigastric artery is incorrect?
   a. The inferior epigastric artery can be injured during laparoscopic port insertion.
   b. An inguinal hernia medial to the inferior epigastric artery is described as an indirect hernia.
   c. It supplies the rectus abdominis muscle.
   d. It supplies the medial aspect of the anterolateral abdominal wall.
   e. It anastomoses with the superior epigastric artery.

7. Pepsinogen is an important enzyme involved in food digestion. Which of the following cells found in the gastric wall secrete pepsinogen?
   a. Parietal cells
   b. D-cells
   c. Enterochromaffin-like cells
   d. Goblet cells
   e. Chief cells

8. Which part of the nephron tubercle is impermeable to water?
   a. The proximal tubule
   b. The descending limb of the loop of Henle
   c. The ascending limb of the loop of Henle
   d. The distal tubule
   e. The collecting duct

9. Which of the following premalignant conditions is incorrectly matched with its associated malignant tumour?
   a. Epithelial hyperplasia of the breast – carcinoma of the breast
   b. Xeroderma pigmentosum – skin cancer
   c. Ulcerative colitis – squamous cell carcinoma of the anus
   d. Cirrhosis of the liver – hepatocellular carcinoma
   e. Paget disease – osteogenic sarcoma

10. A 25-year-old soldier presents to the emergency department looking anxious, with a 5-day-old wound to the right shoulder, which is rapidly increasing in size. On examination he is hypotensive, feverish, with a 2-cm open wound that is warm and red over his right deltoid. There are surrounding erythema and serosanguineous discharge. You manage to palpate surgical emphysema

over the wound. Which of the following organisms is most likely to cause this clinical picture?

a. *Clostridium difficile*
b. *Clostridium perfringens*
c. *Clostridium tetani*
d. *Staphylococcus aureus*
e. *Clostridium botulinum*

11. Which one of the following structures contributes toward the stability of the ankle joint?

a. Ankle syndesmosis
b. Anterior inferior tibiofibular ligament
c. Deltoid ligament
d. Close apposition of articular surfaces of the tibia and fibula
e. All of the above

12. Concerning antidiuretic hormone (ADH), which of the following statements is correct?

a. It is released by the anterior pituitary gland.
b. It acts mainly on the proximal convoluted tubule.
c. It is stimulated by alcohol.
d. Lack of production causes cranial diabetes insipidus.
e. It causes the production of a high volume of urine.

13. Regarding the cardiac action potential, which of the following statements is incorrect?

a. There is a constant leak of sodium ions out of the cell.
b. The influx of calcium ions lengthens the cardiac action potential.
c. The cell membrane is repolarized by potassium ions flowing out of the cell.
d. Acetylcholine decreases the rate of sodium ion leak.
e. Adrenaline increases the rate of sodium ion leak.

14. A 65-year-old man presents to your outpatient clinic with a 3 cm round lump within the region of the parotid gland. During your history you make a note that he has been a lifelong smoker. Subsequent histological examination reveals an encapsulated mass with narrow cystic spaces lined by a double layer of neoplastic epithelial cells. Which one of the following is the most likely diagnosis?

a. Warthin tumour
b. Mucoepidermoid carcinoma
c. Pleomorphic adenoma
d. Ductal papilloma
e. Canalicular adenoma

15. The following cranial nerves (CNs) are paired with their correct route of exit from the base of the skull except:

a. CN II – optic canal
b. CN IV – superior orbital fissure
c. CN VI – foramen ovale
d. CN XI – jugular foramen
e. CN XII – hypoglossal canal

16. The following statements regarding the anatomy of the facial nerve are true except:
    a. It exits the skull via the stylomastoid foramen.
    b. It provides parasympathetic supply to the sublingual gland.
    c. It supplies the platysma muscle.
    d. It supplies the stapedius muscle.
    e. It supplies sensation to the posterior two-thirds of the tongue.

17. While performing an endoscopy on a patient with long-term gastro-oesophageal reflux disease (GORD) you notice an area of erythema around the distal third of the oesophagus. Which of the following pathological processes has most likely occurred?
    a. Neoplasia
    b. Hyperplasia
    c. Heteroplasia
    d. Dysplasia
    e. Metaplasia

18. The following tumour markers are correctly paired with an associated neoplasia except:
    a. Ca 15-3: Breast cancer
    b. Calcitonin: Parathyroid carcinoma
    c. Ca 19-9: Advanced colorectal carcinoma
    d. Vanillylmandelic acid: Pheochromocytoma
    e. Antidiuretic hormone: Oat cell tumour

19. Following history and clinical examination, you are suspicious that your patient has a bone tumour. On reviewing the radiograph of the distal femur you can see that the periosteum has been lifted up and reactive new bone is growing underneath; you identify this appearance as Codman's triangle. Which bone tumour is this sign characteristically associated with?
    a. Osteochondroma
    b. Osteosarcoma
    c. Chondrosarcoma
    d. Osteochondroma
    e. Enchondroma

20. What does the Y descent represent on the Jugular Venous Pressure (JVP) waveform?
    a. Closing of the tricuspid valve
    b. Atrial contraction
    c. Start of ventricular systole
    d. Closing of the mitral valve
    e. Opening of the tricuspid valve

21. On the general surgical ward you are managing a patient who needs to be nil by mouth for several days. Which statement regarding fluid secretions and absorption in the gastrointestinal tract is correct in order to aid your fluid management regimen?
    a. A total of 2.5 L of saliva is secreted per day.
    b. The small bowel absorbs 4–5 L per day.

c. One litre of bile is secreted per day.

d. A total of 300 mL of fluid is secreted in faeces.

e. The small intestine secretes 1.5 L of fluid per day.

22. Which of the following statements is correct regarding the anatomy of the submandibular gland?

a. The submandibular duct arises superiorly from the gland.

b. The superficial lobe of the gland lies between the mylohyoid and the posterior belly of the digastric muscle.

c. The gland is separated from the parotid gland by the stylomandibular ligament.

d. The gland lies superior to the lingual nerve.

e. The gland lies inferior to the hypoglossal nerve.

23. An 18-year-old is brought into the accident and emergency department with a superficial knife stab wound on the side of his right chest wall. His airway, breathing and circulation are unremarkable. On further assessment he is unable to raise his right arm above the horizontal position. Also, when he presses his hands against a wall, his right scapula protrudes away from the chest wall. Which of the following nerves is most likely damaged in this situation?

a. Suprascapular nerve

b. Upper subscapular nerve

c. Lower subscapular nerve

d. Long thoracic nerve

e. Thoracodorsal nerve

24. Regarding wound healing on the skin, the following statements are true except:

a. A Keloid scars are common in Black Africans.

b. A Wounds closed surgically heal by primary intention.

c. A Wounds that heal by secondary intention involve centripetal growth of epithelium.

d. A Hypertrophic scar usually does not extend beyond the wound edges.

e. A Keloid scar usually settles spontaneously in up to 18 months.

25. A 24-year-old woman is admitted as an emergency with appendicitis. While awaiting her procedure she is made nil by mouth (NBM) and is put on intravenous fluids. The first bag of fluids put up is 1 L of normal saline. How much sodium (Na^+) is in this bag?

a. 114 mmol/L

b. 124 mmol/L

c. 134 mmol/L

d. 144 mmol/L

e. 154 mmol/L

26. Regarding the regulation of gastric secretion, the following statements are true except:

a. Somatostatin inhibits gastrin secretion.

b. The majority of gastric secretions are produced during the gastric phase.

c. Secretin from the duodenal mucosa further stimulates gastrin release from the stomach.

d. Vagal activity stimulates gastric secretion in the cephalic phase.

e. Fatty food in the duodenum leads to the release of cholecystokinin.

27. Different nerves are used for different functions. Which of the following nerve types are used to associated with transmitting pain, touch and temperature?
a. Aα
b. Aβ
c. Aδ
d. B
e. C

28. A 22-year-old horse rider was thrown off a horse and landed on his left shoulder and head, stretching his neck. On examination there is loss of shoulder abduction and lateral rotation as well as loss of elbow flexion and supination. Which nerve roots are likely to be damaged?
a. C5–C6
b. C7
c. C7–C8
d. C8
e. T1

29. A 47-year-old man underwent intramedullary nailing for a mid-shaft fracture of tibia 3 h ago. The ward nurses are concerned as he is in a lot of pain. On examination, he has no neurovascular deficit. He complains of excruciating pain on passive extension of the big toe. Passive dorsiflexion and plantar flexion of the ankle do not cause as much pain. Which of the following is the likely diagnosis?
a. Compartment syndrome of the deep posterior compartment of the leg
b. Compartment syndrome of the superficial posterior compartment of the leg
c. Compartment syndrome of the anterior compartment of the leg
d. Compartment syndrome of the lateral compartment of the leg
e. Compartment syndrome of the medial compartment of the leg

30. A 74-year-old male presents to the clinic with a long history of bilateral leg ulceration. Which of the following statements regarding venous ulcers is correct?
a. Elevation aids in treatment.
b. Two-layer compression bandages are the optimal management of venous ulcers.
c. Any concomitant arterial disease should be corrected after the venous ulcers are treated.
d. Venous ulcers are typically found in the pressure-bearing area.
e. Venous ulcers are usually associated with reduced or absent pedal pulses.

31. A 52-year-old woman presents with acute left-sided loin to groin pain on a background of polyuria and generalized skeletal aches. On examination, she has a serum calcium of 3.1 mmol/L with a raised parathyroid hormone (PTH)

concentration of 150 ng/L. A plain kidney, ureter and bladder (KUB) film shows a stone in the left ureter. Which of the following types of renal stone is most likely to be the culprit in this case?

a. Calcium oxalate
b. Uric acid
c. Struvite
d. Cystine
e. Calcium phosphate

32. A 46-year-old female presents to the general surgical clinic with a 9-week history of a left-sided neck lump. Following thorough investigation and discussion at the local multidisciplinary meeting, a hemithyroidectomy is performed. The lesion histologically represents a follicular carcinoma. Which of the following statements regarding follicular carcinoma is correct?

a. Radiation exposure is a risk factor for its development.
b. Lymph node metastases are typical.
c. It has a prevalence of approximately 5% of thyroid carcinomas.
d. It has a 5-year survival rate of approximately 70%.
e. It is diagnosed by ultrasound and fine-needle aspiration cytology.

33. Which one of the following statements regarding magnesium homeostasis is correct?

a. Dietary magnesium is mainly absorbed in the large bowel.
b. The major site for magnesium transport is in the thick ascending loop of Henle.
c. Loop diuretics decrease magnesium loss.
d. Hypermagnesaemia promotes magnesium reabsorption in the kidney.
e. Hypercalcaemia promotes magnesium reabsorption in the kidney by an unknown mechanism.

34. Before performing a mastectomy for breast cancer, knowledge of the surface anatomy and arterial supply to the breast is required. Which one of the following statements regarding the anatomy of the breast is correct?

a. The breast is supplied only by the internal thoracic and lateral thoracic arteries.
b. The breast is supplied completely by the branches of the subclavian artery.
c. The breast is supplied in part by the intercostal arteries.
d. The breast extends vertically from the 2nd to the 4th ribs.
e. About 75% of lymph drains into the parasternal lymph nodes.

35. The axillary artery runs from the first rib to the inferior border of teres major. Which of the following arteries is a direct branch of the axillary artery?

a. Vertebral artery
b. Internal thoracic artery
c. Posterior circumflex humoral
d. Costocervical trunk
e. Dorsal scapula artery

36. The following statements regarding apoptosis are true except:

a. It can be physiological or pathological.
b. It is a regulated process.

c. Cell DNA is cleaved by enzymes.
d. Cell membrane integrity remains intact.
e. It is energy independent.

37. An 85-year-old man is admitted following a significant lower gastrointestinal haemorrhage. A blood transfusion is commenced; however, he shortly develops an acute transfusion reaction. Which of the following hypersensitivity reactions is associated with this type of reaction?
   a. Type I
   b. Type II
   c. Type III
   d. Type IV
   e. Type V

38. Which of the following statements concerning saliva is correct?
   a. The saliva from the submandibular glands contains more protein than the saliva from the parotid gland.
   b. The parotid glands produce a highly mucinous saliva.
   c. The volume of saliva produced each day is approximately 300 mL.
   d. Saliva is hypotonic to plasma at all times.
   e. The basal rate of saliva production is greater from the parotid glands than from the submandibular gland.

39. Which of the following statements regarding cerebrospinal fluid (CSF) is correct?
   a. The total volume is 100 mL.
   b. The rate of production is approximately 250 mL/day.
   c. Normal CSF pressure is 5 kPa.
   d. CSF is only produced in the lateral and third ventricles.
   e. CSF is absorbed by the spinal villi in the lumbar region.

40. What is incarceration of a Meckel's diverticulum into an inguinal hernia otherwise known as?
   a. De Garengeot hernia
   b. Amyand hernia
   c. Richter hernia
   d. Spigelian hernia
   e. Littre hernia

41. When performing a laparoscopic cholecystectomy the surgeon identifies the cystic artery within Calot's triangle. Which of the following structures make up the triangle?
   a. Cystic artery, cystic duct and common hepatic duct
   b. Cystic duct, right hepatic artery and liver
   c. Cystic duct, common hepatic duct and liver
   d. Cystic vein, cystic duct and common hepatic duct
   e. Liver, cystic artery and right hepatic artery

42. The axillary artery is conventionally divided into three parts, each giving off its own branches. The third part of the axillary artery divides into which of the following branches?
    a. Subscapular, circumflex humeral and lateral thoracic arteries
    b. Posterior circumflex humeral and lateral thoracic arteries
    c. Subscapular, anterior circumflex and posterior circumflex humeral arteries
    d. Anterior and posterior circumflex humeral arteries
    e. Superior thoracic and subscapular arteries

43. A 20-year-old woman attends accident and emergency with signs of ischaemia in her cerebral and ophthalmic arteries. Which of the following arterial diseases is most likely the cause?
    a. Kawasaki disease
    b. Polyarteritis nodosa
    c. Buerger's disease
    d. Temporal arteritis
    e. Takayashu disease

44. Concerning the defecation reflex, which of the following statements is correct?
    a. It is triggered when distended rectal walls reach a pressure of 80 mmHg.
    b. Afferent impulses pass to sacral segments 1 and 2.
    c. Efferent impulses activate post-ganglionic parasympathetic nervous system neurons of the myenteric plexus.
    d. Sympathetic stimulation leads to relaxation of the internal anal sphincter.
    e. Conscious resistance to defecate leads to inhibition of the pudendal nerve.

45. The grey matter in the spinal cord is organized into 10 laminae on each side. Which number lamina contains the alpha motor neurons?
    a. I
    b. IV
    c. X
    d. V
    e. IX

46. Which of the following tumour suppressor genes is correctly paired with its correct chromosome of origin?
    a. APC – chromosome 5
    b. p53 – chromosome 13
    c. Retinoblastoma – chromosome 17
    d. NF1 – chromosome 11
    e. WT1 – chromosome 17

47. At a follow-up clinic you note a positive Trendelenburg test in a 74-year-old lady following a hip replacement. Injury to which of the following nerves is the most likely explanation?
    a. Superior gluteal
    b. Inferior gluteal
    c. Obturator

d. Tibial

e. Femoral

48. Which of these statements about the anatomical snuffbox is correct?
    a. The radial border is formed by the tendon of flexor pollicis longus.
    b. The radial border is formed by the tendon of abductor pollicis brevis.
    c. The cutaneous branch of the radial nerve lies in the roof of the snuffbox.
    d. The cephalic vein begins in the floor of the snuffbox.
    e. The radial artery lies in the roof of the snuffbox.

49. In acute inflammation, such as when the body responds to a microbial infection, which one of the following statements is incorrect?
    a. Neutrophils marginate in response to chemical mediators such as histamine.
    b. Bradykinin is a vasodilator.
    c. Bradykinin is a chemical mediator of pain.
    d. Intercellular adhesion molecule-1 (ICAM-1) is important in adhesion to the vascular endothelium.
    e. There is decreased vascular permeability.

50. A 38-year-old woman presents to your ear, nose and throat (ENT) clinic complaining of a 1-month history of repeated attacks of vertigo, which are particularly severe when she turns over in bed. You conduct the Hallpike positional manoeuvre, which confirms your diagnosis. Which of the following is the cause of her vertigo?
    a. Benign positional paroxysmal vertigo (BPPV)
    b. Acute labyrinthitis
    c. Ménière's disease
    d. Cervical spondylosis
    e. Labyrinthine fistula

51. Concerning bone physiology, which one of the following statements is true?
    a. Once matured, bones are no longer metabolically active.
    b. Osteoblasts are responsible for bone resorption.
    c. The inorganic component of bone is referred to as osteoid.
    d. Thyroxine is involved in bone remodelling.
    e. Immobility does not cause bone mass to be lost.

52. Mineralocorticoid deficiency can cause the following conditions except:
    a. Increased urinary sodium (Na^+) loss
    b. Increased urinary potassium (K^+) loss
    c. Metabolic acidosis
    d. Postural hypotension
    e. Buccal pigmentation

53. Which of the following subtypes of malignant melanoma is more common in darker-skinned individuals?
    a. Lentigo maligna melanoma
    b. Nodular melanoma
    c. Superficial spreading melanoma

d. Acral lentiginous melanoma
e. Amelanocytic melanoma

54. Which one of the following is characteristic of necrosis in comparison with apoptosis?
a. The plasma membrane remains intact.
b. There is cell shrinkage.
c. There is an inflammatory response.
d. It typically involves single cells rather than groups of cells.
e. It is a physiological process.

55. Which of the following muscles is not attached to the scapula?
a. Serratus anterior
b. Rhomboid major
c. Pectoralis minor
d. Omohyoid
e. Subclavius

56. Which of the following statements is correct regarding the anatomy of the adrenal gland?
a. The superior adrenal artery is derived from the renal artery.
b. The middle adrenal artery is derived from the abdominal aorta.
c. The inferior adrenal artery is derived from the inferior phrenic artery.
d. The adrenal gland is usually drained by three adrenal veins.
e. The spleen is at risk with right-sided adrenalectomy.

57. Acute inflammation is characterized by which one of the following?
a. Plasma cells
b. Lymphocytes
c. Macrophages
d. Slow reaction to tissue injury
e. Innate immune response

58. A young woman presents to the surgeons late at night following a recent open appendicectomy. Her wound appears red and inflamed with a mottling of the surrounding skin. In addition to the mottling there are several black spots present sporadically located up to 6 cm away from the scar. She is febrile (temperature 38.9°C) and unwell. Which of the following is the best management option?
a. Theatre immediately
b. Observe on the ward
c. Oral antibiotics
d. Intravenous antibiotics
e. a and d

59. A 57-year-old patient has an uneventful open inguinal hernia repair. After 3 months of normal healing, approximately how strong will the resultant scar be as a percentage of the original undamaged skin?
a. 50–60%
b. 60–70%

c. 70–80%

d. 80–90%

e. 90–100%

60. With regard to the epidermis, in which layer are the melanin-producing melanocytes located?

a. Stratum corneum

b. Stratum lucidum

c. Stratum granulosum

d. Stratum spinosum

e. Stratum basale

61. In theatre your registrar asks you to perform an open appendicectomy. Which of the following incisions is commonly used for the operation?

a. Right Kocher's

b. Pfannenstiel

c. Lanz

d. Right paramedian

e. Maylard incision

62. Concerning the course of the thoracic duct, which of the following statements is correct?

a. It arises at L3.

b. It passes through the left crus of the diaphragm.

c. It ascends anterior to the oesophagus.

d. It crosses the midline from right to left at T5.

e. It drains into the right internal jugular vein.

63. A 76-year-old woman presents to the accident and emergency department with a peritonitic abdomen. She is taken for an immediate laparotomy. A pelvic mass is biopsied and several days later histology suggests a Krukenberg tumour. Which of the following is the most likely source of the primary tumour?

a. Pancreatic carcinoma

b. Gastric carcinoma

c. Ovarian carcinoma

d. Lung carcinoma

e. Breast carcinoma

64. When analyzing a spirogram, the expiratory reserve volume is defined as which one of the following?

a. The volume of gas remaining in the lungs after maximal expiration

b. The volume of gas that can be expired after maximal inspiration

c. The maximum volume of gas that can be expired during forced breathing excluding the tidal volume

d. The maximum volume of gas that can be expired during forced breathing including the tidal volume

e. The volume of gas remaining in the lungs after a normal tidal expiration

65. A pulmonary artery catheter is a multilumen flow-directed catheter passed through the right side of the heart and into the pulmonary artery. Which of the following physiological parameters is not measured directly by such a catheter?
    a. Ejection fraction
    b. Pulmonary vascular resistance
    c. Mixed venous oxygen saturation
    d. Mean arterial pressure
    e. Mean pulmonary artery pressure

66. Which of the following statements relating to cholinergic receptors is true?
    a. Nicotine depresses acetylcholine release from parasympathetic nerve endings.
    b. Muscarinic receptors are present in most involuntary organs.
    c. Muscarinic receptors can only be activated by muscarine.
    d. Only nicotinic receptors can be activated by acetylcholine.
    e. Muscarinic receptors are mainly found in the skeletal muscle.

67. Which one of the following statements regarding the borders of the popliteal fossa is correct?
    a. Superolateral and superomedial borders are formed by the lateral and medial heads of the gastrocnemius, respectively.
    b. The superomedial border is formed by semimembranosus and semitendinosus.
    c. Semimembranosus is superficial to semitendinosus.
    d. The inferolateral border is formed by the biceps femoris.
    e. The roof is formed by the popliteal surface of the femur.

68. A 23-year-old woman is referred to the Ear, nose and throat (ENT) clinic with a lump in her neck. The ENT senior house officer notes that there is a lump arising from the posterior triangle of the neck. Which of the following structures form the boundaries of the posterior triangle of the neck?
    a. Posterior border of sternocleidomastoid, the clavicle and anterior border of trapezius
    b. Inferior border of mandible, anterior border of trapezius and anterior border of sternocleidomastoid
    c. Anterior midline of neck, posterior border of sternocleidomastoid and inferior border of mandible
    d. Styloid process, suprasternal notch and posterior border of sternocleidomastoid
    e. Digastric muscle inferior border of mandible and anterior border of trapezius

69. Which one of the following conditions is a cause of primary lymphoedema?
    a. Milroy disease
    b. Cancer
    c. Tuberculosis
    d. Radiotherapy
    e. Surgery

70. Which one of the following statements regarding deep vein thrombosis (DVT) is correct?
    a. If a DVT is present, it usually produces a negative Homan's sign.
    b. Incidence can be increased in the operating theatre with the use of pneumatic calf compression.
    c. It can be mistaken for a torn gastrocnemius muscle.
    d. Incidence is increased with prophylactic low-molecular-weight heparin (LMWH) injections.
    e. There is an insignificant risk of pulmonary embolism.

71. Which one of the following statements regarding the pathology of the spleen is incorrect?
    a. The spleen is derived from the mesoderm.
    b. The majority of the normal spleen consists of red pulp.
    c. White pulp is important in antibody synthesis.
    d. White pulp hypertrophies in myeloid leukaemia.
    e. The marginal zone is the area separating red from white pulp.

72. A 30-year-old man involved in a road traffic accident is brought into the resuscitation area of an accident and emergency department. He was in the passenger seat of a car that was hit from the side, causing the door to crush into his left side, which resulted in injury to the lateral aspect of his left knee. X-rays show a fractured left neck of the fibula. Which one of the following would you most likely expect to find on examination?
    a. Loss of foot inversion
    b. Loss of ankle plantar flexion
    c. Loss of ankle dorsiflexion
    d. Paralysis of tibialis posterior
    e. Trendelenburg gait

73. A 38-year-old man sustained a severe fracture of his left elbow, which damaged the ulnar nerve behind the medial epicondyle of the humerus. A month later, he still has a total ulnar nerve paralysis. Which clinical sign is most likely to be present on examination?
    a. Sensory loss over the ulnar 3½ digits on the ulnar side of the hand
    b. Inability to grip a sheet of paper between his fingers when the hand is placed flat on the table
    c. Excessive sweating over the ulnar border of the left hand
    d. Index and middle fingers on the affected side are held in the claw position
    e. Marked wasting of the thenar eminence

74. A 16-year-old girl is brought into hospital after being struck by a car while riding her bike. The girl wore a helmet that left a bullseye impression on the car windscreen. On examination the patient is confused and does not know where she is. She opens her eyes to speech and localizes to pain. Which of the following is her Glasgow Coma Scale (GCS)?
    a. 10
    b. 11

c. 12
d. 13
e. 14

75. A 55-year-old male presents to the accident and emergency department with epistaxis. His initial observations are within normal range. Which of the following management options should be undertaken first?
    a. Sphenopalatine artery ligation
    b. Application of Merocel packs
    c. Immediate cautery of bleeding points
    d. Sucking on an ice cube and compression
    e. Ear, nose and throat (ENT) referral

76. Which of the following statements regarding the hamstring muscles is correct?
    a. The hamstring muscles arise from the anterior superior iliac spine.
    b. Semimembranosus inserts on the lateral condyle of the tibia.
    c. The short head of biceps femoris originates from the linea aspera.
    d. All three muscles are supplied by the femoral nerve.
    e. The hamstring compartment receives its blood supply from only the profunda femoris artery.

77. An 85-year-old man undergoes a right hemicolectomy for a right-sided colonic cancer. A preoperative computed tomography (CT) scan showed no evidence of Metastasis. The postoperative histopathology report states the tumour is invading through the intestinal wall into adjacent structures and the apical lymph node is involved. Which Dukes' stage is this?
    a. Stage A
    b. Stage B
    c. Stage C1
    d. Stage C2
    e. Stage D

78. A 60-year-old man is scheduled to have a total gastrectomy for Zollinger–Ellison syndrome. He has been informed preoperatively that he will require lifelong intramuscular injections of vitamin B_{12}. Absence of which cell type is responsible for the vitamin replacement requirement?
    a. Goblet cells
    b. Mucous neck cells
    c. Parietal cells
    d. G-cells
    e. Chief cells

79. Which of the following conditions is associated with a metabolic acidosis and a high anion gap?
    a. Ketoacidosis
    b. Diarrhoea
    c. High-output ileostomy
    d. Increased renal bicarbonate loss
    e. Decreased renal hydrogen ion excretion

80. Concerning action potentials, which of the following statements is correct?
    a. The equilibrium potential of an ion is calculated by the Goldman equation.
    b. The typical value of the resting membrane potential for a neuron is 70 mV.
    c. An action potential is a rapid hyperpolarization followed by subsequent depolarization.
    d. For any individual cell, each action potential is of the same amplitude and propagated at the same speed.
    e. The resting membrane potential of a cell is calculated by the Nernst equation.

81. Which of the following is an acute-phase protein?
    a. Fibrinogen
    b. Leukotriene C_4 (LTC_4)
    c. Interleukin-1 (IL-1)
    d. Interleukin-12 (IL-12)
    e. Interferon-γ (IFN-γ)

82. Which one of the following statements is correct concerning the portal vein?
    a. It carries blood from three major veins: the superior and inferior mesenteric vein and the left gastric vein.
    b. It is formed posterior to the head of the pancreas.
    c. It lies posterior to the bile duct in the free edge of the lesser omentum.
    d. At the porta hepatis the portal vein divides into four branches.
    e. It lies anterior to the hepatic artery in the free edge of the lesser omentum.

83. Which of the following structures is found at the transpyloric plane of Addison?
    a. Fundus of stomach
    b. Tail of pancreas
    c. Inferior mesenteric artery branching from aorta
    d. Upper border of L3
    e. Duodenojejunal junction

84. A 65-year-old Afro-Caribbean man comes to see you in clinic complaining of progressive lower back pain with increasing tiredness and shortness of breath. He has mentioned in the last few days his legs have become discoordinated and he has had difficulty passing urine and opening his bowels. Emergency scans diagnosed spinal cord compression. Prostate-specific antigen (PSA) levels are normal. Which of the following investigations would confirm the diagnosis?
    a. A computed tomography (CT) scan of his spine
    b. Urine sample
    c. Ultrasound scan (USS) of the abdomen
    d. Chest X-ray
    e. Colonoscopy

85. Low molecular weight heparin (LMWH) is used commonly in surgical patients. When compared with unfractionated heparin, which one of the following statements is correct?
    a. Unfractionated heparin requires a once-daily infusion.
    b. Unfractionated heparin does not require regular activated partial thromboplastin time (APPT) monitoring.

   c. Unfractionated heparin contains only low-molecular-weight polysaccharides.

   d. LMWH has a higher risk of heparin-induced thrombocytopenia.

   e. LMWH reduces the risk of extension or recurrence of DVT by 38% compared with unfractionated heparin.

86. A splenectomy is indicated for all but which one of the following conditions?

   a. Some cases of traumatic splenic injury

   b. Idiopathic thrombocytopenic purpura (ITP)

   c. Sickle cell disease

   d. Autoimmune haemolytic anaemia

   e. Hereditary spherocytosis

87. Which of the following statements regarding calcium homeostasis is true?

   a. Vitamin D stimulates osteoclasts.

   b. Vitamin D reduces calcium and phosphate absorption through the terminal ileum.

   c. Calcitonin is secreted from the chief cells of the parathyroid gland.

   d. Parathormone stimulates 1α-hydroxylase.

   e. Parathormone inhibits collagen synthesis by osteoblasts.

88. Which one of the following molecules is used for cell signalling?

   a. CO_2

   b. O_2

   c. NO

   d. N_2

   e. H_2CO_3

89. The inguinal canal is occupied by the spermatic cord in males and the round ligament of the uterus in females. Which one of the following statements regarding the inguinal canal is correct?

   a. The floor of the inguinal canal consists of the transversalis fascia and conjoint tendon.

   b. The posterior wall of the inguinal canal consists of the inguinal ligament and lacunar ligament.

   c. The roof of the inguinal canal consists of the internal oblique and transversalis muscles.

   d. The anterior wall of the inguinal ligament consists of the inguinal ligament.

   e. Indirect inguinal hernias protrude through Hesselbach's triangle.

90. Which of the following muscles are supplied by the radial nerve?

   a. Supinator

   b. Extensor carpi ulnaris

   c. Brachioradialis

   d. All of the above

   e. b and c only

91. Which one of the following statements is true regarding folate deficiency?

   a. Folate deficiency leads to a microcytic anaemia.

   b. Folate is normally absorbed in the terminal ileum.

c. The main cause of deficiency is due to an increase in requirement of folate.

d. Methotrexate blocks utilization of folate.

e. Haemolysis causes a decrease in folate use.

92. All of the following are involved in the intrinsic pathway of clotting except:

    a. Factor XII
    b. Factor XI
    c. Factor IX
    d. Factor VII
    e. Calcium

93. Which one of the following statements correctly defines pulse pressure?

    a. Difference between the systolic and diastolic blood pressure
    b. Sum of the systolic and diastolic blood pressure
    c. Difference between the systolic and stroke volume
    d. Heart rate multiplied by stroke volume
    e. Cardiac output multiplied by systemic vascular resistance

94. Concerning the rotator cuff muscles, which of the following statements is correct?

    a. Teres minor is an external rotator of the shoulder.
    b. Abduction of the shoulder is initiated by subscapularis.
    c. Supraspinatus inserts into the superior aspect of the lesser tuberosity of the humerus.
    d. Subscapularis inserts into the greater tuberosity of the humerus.
    e. Infraspinatus is an internal rotator of the shoulder.

95. The rotator cuff consists of the tendinous insertions of supraspinatus, infraspinatus and which other two muscles?

    a. Teres major and subscapularis
    b. Deltoid and teres minor
    c. Rhomboid minor and levator scapulae
    d. Teres minor and subscapularis
    e. Teres major and teres minor

96. An 18-year-old man is brought into the emergency department following a shooting. He is noted to have multiple internal injuries and is transfused 12 units of blood to stabilize him on his way to theatre. The anaesthetist notices changes in his electocardiogram trace as he is taken into theatre. Which one of the following is the most likely electrolyte abnormality identified?

    a. Low sodium and high phosphate
    b. High sodium and low potassium
    c. Low calcium and high potassium
    d. High calcium and high sodium
    e. Low magnesium and raised urea

97. Which of the following factors has the greatest relative risk (RR) of venous thrombosis?

    a. Use of the oral contraceptive pill (OCP)
    b. Homozygous factor V Leiden

c. Homozygous prothrombin gene mutation
d. Heterozygous antithrombin III deficiency
e. Heterozygous protein C deficiency

98. A 31-year-old obese smoker with heterozygous Christmas disease fractures his femur after crashing his motorcycle. He is bed-bound in traction initially and then undergoes a 2-h operation to fix the fracture. Owing to postoperative complications he remains in bed for a further 5 days. Nine days after his injury he develops a deep vein thrombosis (DVT) in his calf. Which of the following have increased his risk of developing a DVT?
    a. Obesity
    b. Smoking
    c. Christmas disease
    d. All of the above
    e. a and b only

99. Which of the following regarding the regulation of respiration is correct?
    a. The pneumotaxic centre is found in the midbrain.
    b. The apneustic centre in the pons tends to shorten inspiration.
    c. Peripheral chemoreceptors in the carotid bodies respond to levels of PCO_2.
    d. The Hering–Breuer reflex prevents overinflation of the lungs.
    e. Central chemoreceptors respond to changes in the arterial PO_2.

100. Concerning the loop of Henle and proximal convoluted tubule of the nephron, which of the following statements is correct?
    a. A small amount of water and sodium is absorbed from the thick ascending limb.
    b. The thin descending limb is the major site for reabsorption of solutes.
    c. The first half of the proximal convoluted tubule absorbs phosphate and lactate.
    d. Approximately 10% of filtered solutes are reabsorbed by the proximal convoluted tubule.
    e. The thin descending limb is impermeable to water.

101. The recurrent laryngeal nerve is an important structure that must be avoided when operating on the thyroid gland. Which one of the following statements regarding the recurrent laryngeal nerve is true?
    a. The right recurrent laryngeal nerve passes inferior to the right main bronchus.
    b. The left recurrent laryngeal nerve passes arches under the left subclavian artery and then ascends to the pharynx.
    c. The laryngeal nerves are derived from the hypoglossal nerve.
    d. The recurrent laryngeal nerve enters the larynx by passing deep to the inferior border of the inferior constrictor muscle of the pharynx.
    e. The recurrent laryngeal nerves descend in the tracheo-oesophageal groove.

102. A 28-year-old male undergoes an oesophagogastroduodenoscopy for persistent epigastric discomfort. He is diagnosed as having moderate gastritis and is *Helicobacter pylori* positive. The following statements regarding *H. pylori* are true except:
    a. It can be transmitted iatrogenically.
    b. It can lead to peptic ulceration.
    c. It is Gram-positive bacteria.
    d. It can be diagnosed with a biopsy.
    e. It produces the urease enzyme.

103. A 35-year-old woman is admitted for an elective laparoscopic cholecystectomy. Her operation is prolonged and is complicated by damage to the common bile duct. Two days after her operation is noted as having a swollen calf and becomes cold and clammy, with tachypnoea and tachycardia associated with central chest and epigastric pain. Her blood gas on air shows pH 7.48, PCO_2 3.5 kPa, PO_2 7.3 kPa, HCO_3^- 24 mmol/L. Her electrocardiogram and blood results are pending. Which one of the following is the most likely diagnosis?
    a. Pancreatitis
    b. Pneumonia
    c. Pulmonary embolism
    d. Tietze syndrome
    e. Myocardial infarction

104. A 50-year-old man undergoes an emergency laparotomy for an upper gastrointestinal haemorrhage. At surgery a bleeding duodenal ulcer is found to be the cause of the haemorrhage. Which of the following vessels is the likely cause of bleeding?
    a. Short gastric artery
    b. Left gastric artery
    c. Right gastric artery
    d. Gastroduodenal artery
    e. Right gastroepiploic artery

105. An 83-year-old woman presents with a 3-month history of swelling just inferior to the left ear lobule. The lump is 1 cm in diameter, soft and painless to touch. There is no evidence of facial nerve involvement. Of note, you find a small lump in similar position on the contralateral side. Which one of the following is the most likely diagnosis?
    a. Pleiomorphic adenoma
    b. Adenolymphoma
    c. Adenoid cystic carcinoma
    d. Sialadenitis
    e. Chronic parotitis

106. Which statement regarding the regulation of sodium and water reabsorption is incorrect?
    a. Antidiuretic hormone is produced in the supraoptic nucleus of the hypothalamus.
    b. Aldosterone stimulates resorption of sodium from the distal tubule.

c. Atrial natriuretic peptide increases glomerular filtration.

d. Renin release is stimulated by a reduction in sodium levels.

e. Antidiuretic hormone secretion is stimulated by an increased arterial pressure.

107. Concerning the physiological effects of thyroid hormones, which of the following statements is correct?

a. Triiodothyronine (T_3) increases oxygen consumption in all metabolically active tissues.

b. Thyroxine (T_4) decreases oxygen consumption in the anterior pituitary gland.

c. The plasma levels of thyroid hormones share a reciprocal relationship with the appearance of uric acid in the urine.

d. Excessively high thyroid hormone levels result in excess conversion of vitamin A to carotene.

e. Hyperthyroidism leads to the accumulation of polysaccharides and hyaluronic acid in tissues.

108. Which one of the following statements is correct regarding apertures of the diaphragm?

a. The aperture at T10 is in the central tendon of the diaphragm.

b. The aperture at T12 is at the right crus of the diaphragm.

c. During inspiration the inferior vena cava dilates facilitating blood flow to the heart.

d. Blood flow of the aorta is affected by diaphragmatic contraction.

e. The opening at T8 is posterior to the diaphragm.

109. The endothelial cells in all of the following produce thrombomodulin except:

a. Hepatic circulation

b. Cutaneous circulation

c. Cerebral microcirculation

d. Renal circulation

e. Pulmonary circulation

110. A 72-year-old woman presents with central abdominal pain radiating toward her back over the past 3 h, with several episodes of vomiting and absolute constipation. She has a past history of atrial fibrillation, for which she is on warfarin, and had a cholecystectomy 20 years ago. She has never smoked or drank alcohol. She is clinically dehydrated, with generalized guarding and rebound of the abdomen. Her white cell count is raised at 19×10^9/L and she has a C-reactive protein (CRP) of 231. Liver function tests are normal. Her blood gas shows on 15 L O_2: pH 7.27, PCO_2 3.4 kPa, PO_2 14.6 kPa, lactate 7.3, HCO_3^- 14 mmol/L, base excess (BE) 5.4 mmol/L. Which one of the following is the most likely diagnosis?

a. Infarcted bowel

b. Pancreatitis

c. Pulmonary embolism

d. Pneumonia

e. None of the above

111. An accident and emergency registrar refers a patient with an injured axillary nerve. In which of the following scenarios is this nerve characteristically damaged?
    a. Posterior dislocation of the humerus
    b. Anterior dislocation of the humerus
    c. Fracture of the surgical neck of the humerus
    d. Distraction injury of the neck and shoulder
    e. Fracture of the clavicle

112. A patient undergoes a radical parotidectomy for a malignant parotid tumour, at which time it is found necessary to perform a total division of the left facial (VII) nerve. Postoperatively, which is the most likely sequela?
    a. Maintenance of left sided forehead wrinkling.
    b. Numbness over the cheek on the left side
    c. Ptosis of the upper eyelid on the left side
    d. Loss of taste sensation over the anterior two-thirds of the tongue on the left side
    e. Tendency for food and fluids to collect in the buccal sulcus after meals

113. A 65-year-old man who has been investigated by the general practitioner (GP) for lethargy and tiredness is referred to the surgeons with a right upper quadrant mass. The GP was concerned he had a possible small bowel cancer. On examination you note the patient to have oral ulcerations with a marked hepatosplenomegaly. The patient also has multiple masses that can be felt in his neck and supraclavicular fossa. You order a blood test, which provisionally supports your primary diagnosis, after which you obtain a bone marrow biopsy. Which of the following results would practically confirm your diagnosis?
    a. Owl eye nuclei
    b. Auer rods
    c. Reed–Sternberg cells
    d. Lymphoblasts
    e. Aplastic bone marrow

114. Which one of the following is not a recognized treatment option for basal cell carcinoma?
    a. Curettage and cautery
    b. Watch and wait
    c. Cryotherapy
    d. Surgical excision
    e. Sentinel node biopsy

115. Which one of the following conditions results in decreased affinity of haemoglobin for oxygen?
    a. The arterial PCO_2 is decreased.
    b. The concentration of hydrogen ions is decreased.

c. The temperature is increased.
d. The arterial carbon monoxide is increased.
e. The concentration of 2,3-diphosphoglycerate (2,3-DPG) is decreased.

116. A 30-year-old male office worker is brought to hospital after being stabbed in the abdomen. He is of average weight and is normally generally fit. You note that he is anxious but conscious with a slightly raised respiratory rate. You are given the following observations by the paramedic crew: blood pressure 120/105 mmHg, heart rate 105 bpm, urine output of 20 mL in the last hour. Which (if any) class of shock is he currently in?
    a. Not shocked
    b. Class I
    c. Class II
    d. Class III
    e. Class IV

117. Which of the following statements regarding incomplete spinal cord injuries is correct?
    a. Anterior cord syndrome occurs in syringomyelia.
    b. Central cord syndrome involves preservation of pain and temperature below the lesion.
    c. Cauda equina syndrome is an upper motor neuron lesion.
    d. Posterior cord syndrome is commonly seen in hyperflexion injuries.
    e. Brown–Sequard syndrome involves loss of pain and temperature on the opposite side below the lesion.

118. Which of the following muscles initiates shoulder abduction?
    a. Deltoid
    b. Supraspinatus
    c. Infraspinatus
    d. Trapezius
    e. Subscapularis

119. Which of the following clinical features are not associated with carpal tunnel syndrome?
    a. Nocturnal and early morning exacerbation of symptoms
    b. Paraesthesia to thumb, index and middle fingers
    c. Wasting of thenar muscles
    d. Inability to perform Froment's test
    e. Aching up the forearm up to the elbow

120. Which of the following increases the physiological dead space in the respiratory system?
    a. Standing position
    b. Neck flexion
    c. Hyperventilation
    d. Hypotension
    e. Bronchoconstriction

121. You are concerned about myocardial ischaemia in a postoperative patient who is complaining of chest pain. The electorcardiogram shows tachycardia and isolated ST segment depression in leads V1 and V2. Which coronary artery is most likely to be responsible?
    a. Circumflex coronary artery
    b. Left anterior descending coronary artery
    c. Posterior descending coronary artery
    d. Left main stem coronary artery
    e. Right coronary artery

122. Which of the following statements about the axillary artery is incorrect?
    a. It starts at the lateral border of the 1st rib.
    b. It ends at the lower border of the teres minor.
    c. It is divided into three parts by pectoralis minor.
    d. It gives off the subscapular artery.
    e. The axillary vein lies medial to it.

123. The human body has different skeletal muscle fibres. Regarding muscle fibres, which of the following statements are true?
    a. Type IIb fibres have a high oxidative capacity.
    b. Type I fibres can reach a peak tension in less than 10 ms.
    c. Type IIb fibres have a high concentration of mitochondria.
    d. Type I fibres have a low myosin ATPase content.
    e. White fibres have a low twitch rate.

124. Which of the following statements regarding the vagus nerve is correct?
    a. The vagus nerve does not innervate muscles in the pharynx.
    b. Activation of the vagus nerve stimulates chief cells in the stomach.
    c. Stimulation of the vagus decreases intestinal motility.
    d. The vagus nerve innervates the descending colon.
    e. The vagus nerve does not innervate the skin.

125. Which of the following statements concerning inotropes is correct?
    a. Adrenaline is predominantly an α_1 receptor agonist.
    b. Dobutamine is predominantly a β_1 receptor agonist.
    c. Isoprenaline acts on both α_1 and α_2 receptor.
    d. Nitrates have weak inotropic effects.
    e. Dopamine predominantly causes α agonism at low doses.

126. Concerning the blood supply/drainage of the heart, which of the following statements is correct?
    a. The anterior interventricular artery arises from the right coronary artery.
    b. The circumflex artery arises from the left coronary artery.
    c. The posterior interventricular artery forms an anastomosis with the marginal artery.
    d. The anterior cardiac veins always drain into the coronary sinus.
    e. The small cardiac vein always drains directly into the right atrium.

127. Which of the following statements regarding stretch reflexes is true?
    a. The reflexes require a minimum of three nerves.
    b. Stretch reflexes are not present in postural muscles.
    c. The reflex is initiated by actively stretching the muscle spindles.
    d. The stretch reflex is most easily demonstrated in flexor muscles.
    e. The reflex results in an isotonic muscle contraction.

128. Which of the following is the correct boundary of the omental foramen (epiploic foramen or foramen of Winslow)?
    a. Anteriorly the hepatic artery
    b. Posteriorly the hepatic vein
    c. Superiorly the quadrate lobe of the liver
    d. Inferiorly the hepatic vein
    e. None of the above

129. Concerning the blood supply/drainage of the heart, which of the following statements is correct?
    a. The anterior interventricular artery arises from the right coronary artery.
    b. The circumflex artery arises from the left coronary artery.
    c. The posterior interventricular artery forms an anastomosis with the marginal artery.
    d. The anterior cardiac veins always drain into the coronary sinus.
    e. The small cardiac vein always drains directly into the right atrium.

130. Which of the following statements relating to antidiurectic hormone (ADH) is true?
    a. ADH stimulates aquaporins in the distal tubule.
    b. Decreased blood volume leads to decreased ADH secretion.
    c. Increased osmolality leads to an increased urine volume.
    d. Changes in osmolality are detected in the hypothalamus.
    e. The stretch receptors involved in ADH secretion are found in the aortic arch.

131. Which of the following statements is correct concerning Ca^{2+} metabolism?
    a. Hypercalcaemia increases secretion of parathormone (PTH).
    b. Calcitonin reduces serum Ca^{2+} levels.
    c. Calcitonin plays a key role in daily regulation of Ca^{2+}.
    d. Low Ca^{2+} levels will lead to decreased permeability of Na^+ channels in nerve cells.
    e. High Ca^{2+} levels are usually found in secondary hyperparathyroidism.

132. Which of the following statements regarding the right atrium is false?
    a. Forms the right heart border
    b. Has the coronary sinus opening above the septal cusp of the tricuspid valve
    c. Has a posterior wall formed by the interatrial septum
    d. Lies in front of the left atrium
    e. Has the sinoatrial (SA) node medial to the sulcus terminalis

133. During a total mastectomy in a 65-year-old woman, the consultant surgeon performs a level II axillary dissection. Which one of the following statements is correct?
    a. Level II clearance extends up to the lateral border of pectoralis minor.
    b. Level II clearance extends up to the first rib.
    c. Level II clearance extends up to axillary vein.
    d. The intercostobrachial nerve supplying the latissimus dorsi muscle can be damaged.
    e. The thoracodorsal nerve passes along the posterior wall of the axilla.

134. Which of the following statements regarding calcium metabolism is incorrect?
    a. Parathormone (PTH) is secreted by the parathyroid glands.
    b. Calcitonin is produced by the parafollicular cells of the thyroid gland.
    c. Calcitonin acts to decrease calcium levels.
    d. PTH binds to osteoclasts increasing their expression of receptor activator of nuclear factor kappa B ligand (RANKL).
    e. Calbindin is important in intestinal calcium absorption.

135. Which of the following structures is located in the anterior mediastinum?
    a. Thymus gland
    b. Oesophagus
    c. Aorta
    d. Heart
    e. Trachea

CHAPTER 10
PRACTICE PAPER

Answers

1. c. The oesophagus traverses the mid-portion of the diaphragm, which corresponds to the level of T10. The oesophagus is accompanied by the left and right vagus nerves, which, at this point, are named the anterior and posterior gastric nerves, respectively. The left and right vagus nerves rotate anticlockwise because they follow the rotation of the gut. Other structures passing through at this level include the oesophageal branches of the left gastric vessels and a few lymphatic vessels.

2. e. An abscess is a localized tissue collection of pus, surrounded by a 'pyogenic membrane'. This is not a true membrane but rather a wall of fibrin, capillaries, neutrophils and fibroblasts. A pre-existing pilonidal sinus gives rise to a pilonidal abscess and is generally colonised with coliforms. A psoas abscess is most frequently caused by *Staphylococcus aureus*, tuberculosis and other rare microorganisms. A sterile abscess is defined as an abscess devoid of microorganisms which may occur following sterilization of a septic abscess with antibiotics. Pus contains a mixture of dead and live neutrophils, fibrin, lipid, coagulation and complement factors.

3. b.

Virus	Type	Tumour
Epstein–Barr	DNA	Burkitt's lymphoma, nasopharyngeal cancer, lymphoma
Human herpes virus-8	DNA	Kaposi's sarcoma
Human T-cell leukaemia	RNA	T-lymphoblastic leukaemia
Hepatitis B	DNA	Hepatocellular carcinoma
Human papilloma	DNA	Cervical, anal carcinoma

4. a. Symptoms of hyperkalaemia can be quite non-specific and include malaise and weakness. There may be mild hyperventilation in response to a metabolic acidosis. Ultimately, the patient may develop a cardiac arrhythmia and die. Hyperkalaemia causes the cardiac cell membranes to become hyperpolarized, which leads to decreased cardiac excitability and then in turn hypotension, bradycardia and asytole. Causes include renal insufficiency, medications (such as angiotensin-converting enzyme [ACE] inhibitors and non-steroidal anti-inflammatory drugs [NSAIDs]), mineralocorticoid deficiency, rhabdomyolysis and massive blood transfusions. The electrocardiogram (ECG) changes are reduced P waves, broadening of the QRS complex, sinusoidal ST segment and peaked T waves. If these changes occur, or the plasma level is >7.0 mmol/L, emergency treatment should be started. This includes continuous cardiac monitoring, stopping any causative infusions, calcium gluconate, an insulin/dextrose infusion, salbutamol nebulizer and ultimately haemodialysis.

5. e. There are five areas of portosystemic communication: the lower end of the oesophagus, the upper end of the anal canal, the periumbilical region, the retroperitoneal areas and finally between the portal branches of the liver and veins of the diaphragm across the bare area of the liver.

Sites of portosystemic anastomoses

Site	Portal circulation	Systemic circulation
Lower oesophagus	Oesophageal branches of left gastric vein	Azygous vein
Periumbilical	Vein of ligamentum teres	Superior/inferior epigastric veins
Upper anal canal	Superior rectal vein	Middle/inferior rectal veins
Retroperitoneal	Right/middle/left colic veins	Renal/lumbar/phrenic veins
Bare area of liver	Hepatic/portal veins	Inferior phrenic veins

6. b. The inferior epigastric artery arises from the external iliac artery above the inguinal ligament. It runs obliquely, medial to the deep inguinal ring, piercing the transversalis fascia. It runs superiorly entering the rectus sheath below the arcuate line, running deep to the rectus abdominis. It supplies the rectus abdominis muscle and the medial aspect of the anterolateral abdominal wall. Superiorly, it anastomoses with the superior epigastric artery, a branch of the internal thoracic artery, above the umbilicus. The inferior epigastric artery is a landmark in distinguishing between inguinal hernias, with indirect hernias originating lateral to the vessel, and direct hernias originating medially to the artery.

Care must be taken during port placement in laparoscopic surgery as the vessel can easily be punctured.

7. e. Microscopic examination of the gastric mucosa shows that it is deeply folded. The folds create gastric glands, which open out at gastric pits into the stomach lumen. The exocrine gastric cells are found within the gastric glands. There are a number of secretory cells, which secrete different products into the lumen of the gastric glands and into the blood:

- *Parietal (oxyntic) cells* – hydrochloric acid and intrinsic factor
- *D-cells* – somatostatin
- *Enterochromaffin-like cells* – histamine and serotonin
- *Goblet cells* – mucus
- *Chief (peptic) cells* – pepsinogen
- *G-cells* – gastrin

8. c. For water to be reabsorbed it must move passively down a concentration gradient. The hypertonicity required is created by the high ion concentrations within the medulla. High ion concentrations can be established via the countercurrent multiplier mechanism. In the descending limb of the loop of Henle, water is absorbed and NaCl is passively added to the ultrafiltrate. Consequently, the ultrafiltrate is concentrated over four times from the start of the descending loop. In the ascending loop Na^+ is actively reabsorbed (Cl^- passively follows) but this area is impermeable to water. This leads to a decrease in the osmolality of the ultrafiltrate and an increase in the osmolality of the surrounding medullary parenchyma. The osmolality of the ultrafiltrate entering the loop is approximately 300 mosmol/L, at the bottom of the loop it is about 1400 mosmol/L and then, as it enters the distal tubule, it is around 100 mosmol/L. The U shape of the loop allows repeated cycles of ion pumping and fluid shifts and is significantly more effective at concentrating urine than a parallel system would be.

9. c. A premalignant disease is an identifiable lesion/condition associated with an increased risk of developing malignant tumours. Ulcerative colitis is associated with an increased risk of developing adenocarcinoma of the colon or carcinoma of the bile duct.

10. b. *Clostridium difficile* commonly causes severe diarrhoea. Its increased incidence has been linked to overuse of broad-spectrum antibiotics and can result in pseudomembranous colitis. *Clostridium tetani* is the causative organism for tetanus. *Clostridium botulinum* produces botulinum neurotoxins (causing botulism), which leads to a spreading paralysis. *Staphylococcus aureus* is implicated in skin infections such as cellulitis. In this scenario, the patient is clinically unwell, with evidence of gas under the skin; therefore the most likely organism involved is *Clostridium perfringens*. Local tissue necrosis in gas gangrene is caused by the release of powerful exotoxins. Management includes aggressive surgical debridement, intravenous antibiotics and hyperbaric oxygen therapy.

11. e. The ankle joint is synovial in type and involves the talus of the foot and the tibia and fibula of the lower leg. The ankle joint is stabilized by medial (deltoid) and lateral ligaments. Together, the fibula and tibia create a deep mortice for the upper expanded part of the body of the talus. The talus fits tighter into its socket when the foot is dorsiflexed as the wider surface of the talus moves into the ankle. The syndesomsis and the inferior tibiofibular ligament are also important stabilizers of the ankle.

12. d. Antidiuretic hormone (ADH), also known as vasopressin, is released by the posterior pituitary gland. It functions mainly in the distal tubule and collecting duct by increasing permeability to water, hence retaining water and preventing it from being excreted. This results in the production of low-volume concentrated urine during periods of dehydration. Lack of production of ADH causes cranial diabetes insipidus, whereas the inability of the kidneys to respond to ADH causes nephrogenic diabetes insipidus. ADH is inhibited by alcohol. All these conditions lead to the production of high-volume dilute urine.

13. a. The cardiac action potential differs from that in a somatic nerve. There is a constant sodium ion leak into the cell causing a gradual increase in the resting membrane potential. Upon reaching threshold the voltage-gated sodium channels open resulting in rapid depolarization. An influx of calcium ions prolongs the cardiac action potential. Repolarization occurs by potassium ions flowing out of the cell. Adrenaline increases the rate of sodium ion leak, while acetylcholine decreases the rate of sodium ion leak.

14. a. The histology describes a Warthin tumour (papillary cystadenoma lymphomatosum) which is the second most common salivary gland neoplasm. This benign tumour arises almost exclusively in the parotid gland (unlike the other salivary tumours) and is more common in males than females, typically presenting in patients aged 40–60 years. Approximately 10% are multifocal and 10% are bilateral. People who smoke are eight times more likely to develop these tumours than non-smokers. In comparison, pleomorphic adenomas are benign tumours that are derived from a mixture of epithelial and myoepithelial cells. Consequently, these tumours may contain varying quantities of myxoid, hyaline, cartilaginous and even osseous tissue. Pleomorphic adenomas account for 60% of parotid tumours.

15. c. Cranial nerve (CN) I (olfactory nerve) exits from the cribriform plate and is the only CN to exit from the anterior cranial fossa.

- CNs II–VI exit from the middle cranial fossa, and the remaining CNs all exit from the posterior cranial fossa.
- CN II (optic nerve) exits via the optic canal and is covered in all three meningeal layers (pia, arachnoid and dura mater).
- CN III (occulomotor nerve), CN IV (trochlear nerve), CN V (trigeminal nerve – ophthalmic branch) and CN VI (abducens nerve) all exit via the superior orbital fissure. This fissure lies between the greater and lesser wings of the sphenoid bone, and in blowout fractures these structures can be damaged.
- The maxillary branch of CN V exits via the foramen rotundum of the sphenoid bone, whereas the mandibular branch of CN V exits via the foramen ovale, posterior to the foramen rotundum but still part of the sphenoid bone.
- CN VII (facial nerve) exits via the stylomastoid foramen.
- CN VIII (vestibulocochlear nerve) exits via the internal acoustic meatus.
- CN IX (glossopharyngeal nerve), CN X (vagus nerve) and CN XI (accessory nerve) all exit via the jugular foramen, located behind the carotid canal.
- CN XII (hypoglossal nerve) exits via the hypoglossal canal.

16. e. The facial nerve (CN VII) exits the base of the skull via the stylomastoid foramen. It provides motor and proprioceptive supply to the muscles of facial expression, including the platysma. It also supplies the stapedius muscle via the greater petrosal nerve. It supplies taste, whereas the mandibular division of CN V supplies sensation to the anterior two-thirds of the tongue. CN IX supplies taste and sensation to the posterior one-third of the tongue. The facial nerve gives off parasympathetic supply to the submandibular, sublingual and lacrimal glands. It also functions as the efferent limb for the corneal reflex.

17. e.   Patients with gastro-oesophageal reflux disease (GORD) reflux gastric acid into the distal oesophagus. The acid causes inflammation to the oesophagus, and if the exposure is severe and chronic enough, metaplastic transformation may take place. *Metaplasia* is the term used to describe the process where one differentiated cell type is replaced with another. The process is reversible and so, if the irritant is removed, the tissue may return to normal. In this scenario, the metaplastic change is from squamous epithelium to more intestinal, columnar-like epithelium. The process in the oesophagus is called Barrett's oesophagus.

18. b.   Parathyroid carcinoma may lead to an increase in parathyroid hormone (PTH) production. Further examples of tumour markers include:

- *Pituitary:* Adrenocorticotropic hormone (ACTH), growth hormone, prolactin
- *Adrenal:* Cortisol
- *Carcinoid:* 5-Hydroxyindoleacetic acid (5-HIAA)
- *Oat cell:* ACTH, antidiuretic hormone
- *Prostate:* Prostate-specific antigen (PSA)
- *Hepatic:* α-Fetoprotein (AFP) (**Note**: Also cirrhosis, pregnancy, hepatitis, neural tube defect)
- *Colorectal:* Carcinoembryonic antigen (CEA), Ca 19-9 (advanced)
- *Testicular teratoma:* β-hCG, CEA, AFP
- *Testicular seminoma:* Placental alkaline phosphatase
- *Breast:* Ca 15-3
- *Pancreatic:* Ca 19-9
- *Thyroid:* Thyroglobulin, calcitonin (medullary carcinoma)
- *Phaeochromocytoma:* Vanillylmandelic acid

19. b.   Radiographs of osteosarcomas usually show a large, destructive, mixed lytic and blastic mass within the metaphyseal region of the long bones or the limbs. As the tumour grows it penetrates through the cortex and lifts the periosteum. A periosteal reaction results in reactive new bone formation, and the triangle of new bone formed between the cortex and raised ends of the periosteum is known as Codman's triangle. Eventually, the tumour expands through the periosteum and penetrates the surrounding soft tissue causing streaks of calcification resulting in a 'sun ray' appearance.

20. e.   The jugular venous pressure (JVP) is identified in the neck by observing a double pulsation in the internal jugular vein. The pressure within the internal jugular results from cyclical atrial contraction and dilatation. Below is an explanation of the waveform:

- *A wave:* Represents atrial systole and is absent in atrial fibrillation and is increased in tricuspid or pulmonary stenosis. During complete heart block atrial contraction may occur at a time when the tricuspid valve is closed causing 'cannon' waves.
- *C wave:* Represents closure of the tricuspid leaflets in the right atrium at the start of ventricular systole.
- *X descent:* The pressure inside the atrium drops as a result of the atrium relaxing and the tricuspid valve moving down during ventricular systole.

- *V wave:* The rise in atrial pressure is caused by rapid blood filling prior to opening of the tricuspid valve.
- *Y descent:* The tricuspid valve opens and blood passively flows into the right ventricle.

21. e. Mouth – 0.8–1.5 L saliva secreted; stomach – 2–3 L gastric juices secreted; gallbladder – 500 mL bile secreted; pancreas – 1.5 L juices secreted; small bowel – 8–9 L fluid absorbed, 1.5 L fluid secreted; large bowel – 1 L fluid absorbed, 100 mL excreted in faeces. The fluid balance of a patient needs to factor in the absorption and secretion of all parts of the gastrointestinal tract in order to maintain a positive net balance.

22. c. The submandibular duct (of Wharton) arises anteriorly, travelling lateral to the tongue, and opens in the papilla lateral to the frenulum anteriorly – it is crossed by the lingual nerve, which lies lateral to the duct at first, but then crosses underneath it to lie medially. The superficial lobe of the gland lies between the mylohyoid and the angle of the mandible. The submandibular gland is separated from the parotid gland posteriorly by the stylomandibular ligament. The lingual nerve lies superior to the submandibular gland; conversely, the hypoglossal nerve lies inferiorly – both of these nerves are at risk of damage during submandibular gland excision, as is the marginal mandibular branch of the facial nerve.

23. d. The nerve injured is most likely to be the long thoracic nerve, which supplies the serratus anterior muscle. This nerve courses superficially over the serratus anterior muscle; hence it is vulnerable to injury especially when the limbs are elevated. The arm cannot be completely abducted above the horizontal position because the serratus anterior is unable to rotate the glenoid cavity superiorly. Also, the scapula moves laterally and posteriorly, a condition termed 'winged scapula' whenever the long thoracic nerve is damaged.

24. e. Wound healing on the skin naturally depends on the size of the wound itself and the nature of the healing process. Wounds that are surgically incised and closed have their edges approximated closely together and heal by primary intention. They can take up to 2 weeks to heal. When there is gross tissue loss or surgical wound infection, the wound may be left open to heal by secondary intention. Granulation tissue forms at the base of the wound and re-epithelialization occurs from the edges to cover the defect. Two known abnormalities of wound healing are keloid and hypertrophied scars. In keloid scarring there is excessive collagen and fibroblast production. The scarring usually extends beyond the wound itself and usually does not settle. Hypertrophied scars do not extend beyond the wound edges, take around 3 weeks to develop and usually settle spontaneously within 18 months.

25. e. The daily requirement of an adult's fluid intake equates to 3 L/day for an average adult. If an individual is placed nil by mouth (NBM) this requirement is easily achieved with three bags of intravenous fluids each run over 8 h. One litre of normal saline contains 154 mmol/L of Na^+. The average adult requires 100 mmol/L of Na^+ per day, as well as 60 mmol/L of potassium per day.

You may add 20 mmol/L of potassium to each bag prescribed over the day in order to achieve this required amount.

26. c.   Gastric secretion is divided into three phases. In the cephalic phase, the sight, smell, taste or thought of food stimulates the stomach to secrete hydrochloric acid via vagal stimulation. Vagal activity also stimulates gastrin secretion from G-cells, which in turn stimulates further acid secretion. Food entering the stomach stimulates the gastric phase. It is the predominant phase of acid secretion and accounts for about 60% of all secretions. The intestinal phase begins when chyme enters the duodenum. Highly acidic solutions stimulate the release of secretin, which is an inhibitor of gastrin and a potent stimulus for the release of bile and pancreatic juice. Fatty food in the duodenum also stimulates cholecystokinin, which stimulates contraction of the gallbladder and inhibits gastrin secretion.

27. c.   Peripheral nerves are divided into three broad groups, A, B and C (group A is further subdivided four times), according to the speed of conduction of a nerve. The speed of conduction is governed by two factors: its diameter and whether the axon is myelinated or not. Group A fibres are all myelinated. Group B fibres are smaller but remain myelinated. These nerves are found in visceral nerves (pre-ganglionic autonomic). Group C fibres are small and not myelinated. The table below classifies the different nerve fibres.

Type	Function	Diameter (μm)	Conduction velocity (m/s)	Myelin
Aα	Motor proprioception	12–20	70–120	Yes
Aβ	Touch and pressure	6–13	30–90	Yes
Aγ	Muscle spindles	3–6	15–40	Yes
Aδ	Pain, touch and temperature	1–5	12–30	Thin
B	Pre-ganglionic autonomic	1–3	3–15	Yes
C	Pain (dull ache), post-ganglionic	0.5–1	1	No

28. a.   This patient has injured the superior part of his brachial plexus because of an excessive increase in the angle between the neck and shoulder. This gives a characteristic appearance of a 'waiter's tip' position of the affected arm, and the condition known as Erb palsy. C5 and C6 nerve roots combine to form the superior trunk of the brachial plexus.

29. a.   In compartment syndrome, pain is worsened by passive stretching of the affected compartment. In this case the muscle being stretched is flexor hallucis longus. This muscle is in the deep posterior compartment of the leg, along with the flexor digitorum longus and tibialis posterior. The anterior compartment contains the tibialis anterior, extensor hallucis longus, extensor digitorum longus and peroneus tertius. The superficial posterior compartment contains the gastrocnemius, plantaris and soleus. The lateral compartment contains the peroneus longus and brevis. There is no medial compartment of the leg.

30. a. Venous ulcers are typically found in the gaiter area, with a sloping edge with sloughy base and a moderate degree of exudate. It is important to exclude coexisting ischaemia with venous ulcers, and treat if present, as treatment of venous ulcers is by elevation and four-layer bandaging with regular dressings, and can compromise blood supply to the area further. The surrounding skin can be hyperpigmented with lipodermatosclerosis.

31. e. The most common form of renal stone is from calcium oxalate, occurring in 80% of cases. These stones can sometimes be seen on plain KUB X-ray films. Calcium phosphate stones are generally associated with primary hyperparathyroidism as in this case (high PTH and high calcium levels). Uric acid forms 10% of cases and produces radiolucent stones. Struvite stones are associated with urea-splitting bacteria and form in an alkaline urine. They account for 10% of urinary calculi. Cystine stones are associated with patients suffering from cystinuria, a condition where patients accumulate cystine in their urine.

32. d. Follicular carcinoma is the second most common carcinoma of the thyroid, with a prevalence of approximately 15% (following papillary carcinoma, with a prevalence of approximately 80%). Spread is typically haematogenous; lymphatic spread is unusual. It has a 5-year survival rate of approximately 70%. It is diagnosed by ultrasound and excision biopsy to demonstrate extracapsular spread; fine-needle aspiration cytology is unable to differentiate between follicular carcinoma and change follicular adenoma. Follicular carcinoma is often an incidental finding at postmortem. Radiation exposure is unrelated to its development.

33. b. Dietary magnesium is absorbed mainly in the duodenum, with body concentration being regulated by the kidneys. Unlike most salts, magnesium is transported in the thick ascending loop of Henle. Therefore, diuretics can increase magnesium loss. Raised magnesium and calcium levels reduce the amount of magnesium reabsorbed by the loop of Henle.

34. c. The breast extends vertically from the 2nd to the 6th ribs. The breast tissue extends toward the axilla and is known as the tail of Spence. It is important to include this area when performing a mastectomy and examination of the breast. The arterial supply to the breast is from the internal thoracic artery, which is a branch of the subclavian artery. The lateral thoracic and thoracoacromial arteries are branches of the axillary artery. Further blood supply to the breast is from the intercostal arteries. Approximately 75% of lymph drains into the axillary lymph nodes.

35. c. Branches of the axillary artery can be classified into three parts with regard to their relation to the pectoralis minor muscle: medial, posterior and lateral to the muscle.

- Medial: Superior thoracic artery
- Posterior: Thoracoacromial artery, lateral thoracic artery
- Lateral: Subscapular artery, anterior and posterior circumflex humoral arteries

The vertebral, internal thoracic and dorsal scapula arteries, along with the costocervical trunk, are branches of the subclavian artery.

36. e. Apoptosis is an energy-dependent process involving cell death by activation of endogenous endonucleases, which digest cell DNA into smaller fragments. It has to be distinguished from cell necrosis, which is invariably pathological. In apoptosis, single unwanted cells are shrunk and phagocytosed by neighbouring cells. Functionally, these include removal of cells with damaged DNA or virally infected cells or elimination of cells in embryonal development during morphogenesis. Mediators of apoptosis include p53, bcl-2 and fas (CD 95).

37. b. Hypersensitivity is an altered immunological response in which a severe and harmful reaction occurs to extrinsic antigens. Type I involves an immediate hypersensitivity or allergy due to overproduction of immunoglobulin E (IgE) on mast cells or basophils associated with bee stings, antibiotics and so forth. Type II involves circulating antibodies (IgG/IgM) reacting with antigens on cell surfaces. Examples of this type include transfusion reactions and rhesus incompatibility. Type III involves the deposition of immune complexes in the tissues, for example autologous or microbial antigens. Type IV is a delayed hypersensitivity mediated by T-cells, for example microbial agents – tuberculosis (TB), viruses. Type V reactions are caused by some IgG antibodies stimulating cells against which they are directed. This is seen in Graves disease where the thyroid-stimulating hormone (TSH) receptor antibody results in prolonged hypersecretion of thyroid hormone.

38. d. The saliva produced by the submandibular glands contains a comparatively low concentration of protein compared to the parotid gland. However, the reverse is true for the viscosity of saliva production, with the saliva from the submandibular glands being more viscous than that from the parotid gland. The high viscosity is due to the high mucin content. The basal rate of saliva production is higher from the submandibular gland than from the parotid gland, but this relationship is reversed during stimulation. The volume of saliva produced each day ranges from 500 to 1500 mL. The saliva is hypotonic to plasma at all times, and when flow rates are at their highest, the tonicity of saliva does not exceed 70% of plasma tonicity.

39. e. Cerebrospinal fluid (CSF) lies in the subarachnoid space surrounding the brain and spinal cord. It has two main functions, acting as a 'hydraulic' cushion protecting the brain from trauma and providing a stable ionic environment for cerebral function. The total volume of CSF is around 140 mL, where 40 mL surrounds the brain and 100 mL surrounds the spinal cord. Approximately 500 mL of CSF is produced by the choroid plexus in the lateral, third and fourth ventricles per day. The CSF circulates around the subarachnoid space and is reabsorbed into the venous sinuses predominantly by the arachnoid villi, but CSF is also absorbed by the spinal villi in the lumbar region. Absorption of CSF is constant to maintain a pressure of 0.5–1 kPa.

40. e. Littre hernia is incarceration of a Meckel's diverticulum within a hernial sac. De Garengeot hernia is incarceration of the vermiform appendix within a femoral hernia. Amyand hernia is incarceration of the vermiform appendix within an inguinal hernia. Richter hernia is a hernia involving only one sidewall of the bowel, which may result in bowel strangulation without the signs of bowel obstruction. Spigelian hernia is a hernia occurring between the rectus abdominis muscle medially and the semilunar line laterally. This most commonly occurs below the arcuate line.

41. c. The cystic artery is usually a branch of the right hepatic artery. It runs through Calot's triangle formed by the cystic duct, common hepatic duct and liver. A number of variations in the origin of the cystic artery are found, from the common hepatic artery, left hepatic artery or even the gastroduodenal artery. Venous return is via small veins in the gallbladder bed, with no accompanying vein to the cystic artery.

42. c. The axillary artery starts at the border of the first rib as a continuation of the subclavian artery, and continues as the brachial artery at the tip of teres minor. The axillary artery is split into three parts, each giving off its own branches:

First part – this extends from the lateral border of the first rib to the superior border of the pectoralis minor muscle, giving off the superior thoracic artery.
Second part – this extends deep to pectoralis minor, giving off the thoracoacromial artery and the lateral thoracic artery.
Third part – this extends from the inferior border of pectoralis minor to the inferior border of teres major, giving off the subscapular, anterior and posterior circumflex humeral arteries.

43. e. Arteritis refers to a group of conditions leading to inflammation of vessel walls. They may involve large, medium or small arteries.

- *Polyarteritis nodosa* – this disease affects small- or medium-sized vessels. The typical lesion is focal necrosis of the vessel wall. Aetiology seems to be caused by antigen–antibody complexes which may be stimulated by certain viral infections, for example hepatitis B.
- *Buerger's disease* – this painful condition commonly affects young men who are heavy cigarette smokers. The disease involves the small arteries of the limbs.
- *Temporal arteritis* – this disease of unknown aetiology affects elderly people causing facial pain and headache. There may also be ocular symptoms, even blindness.
- *Takayashu disease* – this rare disease commonly affects young women involving the cerebral, ophthalmic or carotid arteries.
- *Kawasaki disease* – a condition that affects young children and is associated with fever, rash and red throat.

44. c. The defecation reflex is triggered at an intrarectal pressure of 18 mmHg. Afferent impulses of the reflex pathway pass to sacral segments 1–3. Parasympathetic stimulation leads to relaxation of the internal anal sphincter. Activation of the pudendal nerve leads to increased tone of the external anal sphincter, and is involved in the process of consciously resisting the urge to defecate.

45. e. Alpha motor neurons are large motor neurons of the brainstem and spinal cord. They are responsible for innervating extrafusal muscle fibres. They are located in lamina IX of the spinal cord grey matter.

Laminae of spinal cord are as follows:

- I–VI: Posterior/dorsal horn
  - Lamina I: Marginal nucleus of spinal cord
  - Laminae II: Substantia gelatinosa of Rolando
  - Laminae III/IV: Nucleus proprius

- VII–IX: Anterior/ventral horn
  - Lamina VII: Intermediolateral nucleus, nucleus dorsalis
  - Lamina VIII: Motor interneurons
  - Lamina IX: Motor neurons
- Lamina X: Neurons bordering central canal

46. a. Tumour suppressor genes are normal genes switching off cell proliferation by acting on the cell cycle in G1. Loss of both copies of the tumour suppressor gene is required for cancer to develop.

Tumour suppressor gene	Chromosome	Neoplasms
WT1	11	Wilm's tumour, bladder cancer
Retinoblastoma	13	Retinoblastoma, sarcoma
NF1	17	Neurofibromas
APC	5	Colorectal cancer
p53	17	Lung and breast cancer

47. a. Superior gluteal nerve injury paralyzes the three muscles gluteus medius, gluteus minimus and tensor fascia latae and hence leads to a positive Trendelenburg test. These three muscles, especially the gluteus medius, tilt the pelvis in order to raise the contralateral pelvis during walking, which would otherwise be pulled down by gravity. In the Trendelenburg test, this action of the gluteus medius (superior pelvic tilt of contralateral hip) is absent and we actually observe that there is a downward drop of the unsupported hip because of unopposed action of gravity. This leads to a lurching gait in the patient.

48. c. The anatomical snuffbox lies between the extensor pollicis longus tendon on the ulnar side and the extensor pollicis brevis and abductor pollicis longus tendons on the radial side. The tendons are crossed by the cutaneous branches of the radial nerve in the roof. The cephalic vein begins in the roof of the snuffbox, and the radial artery lies on the floor deep to the tendons. The snuffbox is important clinically as tenderness is associated with fractures of the scaphoid.

49. e. There are four stages of acute inflammation characterized by margination of neutrophil polymorphs, adhesion, emigration and chemotaxis. Neutrophils migrate in response to chemical mediators such as histamine and to components of the complement cascade. Margination of neutrophil polymorphs is assisted by vasodilation. Increased adhesion results from interaction of molecules on the neutrophil and endothelial surface such as B2-integrin and ICAM-1. In acute inflammation there is increased vascular permeability, mediated by histamine, bradykinin nitric oxide and leukotriene B4. Bradykinin is also a chemical mediator of pain.

50. a. Benign positional paroxysmal vertigo (BPPV) occurs as a result of a degenerative condition of the inner ear where calcified particles are dislodged. The attacks of vertigo are short-lived and are brought on by turning the head.

BPPV can occur in cases of chronic otitis media, secondary to head trauma, or spontaneously. The Hallpike positional manoeuvre reproduces the symptoms by rapidly turning the head when it is positioned and held below the rest of the body on the examination couch. Treatment is with the Epley manoeuvre. Ménière's disease is the triad of vertigo, deafness and tinnitus. Acute labyrinthitis causes severe vertigo and loss of hearing.

51. d. Bone is a type of connective tissue that is metabolically active and constantly undergoing remodelling depending on the demands placed on it. It has both organic (osteoid) and inorganic components. The organic component consists of glycoproteins, hyaluronic acid and collagen, whereas the inorganic component consists of ions and minerals. There are four main cell types in bone: osteoprogenitor cells are undifferentiated cells, osteoblasts secrete organic matrix and lay down new bone, osteoclasts reabsorb bone via lytic enzymes and osteocytes are matured bone cells. Bone remodelling is much greater in physically active people, and bone mass can be lost if there is prolonged immobility (disuse osteoporosis). Several hormones are involved in bone remodelling including parathormone, thyroxine, calcitonin and oestrogen.

52. b. Mineralocorticoid deficiency can be a feature of Addison disease, where there is destruction of the adrenal cortex. This is mainly caused by autoimmune destruction but infection (e.g. tuberculosis) and malignancy (metastasis) can also be a cause. Mineralocorticoid (aldosterone) is produced by the zona glomerulosa of the adrenal cortex. It causes Na^+ and hence water retention in the body, thereby increasing blood pressure. When deficient, the body is unable to retain Na^+, and this results in increased urinary Na^+ loss and water loss, leading to hypotension (orthostatic). Loss of Na^+ is compensated by retaining K^+ and H^+, reducing urinary K^+ loss and leading to metabolic acidosis. Hyperpigmentation occurs because of overproduction of adrenocorticotropic hormone (ACTH), which is cleaved into melanocyte-stimulating hormone.

53. d. Melanomas are malignant neoplasms of epithelial melanocytes primarily arising in the skin. Predisposing factors include excessive sun exposure, fair complexion, family history and an increased number/changing moles. Over 50% arise *de novo*. There are five subtypes recognized. Superficial spreading is the most common, occurring mostly on the lower limb or trunk. Lentigo maligna are commonly found on the face in elderly patients. Acral lentiginous are more common in darker-skinned people, found mostly on the palms or soles and mucous membranes. Nodular melanomas usually occur on the trunk and invade early.

54. c. Apoptosis involves single cells, whereas necrosis involves groups of cells. The plasma membrane remains intact with apoptosis, but with necrosis there is loss of membrane integrity. With apoptosis there is cell shrinkage, fragmentation and formation of characteristic apoptotic bodies, whereas in necrosis there is cell swelling and lysis with phagocytosis of cell remnants by neutrophils. Apoptosis has no inflammatory response, and the cell remnants are phagocytosed by neighbouring cells. Apoptosis can be seen in pathological and physiological conditions, whereas necrosis is typically a pathological condition.

55. e. Seven muscles attach the scapula to the chest wall and maintain normal scapular control. The two main muscles are trapezius and serratus anterior. The other five are levator scapulae, rhomboids major and minor, pectoralis minor and omohyoid. Winging of the scapula is caused by partial or complete paralysis of the serratus anterior muscle, supplied by the long thoracic nerve. The rotator cuff muscles also originate from the scapula and are involved in shoulder movements.

56. b. The adrenal gland is usually supplied by three adrenal arteries: superior, middle and inferior. These are derived from the inferior phrenic artery, abdominal aorta and renal artery, respectively. The adrenal gland drains into one adrenal vein. On the left, the adrenal vein empties into the left renal vein, and on the right, it empties into the inferior vena cava. The adrenal gland consists of the cortex and medulla. The cortex can be divided into the zona glomerulosa (mineralocorticoids), fasciculate (glucocorticoids) and reticularis (gonadocorticoids), where the zona glomerulosa forms the outer layer and the zona reticularis the inner layer.

57. e. When comparing acute with chronic inflammation, acute inflammation is characterized by the presence of neutrophils and an innate immune response, rapid onset with prominent vasodilation and an increase in vascular permeability, lasting hours to weeks. Chronic inflammation is characterized by the presence of lymphocytes and macrophages, and cell-mediated immunity with a slow prolonged response.

58. e. The patient is likely suffering from necrotizing fasciitis (a rare infection of the deeper layers of the skin and subcutaneous tissues). This would be an unusual complication of an appendicectomy but can occur. Laboratory tests and diagnostic investigations can be useful, but the diagnosis is mainly clinical. The optimum treatment is to resuscitate the patient aggressively and take the patient to theatre for aggressive surgical debridement as soon as possible.

59. c. After 3 months the scar is 70–80% of the tensile strength of unwounded skin. After this time there is little further increase in strength. After 1 week, the strength of the wound is approximately 10% that of the original skin. Over the next 4 weeks the tensile strength rapidly increases but then starts to decrease so that it reaches a plateau of 70–80% at 3 months. During the first 2 months, the relative excess of collagen deposition compared with collagen resorption increases wound strength. Over the third month collagen synthesis stops and further tensile strength is gained by remodelling the already laid down collagen to increase cross-linking and fibre size.

60. e. The stratum spinosum is also known as the prickle layer of the epidermis because of its desmosomal connections with adjacent cells. It is important in bipolar lipid production to reduce water evaporation. The stratum corneum is the outermost layer of the epidermis and consists of keratin-filled anuclear cells. The thickness of this layer is determined by what it is exposed to. For example, on the plantar surface of the feet the skin is subject to greater insult than the skin on the dorsal surface, and so will have a thicker protective stratum corneum. Melanocytes are found in the stratum basale.

61. c. A Lanz or gridiron incision is used for appendicectomy. The Lanz incision is made horizontally over McBurney's point within the skin crease. It gives a better cosmetic result. Right Kocher's or subcostal is used to access the liver, gallbladder and biliary tree. Pfannenstiel is a transverse incision just above the pubic symphysis, for caesarean section and benign pathology hysterectomy. A modified version of this is the Maylard incision which allows wider access to the pelvis by sectioning the rectus abdominis muscles transversely as opposed to the vertical incision of the linea alba of a Pfannenstiel incision.

62. d. The thoracic duct arises between L1 and L2 as the cysterna chyli. It passes through the right crus of the diaphragm. It ascends posterior to the oesophagus. It crosses the midline from right to left at T5. It drains into the left brachiocephalic vein (at the confluence of the internal jugular and subclavian veins).

63. b. Gastric carcinoma is now the second most common carcinoma in the UK. It often presents late and so is a difficult disease to treat. The majority are adenocarcinomas with 2–8% being lymphomas. Gastrointestinal stromal tumour (GIST) and neuroendocrine tumours are less common. Spread is local, blood-borne, lymphatic and transcoelomic, which can occur throughout the peritoneal cavity, and preferentially to the ovaries, where it is known as a Krukenberg tumour. Treatment of choice is surgery, in which case early diagnosis is essential. Distal tumours are treated by subtotal gastrectomy and proximal tumours by total gastrectomy.

64. c. A spirogram is a useful test to perform as part of a pre-assessment before theatre. The expiratory reserve volume is defined as the maximum volume of gas that can be expired during forced breathing in addition to the tidal volume. The tidal volume is the volume of air inspired or expired in a normal breath. The residual volume is the volume of gas remaining in the lungs after maximal expiration. The functional residual capacity is the volume of gas remaining in the lungs after a normal tidal expiration; therefore, the expiratory reserve volume is the difference between the functional residual capacity and the residual volume. The inspiratory reserve volume is the maximum volume of gas that can be inspired during forced breathing in addition to the tidal volume. The vital capacity is the volume of gas that can be expired after maximal inspiration.

65. b. Pulmonary artery catheters are useful in calculating a number of cardiovascular parameters in the critically ill for both assessment and therapeutic guidance. Indications include inotropic support, suspicion of acute respiratory distress syndrome (ARDS), septic shock and multiorgan failure. Direct measurements include mean arterial pressure, heart rate, cardiac output, ejection fraction and mixed venous oxygen saturation. Derived variables include cardiac index, stroke volume systemic and pulmonary vascular resistance and oxygen delivery/consumption.

66. b. All somatic motor neurons, pre-ganglionic neurons and most post-ganglionic parasympathetic neurons are cholinergic; that is, they use acetylcholine (ACh) as their neurotransmitter. The effects of ACh on an organ depend on the type of the cholinergic receptor, either nicotinic or muscarinic. They are named thus because of the fact that nicotine, from tobacco plants, and muscarine, from poisonous mushrooms, are able to stimulate the two different types of receptor, respectively. Nicotinic receptors are found in the neuromuscular junction of skeletal muscle fibres and in autonomic ganglia. Muscarinic receptors are found in smooth muscle, exocrine glands and the heart. These receptors are further differentiated by the action of tubocurarine, which specifically blocks nicotinic receptors, and atropine, which specifically blocks the muscarinic receptors.

67. b. The inferolateral and inferomedial borders are supplied by the lateral and medial heads of the gastrocnemius, respectively. The superomedial border is formed by the semimembranosus and the semitendinosus, with the superolateral border formed by the biceps femoris. The semimembranosus is deep to the semitendinosus. The roof is formed by skin and fascia and the floor is formed by the popliteal surface of the femur.

68. a. The neck is divided into anterior and posterior triangles by the sternocleidomastoid muscles.

Anterior triangle boundaries:

- Medially: The midline
- Laterally: Anterior border of sternocleidomastoid
- Superiorly: Lower border of mandible

Posterior triangle boundaries:

- Anteriorly: Posterior sternocleidomastoid
- Posteriorly: Anterior border of trapezius
- Base: Middle third of the clavicle

69. a. Milroy disease is a congenital hereditary primary lymphoedema caused by aplasia of the lymph trunks resulting in progressive swelling of one or both legs. It is an example of primary lymphoedema. Secondary lymphoedema is where there is a known cause of lymphatic failure. This includes surgical excision, such as during an axillary dissection, or radiotherapy, which causes a block of fibrous tissue so that regenerating lymph vessels are unable to cross through. Infection by *Wuchereria bancrofti* causing elephantiasis, tuberculosis and infiltrative cancer are other causes of secondary lymphoedema.

70. c. Differential diagnosis includes a torn gastrocnemius muscle. Homan's sign involves passive dorsiflexion of the foot causing pain in the calf in cases of deep vein thrombosis (DVT). Risk can be reduced using thromboembolic deterrent stockings, prophylactic low-molecular-weight heparin (LMWH) injections and pneumatic calf compression in theatre.

71. d. The spleen is derived from the mesoderm lying between the 9th and 12th ribs. The spleen is composed of red and white pulp. Red pulp is composed of connective tissue named the cords of Bilroth and is separated from the white pulp by a marginal zone. About 75% of the spleen consists of red pulp, which acts as a mechanical filter of red blood cells, removing antigens and microorganisms. White pulp contains more lymphoid tissue and plays a part in antibody synthesis and removal of antigen-coated organisms. White pulp is known to hypertrophy in conditions such as lymphoid leukaemia causing splenomegaly.

72. c. In a neck of fibula fracture, the common peroneal nerve is most likely to be damaged as it surrounds the neck as part of its course. The common peroneal nerve supplies muscles in the lateral and anterior compartment of the leg, allowing ankle dorsiflexion and foot eversion. If damaged, the patient is unable to dorsiflex or evert the foot, causing a foot drop and a high stepping gait.

73. b. The ulnar nerve (usually) supplies sensation to the skin of the fifth and the ulnar side of the fourth finger. There is sympathetic interruption, with absence of sweating in the affected area. The thenar muscles are supplied by the median nerve and are therefore spared. Although the fourth and fifth digits are held in the clawed position when the nerve is injured at the wrist, a high lesion paralyzes the long flexors to these two fingers and results in the loss (or at least a marked reduction) of this sign. A test for paralysis of the palmar interossei, supplied by the ulnar nerve, is the inability to adduct the fingers and thus to be unable to grip a sheet of paper between them.

74. c. The answer is 12 as she is confused but opening her eyes to speech and localizing to pain. The Glasgow Coma Scale (GCS) offers a reliable, reproducible quantitative assessment of a patient's level of consciousness. It is measured on three scales, with the lowest possible score being 3 and the highest 15.

Eye opening

- 4 – spontaneously
- 3 – to speech
- 2 – to pain
- 1 – not at all

Motor response

- 6 – obeys commands
- 5 – localizes pain
- 4 – withdraws from pain
- 3 – abnormal flexion to pain
- 2 – extension to pain
- 1 – no response

Verbal response

- 5 – orientated
- 4 – confused conversation
- 3 – inappropriate words
- 2 – incomprehensible sounds
- 1 – no verbalization

75. d. Initial management following Airway, Breathing, Circulation (ABC) assessment consists of immediate nasal compression and sucking on an ice cube or lolly for children. There is little evidence that the application of ice packs is beneficial. If bleeding does not stop, then nasal packing is used to achieve an appropriate tamponade. If the bleeding site is visible with minimal blood loss, primary cauterization can be performed. Sphenopalatine ligation is rarely necessary and only happens in patients who fail conservative management.

Ear, nose and throat (ENT) referral is not mandatory if the epistaxis is minor and controlled by simple compression or cautery.

76. c. The hamstring muscles all arise from the ischial tuberosity and insert into the tibia or fibula. They are the semimembranosus, semitendinosus and biceps femoris. Semimembranosus extends from the ischial tuberosity to the medial condyle of the tibia. Semitendinosus arises from the medial aspect of the ischial tuberosity and inserts deep to the gracilis on the upper part of the tibia. The long head of biceps arises with semitendinosus, with the short head arising from the linea aspera. Both heads form one single tendon inserting into the head of the fibula. The hamstring compartment receives its blood supply from the profunda femoris artery, but because of the length of the muscles, they also receive multiple contributions from other arteries proximally and distally.

77. d. The Dukes' classification predates the more modern Tumour, Nodes, Metastasis (TNM) classification. It was put forward by Dr Cuthbert Dukes in 1932 and originally did not include stage D. The classification is:

Stage A: Tumour confined to the bowel wall (not extending beyond muscularis propria)
Stage B: Tumour penetrating the bowel wall
Stage C1: Lymph node involvement but not including the apical node
Stage C2: Lymph node involvement including the apical node
Stage D: Distant metastasis

78. c. The gastric parietal cells produce intrinsic factor, which binds vitamin B_{12} in the stomach, thereby facilitating its absorption in the ileum. Post-gastrectomy patients require replacement because of the absence of these cells. The G-cells are found in the antral mucosa and upper small bowel and secrete gastrin, which stimulates secretion of acid by parietal cells. Goblet cells are found in the bowel, not stomach. Chief cells produce pepsinogen.

79. a. The anion gap = $(Na^+ + K^+) - (HCO_3^- + Cl^-)$. If there is a high anion gap, there is an unmeasured anion present in increased quantities. This can be seen in ketoacidosis and lactic acidosis. A normal anion gap can still be seen in metabolic acidosis. This implies that HCl is being retained, or that $NaHCO_3$ is being lost, which can lead to a hyperchloraemic acidosis. Examples of this are seen in diarrhoea, high output ileostomy and renal tubular acidosis. A fall in albumin level can lead to a decrease in the anion gap.

80. d. The Nernst equation can be used to calculate the equilibrium potential, which is the potential difference at which an ion ceases to flow across the cell membrane along its electrochemical gradient. The typical value of the resting membrane potential for a neuron is –70 mV. An action potential is a rapid depolarization followed by subsequent repolarization to the resting membrane potential. The Goldman equation can be used to calculate the resting membrane potential, which is the potential difference across the cell membrane.

81. a. During times of acute inflammation the body upregulates certain proteins to help overcome the insult, including acute-phase proteins. These proteins are mainly synthesized in the liver and may reach concentrations several hundred-fold above their normal value. The most commonly used acute-phase protein in current clinical practice is the C-reactive protein (CRP). Other well-known proteins are fibrinogen and serum amyloid A (SAA) protein. Upregulation is controlled by cytokines, typically interleukin-6 (IL-6) for CRP and fibrinogen and IL-1 or tumour necrosis factor for SAA. Many acute-phase proteins, such as CRP and SAA, bind to bacterial cell walls and may act as opsonins and fix complement. The rise in fibrinogen causes erythrocytes to form rouleaux (stacks), which gravitate more quickly than individual erythrocytes. This discrepancy allows the measurement of the erythrocyte sedimentation rate (ESR), which is a basic test of a systemic inflammatory response.

82. c.   The portal vein is the main channel of the portal system of veins. It carries blood from three major veins: the superior and inferior mesenteric veins and the splenic vein. The portal vein is formed posterior to the neck of the pancreas. The portal vein ascends in the free edge of the lesser omentum to the liver (posterior to the hepatic artery and bile duct). At the porta hepatis the portal vein divides into right and left branches, which empty their blood into the hepatic sinusoids.

83. e.   The transpyloric plane of Addison is a perpendicular plane found midway between the pubic symphysis and the jugular notch. Structures found at this level include:

- Body of L1 vertebrae
- Duodenojejunal junction
- Hilum of kidneys
- Portal vein formed from anastomosis of splenic and superior mesenteric veins
- Attachment of transverse mesocolon
- Termination of spinal cord
- Gallbladder fundus
- Superior mesenteric artery branching off aorta
- Pancreas neck
- Hilum of spleen
- Pylorus of stomach

84. b.   This man has presented with a history and presentation typical of multiple myeloma (MM), which commonly presents in the 65- to 70-year-old age group, and is more frequent in males and the Afro-Caribbean population. It is a malignant clonal infiltration of B-lymphocyte-derived plasma cells. Owing to bone marrow infiltration by the myeloma, patients often present with problems of anaemia, infection and bleeding. High paraprotein levels, causing hyperviscosity, lead to renal impairment, amyloidosis and renal infarction. MM is also associated with lytic bone lesions, which can cause spinal cord compression. In two-thirds of cases, urine samples contain Bence–Jones proteins, which are free immunoglobulin light chains (kappa or lambda) which are filtered by the kidney. β-2 microglobulin is a prognostic test.

85. e.   Unfractionated heparin requires a continuous intravenous infusion with regular checks on the activated partial thromboplastin time (APPT) to ensure the infusion is running at the correct rate. Unfractionated heparin consists of polymers of varying molecular weights. Low molecular weight heparin (LMWH) is fractionated to contain only short-chain polysaccharides. It is used for deep vein thrombsis (DVT) prophylaxis in surgery, and has also been found to be more efficient at reducing the risk of DVT extending further and reoccurring. LMHW also has a lower risk of heparin-induced thrombocytopenia and, potentially, osteoporosis when compared with unfractionated heparin.

86. c. Traumatic injury to the spleen can be blunt or penetrating. Splenic injury is graded into five types ranging from capsular tear less than 1 cm to a shattered spleen. Conservative treatment is usually reserved for grades 1, 2 and sometimes 3, but will vary depending on the physiological state of the patient. If the patient becomes unstable, or if the injury is greater than grade 3, a splenectomy is performed. Splenectomy is also performed for idiopathic thrombocytopenic purpura (ITP), hereditary spherocytosis and autoimmune haemolytic anaemia. There is little evidence for splenectomy in sickle cell disease during an acute sequestration crisis over a blood transfusion.

87. d. Calcium homeostasis is maintained by parathormone (parathyroid hormone/PTH), calcitonin and vitamin D. PTH is secreted by the chief cells of the parathyroid gland when there is a fall in extracellular calcium. PTH increases plasma calcium by decreasing osteoblast activity, increasing reabsorption from the distal tubule. PTH also reduces phosphate reabsorption in the kidney and stimulates 1α-hydoxylase and thus activates vitamin D. Vitamin D is taken from the diet and ultraviolet radiation also converts cholesterol into Vitamin D_3. Vitamin D increases uptake of calcium and phosphate from the gut and kidney and directly stimulates osteoblasts. Calcitonin is secreted by the parafollicular C-cells of the thyroid gland in response to hypercalcaemia. Calcitonin increases excretion of calcium and phosphate from the kidney and inhibits osteoclast activity.

88. c. Nitric oxide (NO) is especially secreted by nerve terminals in areas of the brain responsible for long-term behaviour and memory. It is synthesized instantly as needed then diffuses out of the presynaptic terminals over a period of seconds rather than being released in vesicular packets. It is also released by the endothelium of blood vessels as endothelium-derived relaxing factor. It diffuses into postsynaptic neurons nearby. In the postsynaptic neuron it usually does not greatly alter the membrane potential but instead changes intracellular metabolic functions that modify neuronal excitability.

89. c. The inguinal canal is approximately 4 cm in length passing from the deep to the superficial inguinal ring. The floor of the inguinal canal consists of the inguinal ligament and lacunar ligament. The posterior wall of the inguinal canal consists of the transversalis fascia and conjoint tendon. The roof of the inguinal canal consists of the internal oblique and transversalis muscle. The anterior wall of the inguinal ligament consists of the external oblique aponeurosis. Hesselbach's triangle lies between the inferior epigastric artery superolaterally, inguinal ligament inferiorly and linea semilunaris of the rectus abdominis medially. Direct hernias typically protrude through this area.

90. d. The radial nerve (C5–T1) supplies the extensor muscles of the arm and forearm. Supinator, supplied by the radial nerve, is the main supinator of the hand when the elbow is fully extended, which inhibits any contribution from biceps brachii. Anconus, a small muscle supplied by the radial nerve, extends the elbow, helps stabilize the elbow joint and abducts the ulna during pronation. Brachioradialis, although a flexor, is supplied by the radial nerve. Brachialis is supplied by the musculocutaneous nerve.

91. d.   Folate is normally absorbed in the diet from the jejunum. The main cause of deficiency is malnutrition, as seen in alcoholics or with regular consumption of overcooked food. Other causes include malabsorption, as seen in coeliac disease and Crohn disease. Increased requirements of folate occur in conditions such as pregnancy, malignancy or haemolysis. Drugs can either block utilization, such as methotrexate, or cause malabsorption, such as anticonvulsants.

92. d.   The initial reaction in the intrinsic pathway is conversion of inactive factor XII to active factor XII (XIIa). This activation, which is catalyzed by high-molecular-weight kininogen and kallikrein, can be brought about *in vivo* by exposure of blood to collagen fibres underlying the endothelium. Active factor XII then activates factor XI, and active factor XI activates factor IX. Activated factor IX forms a complex with active factor VIII, which is activated when it is separated from the von Willebrand factor (vWF). The complex of IXa and VIIIa activates factor X. Phospholipids from aggregated platelets and calcium are necessary for full activation of factor X. The extrinsic pathway is triggered by the release of tissue thromboplastin, a protein–phospholipid mixture that activates factor VII. Factor X can be activated by either of two systems.

93. a.   Pulse pressure is defined as the difference between the systolic and diastolic blood pressure. A narrow pulse pressure is suggestive of significant blood loss or dehydration. However, a narrow pulse pressure can also be caused by aortic stenosis. A high pulse pressure is seen in chronic aortic regurgitation, and in healthy individuals after exercise because of a reduction in peripheral vascular resistance. The cardiac output is calculated by heart rate multiplied by stroke volume. Cardiac output multiplied by systemic vascular resistance is the arterial pressure.

94. a.   All rotator cuff muscles originate from the scapular; their insertion and function can be summarized as follows:

- Supraspinatus
  - Inserts into the superior aspect of greater tuberosity
  - Initiates abduction of the shoulder
- Infraspinatus
  - Inserts into the middle aspect of greater tuberosity
  - Externally rotates the shoulder
- Teres minor
  - Inserts into the inferior aspect of greater tuberosity
  - Externally rotates the shoulder
- Subscapularis
  - Inserts into the lesser tuberosity
  - Internally rotates the shoulder

95. d.   Together, these tendons surround the head of the humerus anteriorly, posteriorly and superiorly, conferring stability to the glenohumeral joint when they contract during movement. Rotator cuff deficiency leads to subluxation of the head of the humerus, leading to impingement against the acromion, which results in weakness of abduction and loss of motion. The supraspinatous tendon, which is the dominant part of the rotator cuff, is most frequently degenerate. It is involved in the abduction of the humerus in conjunction with the much stronger deltoid muscle. It is mainly responsible for the initiation of abduction of the humerus.

96. c. As a result of the large volume of blood transfused, this patient is likely to have a hyperkalaemia and a hypocalcaemia; the latter is secondary to the citrate (the anticoagulant used in blood transfusions) in the blood binding his blood calcium. This can lead to cardiac rhythm abnormalities and electrocardiogram changes.

97. b. Factor V Leiden causes an increased breakdown of protein C, an anticoagulant factor. The relative risk (RR) of the heterozygous state is 6, whereas the homozygous state is 80. Oral contraceptive pill (OCP) use is associated with an RR of 4. Protein C deficiency in the homozygous form results in severe thrombosis at birth; the heterozygous form RR is 7. Homozygous prothrombin gene mutation has an RR of 20. Antithrombin III homozygous is lethal *in utero*; the heterozygous form carries an RR of 5.

98. e. Three factors have been identified that predispose a patient to thrombus formation, known as Virchow's triad: (1) endothelial injury, (2) hypercoagulability and (3) altered blood flow leading to stasis or turbulence. Of the three factors, endothelial injury is the most important. Hypercoagulable states arise through primary (genetic) or secondary (acquired) causes.

- Primary causes: Factor V Leiden, mutation in prothrombin gene, antithrombin III deficiency, protein C and protein S deficiency
- Secondary (high risk): Prolonged bed rest, myocardial infarction, atrial fibrillation, tissue damage, cancer, disseminated intravascular coagulation
- Secondary (low risk): Obesity, smoking, hyperoestrogenic states (pregnancy and oral contraceptive use), nephritic syndrome, sickle cell anaemia
- Christmas disease (haemophilia B) is a deficiency of factor IX and therefore increases bleeding.

99. d. Neurological regulation of respiration is controlled by the inspiratory and expiratory neurons in the medulla oblongata, and the apneustic and pneumotaxic centres in the pons. The apneustic centre prolongs inspiration resulting in short expiratory efforts. The pneumotaxic centre inhibits inspiratory neurons shortening inspiration. Chemical regulation of respiration is by peripheral and central chemoreceptors. The peripheral chemoreceptors are located in the carotid bodies and respond primarily to low levels of PO_2 and in part to arterial pH. The central chemoreceptors are located close to the respiratory centre in the medulla. They are indirectly sensitive to changes in the arterial pH. The Hering–Breuer reflex prevents overinflation of the lungs via stretch receptors.

100. c. The thick ascending limb is impermeable to water. The main structure for the kidney's reabsorption of solutes is the proximal convoluted tubule – approximately 70% of filtered sodium, chloride, potassium, nearly all the amino acids and glucose, as well as phosphate and lactate are reabsorbed here.

Approximately 20% of filtered solutes are absorbed in the thick ascending limb; approximately 20% of filtered water is absorbed in the thin descending limb.

101. d. The recurrent laryngeal nerve supplies the motor and sensory function of the larynx and is of anatomical importance in thyroid surgery. The left recurrent laryngeal nerve passes inferior to the arch of the aorta before ascending again and inserting into the larynx, deep to the inferior border of the inferior constrictor muscle of the pharynx. The right recurrent laryngeal nerve passes inferior to the right subclavian artery. The laryngeal nerves are derived from the vagus nerve and ascend in a groove between the oesophagus and trachea.

102. c. *Helicobacter pylori* is a Gram-negative, spiral, motile and microaerophilic organism. Infection causes an increase in gastric acid secretion, leading to peptic ulceration. It produces the enzyme urease, which breaks down urea into CO_2 and the alkali ammonia, which increases the surrounding pH. It can be transmitted via faecal–oral, oral–oral or iatrogenic routes (endoscopy). Diagnosis is by urea breath test or mucosal biopsy (CLO test). Treatment involves triple therapy with a proton pump inhibitor and two antibiotics.

103. c. The blood gas gives a picture of respiratory alkalosis with hypoxia and hypocapnia. This is typically seen in patients suffering from a pulmonary embolism. Pulmonary embolism can also cause a sinus tachycardia and pleuritic chest pain. Tietze syndrome is a condition of unknown aetiology characterized by chondritis of the costal cartilage. It affects one or more costochondral junctions and resolves over a number of months. Although patients with pneumonia may have a similar blood gas, the clinical scenario depicts pulmonary embolism as the most likely diagnosis.

104. d. The short gastric arteries originate from the splenic artery and run in the gastrosplenic ligament. The left gastric artery originates from the celiac trunk and runs up toward the oesophageal opening in the diaphragm providing branches, and downward in the lesser omentum supplying the lesser curvature of the stomach. The right gastric artery originates from the common hepatic artery and also supplies the lesser curvature anastomizing with the left gastric artery. The gastroduodenal artery also originating from the common hepatic artery passes down behind the first part of the duodenum where it may be eroded by an ulcer. Inferiorly it divides into two branches giving the right gastroepiploic artery which supplies the greater curvature of the stomach.

105. b. Parotid gland tumours account for approximately 80% of all salivary gland tumours; of these, two-thirds are pleiomorphic adenomas. Monomorphic adenomas account for the remaining third, the most common of which is a Warthin tumour, which is an adenolymphoma. These are more commonly bilateral. Weakness of the facial nerve suggests malignant infiltration. Adenoid cystic carcinomas are highly malignant tumours of the parotid gland, often causing facial nerve palsy. Sialadenitis is less common in the parotid gland than in the other salivary glands, and it is unusual for it to be bilateral and painless.

106. e. Antidiuretic hormone is produced in the supraoptic nucleus in the hypothalamus. Stimulation is via osmoreceptors which detect increases in the osmolality of the extracellular fluid. Other stimulating factors include a decrease in circulating volume or reduced arterial pressure. Renin is released from the juxtaglomerular cells in response to a decrease in afferent arteriole pressure or a reduction in sodium. Aldosterone is produced from the adrenal cortex stimulating the reabsorption of sodium and water. Atrial natriuretic peptide is released by the heart in response to an increase in the extracellular fluid via the stretch receptors.

107. b. Triiodothyronine (T_3) and thyroxine (T_4) increase the oxygen consumption in most metabolically active tissues; exceptions include:

- Spleen, lymph nodes
- Testes
- Uterus
- Brain (adult)
- Anterior pituitary (actually decreases as a result of decreased TSH secretion)

Increased thyroid hormones lead to increased nitrogen metabolism (leading to increased uric acid secretion, i.e. a direct relationship). Thyroid hormones are responsible for the conversion of carotene (which results in a yellow tint to the skin) to vitamin A – this explains the finding of carotenaemia in hypothyroid patients. Hypothyroidism leads to the accumulation of polysaccharides and hyaluronic acid in tissues, as thyroid hormones normally metabolize such proteins – this accounts for the characteristic puffiness (myxoedema) seen in hypothyroid patients.

108. c. There are three main apertures in the diaphragm, situated at T8, T10 and T12, through which pass several important structures. Each aperture is described in detail below.

- *T8*: Aperture is in the central tendon, situated to the right of the midline. Passing through is the inferior vena cava and terminal branches of the right phrenic nerve. When the diaphragm contracts during inspiration, the inferior vena cava dilates, facilitating blood flow to the heart.
- *T10*: The aperture is at the right crus of the diaphragm, transmitting the oesophagus, anterior and posterior vagal trunks, and the oesophageal branches of the left gastric artery.
- *T12*: This is an opening posterior to the diaphragm, not piercing it; therefore, blood flow is not affected by contraction of the diaphragm. It transmits the aorta, thoracic duct and azygous vein.

109. c. The endothelium of the blood vessels also plays an active role in preventing the extension of clots. All endothelial cells, except those in the cerebral microcirculation, produce thrombomodulin. This protein binds with thrombin to slow the clotting process. The thrombomodulin–thrombin complex also activates protein C, which acts as an anticoagulant by inactivating activated factors V and VIII.

110. a. The blood gas is consistent with acidosis due to the low pH. There is a low bicarbonate level with a negative base excess, suggesting that this is more of a metabolic acidosis. The history of abdominal pain and atrial fibrillation suggests a small embolus has passed into the arterial system causing bowel infarction.

A metabolic acidosis may also fit with pancreatitis; however, with previous gallbladder surgery, normal liver function tests and no history of alcohol abuse, it is less likely.

111. b.   The axillary nerve is a terminal branch of the posterior cord of the brachial plexus. Its course is to run posterolaterally through the quadrangular space of the arm and around the surgical neck of the humerus. It supplies the deltoid and teres minor muscles and an area of skin overlying the inferior aspect of deltoid, called the 'regimental patch'. The nerve is characteristically damaged in an anterior dislocation of the humerus. Consequently, the sensory aspect of the nerve should be tested before and after reduction. The association is so strong that it is almost seen as negligent if appropriate documentation of its function has not been made.

112. e.   The facial nerve supplies all the muscles needed for facial expression including the occipitofrontalis, which wrinkles the forehead. Frontalis has bilateral cortical representation but in this case there is a lower motor neurone injury leading to weakness. A distressing feature is paralysis of the buccinator muscle, which acts to empty the buccal sulcus during mastication. There are no cutaneous sensory fibres in the facial nerve. The levator palpebrae superioris is supplied by the oculomotor nerve, so the patient can still raise his upper lid. The chorda tympani fibres, which transmit taste from the anterior two-thirds of the tongue, pass from the lingual nerve to the facial nerve just below the skull and therefore remain intact in peripheral injuries of the facial nerve.

113. b.   All these symptoms together are a typical presentation of acute myeloid leukaemia, which has a median age of diagnosis of 65 years and is more common in males. Typically, it can cause gross hepatosplenomegaly with a bone marrow aspirate showing Auer rods, which are almost diagnostic of the condition. Owl eye nuclei represent cytomegalovirus (CMV) infection. Reed–Sternberg cells are used to diagnose Hodgkin lymphoma, but diagnosis is usually gained by lymph node biopsy. Lymphoblasts are seen in acute lymphocytic leukaemia, which occurs predominantly in children. An aplastic bone marrow can be indicative of many other conditions such as progressive myelodysplasia and bone marrow infections.

114. e.   Diagnosis of basal cell carcinoma is made clinically but histological diagnosis can be obtained prior to management. A watch and wait policy is appropriate in certain circumstances due to the slow growth and low metastatic potential, provided the lesion is not in a high-risk area (i.e. the face). This option can be used with the elderly and frail. Curettage and cautery is effective for smaller lesions but gives no information on the size of clearance margins. Cryotherapy treats the lesion but provides no tissue for histology. Surgical excision provides a histological specimen, a closed wound and proof of complete excision. Larger lesions may require coverage with a skin graft or even reconstructive surgery. Sentinel node biopsy is part of the recognized treatment options for melanoma.

115. c.   The relationship between the partial pressure of oxygen and the concentration of oxygen in the blood is known graphically as the oxygen dissociation curve. The curve is sigmoidal in shape and represents the increasing ability of haemoglobin to accept oxygen. The curve plateaus at a PO_2 of around 15–16 kPa. A number of physiological parameters can change the affinity of oxygen, which alters the position of the curve. Shifts in the curve to the right (representing a decrease in affinity) are caused by increases in PCO_2 and hydrogen ions, which is known as the Bohr effect. In addition, increases in blood temperature and 2,3-diphosphoglycerate (2,3-DPG) levels in erythrocytes also shift the curve to the right. A decrease in any of the above parameters will shift the curve to the left.

116. c.   Class II suggests that he has lost 15–30% of his blood volume. This loss may not be obvious as a patient is often able to conceal large volumes of body fluids internally. Class II shock has signs of normal systolic blood pressure but reduced pulse pressure, with a tachycardia, increased respiratory rate and reduced urine output. The table below describes the classes of shock.

For an average 70 kg man	Class I	Class II	Class III	Class IV
Blood loss (mL)	<750	750–1500	1500–2000	>2000
Blood loss (%)	<15%	15–30%	30–40%	>40%
Heart rate	<100	>100	>120	>140
Blood pressure (mmHg)	Normal or increased	Normal	Decreased	Decreased
Respiratory rate	14–20	20–30	30–40	>40
Urine output (mL/h)	>30	20–30	5–15	Negligible
Mental status	Slightly anxious	Mildly anxious	Anxious/ confused	Confused/ lethargic

117. e.

- *Anterior cord syndrome:* Associated with flexion/rotation injuries leading to loss of power below the level of the lesion and loss of pain and temperature below the lesion.
- *Central cord syndrome:* Occurs in syringomyelia and centrally placed tumours. Initially the spinothalamic tract is affected leading to loss of pain and temperature below the lesion. Gradually the lateral corticospinal tract is involved leading to flaccid weakness of the arms.
- *Posterior cord syndrome:* Seen in hyperextension injuries leading to loss of proprioception and profound ataxia.
- *Brown–Sequard syndrome:* Hemisection of the cord leading to paralysis on the affected side below the lesion. There is also loss of proprioception and fine discrimination. Pain and temperature are lost on the opposite side below the lesion.
- *Cauda equina syndrome:* Involves compression of the lumbosacral roots below the conus medullaris. This is a lower motor neuron lesion causing bowel and bladder dysfunction with leg numbness and weakness.

118. b.   The shoulder joint is initially abducted by the supraspinatus muscle, up to 15°. The deltoid muscle then abducts to 90°. Abduction beyond that is by rotation of the scapula by the trapezius and serratus anterior muscle. A painful middle arc (central 30° or so) is caused by supraspinatus tendinitis. It is in this range of movement that the supraspinatus tendon impinges on the acromion and coracoacromial ligament.

119. d. The contents of the carpal tunnel include flexor pollicis longus, the four tendons of flexor digitorum superficialis, the four tendons of flexor digitorum profundus and the median nerve. Any lesion reducing the size of the tunnel will result in compression of the median nerve and hence cause symptoms of carpal tunnel syndrome. Symptoms include paraesthesia, pain and intermittent numbness of the thumb, index and radial half of the ring finger.

To relieve these symptoms, surgical division of the flexor retinaculum (carpal tunnel release) may be necessary. The ulnar nerve does not travel within the carpal tunnel and hence signs of ulnar nerve lesion (inability to perform Froment's test, which tests adductor pollicis) are not indicative of carpal tunnel syndrome.

120. d. The anatomical dead space is defined as the dead space in that portion of the respiratory system which is external to the alveoli and includes the air-conveying ducts from the nostrils to the terminal bronchioles. Factors increasing anatomical dead space are:

- Increasing size of subject
- Standing position
- Increased lung volume
- Bronchodilation

The physiological dead space is defined as the total dead space in the entire respiratory system including the alveoli factors increasing physiological dead space:

- Hypotension
- Hypoventilation
- Emphysema
- Pulmonary embolism
- Positive pressure ventilation

121. c. The coronary artery anatomy is variable, as are the relative territories of myocardium supplied by each of the arteries. ST segment depression across all leads implies ischaemia (angina), whereas isolated ST segment depression in leads V1 and V2 may indicate a posterior myocardial infarction. The most likely artery involved in this case is therefore the posterior descending artery. Either the right coronary or circumflex arteries can supply the posterior descending artery, but it is not possible to identify which from the electrocardiogram alone. Left main stem and left anterior descending artery lesions would cause changes over a much larger area.

122. b. The axillary artery is a continuation of the subclavian artery and it starts from the lateral border of the 1st rib. It ends at the lower border of teres major, becoming the brachial artery. The axillary artery is divided into three parts by the pectoralis minor. The first part gives off one branch, the superior thoracic artery. The second part gives off two branches, the thoracoacromial and the lateral thoracic artery. The third part gives off three branches, the subscapular, anterior and posterior circumflex humeral arteries. The axillary vein lies medial to the axillary artery and drains into the subclavian vein.

123. d. Skeletal muscle fibres are categorized by their time to reach maximum tension. There are three main types: type I, type IIa and type IIb. Type I fibres are postural muscles and are able to sustain contraction for a long time without fatigue. They have a high myoglobin content (hence the red colour) and a rich capillary supply that gives them a high oxidative capacity for aerobic respiration. Soleus muscle is postural in nature and contains type 1 fibres. It reaches peak tension in 80–200 ms. Type IIb fibres are thicker and are designed for anaerobic respiration and consequently have fewer mitochondria and less myoglobin. They have a large store of glycogen and a high concentration of glycolytic enzymes giving them a high myosin ATPase content. Extraocular muscles are type IIb muscle fibres and reach a peak tension in 7–8 ms. The type IIa fibres are a mix as they have a fast twitch rate but also a high oxidative capacity.

124. b. The vagus nerve (CN X) originates in the medulla oblongata and has a wandering (hence the name) course down through the thorax and into the abdomen. Vagal stimulation is parasympathetic and so its effects are related to 'rest and digest' activities. These include increasing intestinal motility, stimulating the chief cells to secrete pepsinogen and indirectly stimulating the parietal cells to secrete hydrochloric acid. The vagus also directly stimulates the G-cells to secrete gastrin and the enterochromaffin-like cells to release histamine. The vagus nerve innervates all the organs, except the adrenal glands, from the neck down to the second segment of the transverse colon. Auricular branches arise from the vagus nerve and supply part of the auricle and the external auditory meatus. The vagus nerve also controls a few skeletal muscles in the pharynx and larynx.

125. b. Adrenaline acts on α, β_1 and β_2 receptors, causing massive peripheral vasoconstriction (via α agonism) and positive inotropic/chronotropic effects (via β_1 receptor agonism). Dobutamine is predominantly a β_1 receptor agonist used primarily in cardiogenic shock. Isoprenaline is both a β_1 and β_2 receptor agonist. Nitrates are not inotropes, in that they do not alter the contractility or rate of contraction of the heart; their principle action is venodilatation, and they are used to reduce peripheral vascular resistance. Dopamine has variable physiological effects in relation to the concentration of dose:

- Small dose: Increased splanchnic blood flow, renal artery dilatation (consequent increased urine output)
- Medium dose: Predominantly β_1 receptor effects
- Large dose: Predominantly α receptor effects

126. b. The blood supply to the heart may be summarized as follows:

- Left coronary artery (arising from the posterior aspect of the aortic sinus) divides into:
  - Anterior interventricular artery (which courses the interventricular groove and forms an anastomosis with the posterior interventricular artery)

- Circumflex artery (which courses the atrioventricular sulcus and forms an anastomosis with the right coronary artery)
- Right coronary artery (arising from the anterior aspect of the aortic sinus) divides into:
  - Posterior interventricular artery (the continuation of the posterior interventricular artery, which courses the interventricular groove and forms an anastomosis with the anterior interventricular artery)
  - Marginal branch (which descends over the anterior aspect of the ventricle)

The anterior cardiac veins always drain directly into the right atrium, whereas the small cardiac veins usually drain into the coronary sinus, but this is variable and sometimes they drain directly into the right atrium.

127. e.   The reflex contraction is possible in all muscles but is most readily seen in extensor muscles, such as the quadriceps. The reflex occurs in response to sensory input and does not require any input from upper motor neurons in the brain. The simplest reflex involves just two nerves, which have just one synapse in the spinal cord. The reflex is produced when a light tap is placed on the muscle tendon. This action stretches the entire muscle and passively stretches the muscle spindles. Sensory impulses are then sent from the spindle via the sensory neuron to the ventral grey matter of the spinal cord. The sensory nerve synapses with an alpha motor neuron and this fast-conducting motor nerve stimulates the muscle to make an isotonic contraction. The contraction of the muscle decreases the stretch of the spindle, thereby reducing the afferent nerve impulses and subsequent contraction.

128. a.   The boundaries of the omental foramen are anteriorly, the portal vein, hepatic artery and bile duct (all in the free edge of the lesser omentum); posteriorly, the inferior vena cava and right crus of the diaphragm; superiorly, the caudate lobe of the liver; and inferiorly, the superior part of the duodenum, portal vein, hepatic artery and bile duct.

129. b.   The blood supply to the heart may be summarized as follows:

- Left coronary artery (arising from the posterior aspect of the aortic sinus) divides into:
  - Anterior interventricular artery (which courses the interventricular groove and forms an anastomosis with the posterior interventricular artery)
  - Circumflex artery (which courses the atrioventricular sulcus and forms an anastomosis with the right coronary artery)
- Right coronary artery (arising from the anterior aspect of the aortic sinus) divides into:
  - Posterior interventricular artery (the continuation of the posterior interventricular artery, which courses the interventricular groove and forms an anastomosis with the anterior interventricular artery)
  - Marginal branch (which descends over the anterior aspect of the ventricle)

The anterior cardiac veins always drain directly into the right atrium, whereas the small cardiac veins usually drain into the coronary sinus, but this is variable and sometimes they drain directly into the right atrium.

130. d. Antidiurectic hormone (ADH), also known as vasopressin, is used in the control of water absorption from the collecting ducts within the kidney. It is produced in the supraoptic nucleus of the hypothalamus and then secreted from the posterior pituitary. ADH stimulates aquaporins (found in the cytoplasm of collecting duct cells) to fuse with the cell membrane. Consequently, the collecting duct becomes more permeable to water and thus more water is absorbed. Changes in blood volume are detected by the stretch receptors in the left atrium and impulses are sent to the hypothalamus to inhibit ADH production. Changes in osmolality are detected by the osmoreceptors in the hypothalamus. Increased osmolality (dehydration) or decreased blood volume increases the secretion of ADH. This results in an increased blood volume and a compensatory decrease in the urine output. The converse is true for decreased osmolality and increased blood volume.

131. b. The metabolism of Ca^{2+} is regulated by two hormones, parathormone (PTH) and calcitonin. PTH is secreted by the parathyroid glands in response to hypocalcaemia and acts to increase plasma Ca^{2+} levels. It stimulates the conversion of vitamin D into its active form 1,25-dihydrocholecalciferol. Activated vitamin D increases plasma Ca^{2+} levels by increasing gut uptake, increasing renal absorption and stimulating bone resorption of Ca^{2+}. Calcitonin is secreted by parafollicular C-cells in the thyroid gland. Calcitonin acts to reduce Ca^{2+} levels by increasing renal loss and increasing bone reuptake. However, the action of calcitonin is thought to be significant only in periods of hypercalcaemia and plays little role in daily regulation of calcium. Low Ca^{2+} levels will lead to increased permeability and increased Na^+ reflux, reducing cell threshold and increasing nerve and muscle activity. Secondary hyperparathyroidism is caused by prolonged low Ca^{2+} levels leading to parathyroid gland hypertrophy.

132. e. The sinoatrial (SA) node lies near the opening of the superior vena cava, at the superior border of the sulcus terminalis. The right atrium forms the right heart border. The orifice of the coronary sinus lies between the opening of the inferior vena cava and the atrioventricular orifice.

133. e. The anterior border of the axilla is pectoralis major, the posterior wall is the latissimus dorsi, the medial wall is the chest wall and the lateral wall is the humerus. A level I axillary clearance extends up to the axillary vein, level II up to the medial border of the pectoralis minor muscle and level III up to the 1st rib. There is a risk of damage to the intercostobrachial nerve, which is a sensory nerve to the axilla and medial aspect of the upper arm. The long thoracic nerve supplying serratus anterior and the thoracodorsal nerve supplying latissimus dorsi can also be damaged. The thoracodorsal nerve passes along the posterior wall of the axilla.

134. d. Parathormone (PTH) is secreted by parathyroid glands and is stimulated by a decrease in calcium and an increase in phosphate. Calcitonin, produced by parafollicular cells of thyroid gland, decreases calcium. PTH increases osteoclastic activity by binding to osteoblasts. Osteoblasts increase their expression of the receptor activator of nuclear factor kappa B ligand (RANKL), which binds to a receptor activator of nuclear factor kappa B (RANK) receptor on the osteoclast.

When RANKL binds with RANK, osteoclastic production increases. PTH increases calcium and magnesium reabsorption from distal tubules and thick ascending limb. It reduces phosphate reabsorption from the proximal tubule altering the calcium–phosphate ratio in circulation. Activated 1,25-dihydroxy-vitamin D increases intestinal calcium absorption via calbindin.

135. a.   The anterior mediastinum is bordered anteriorly by the sternum and posteriorly by the great vessels. It contains the thymus, lymph nodes, fat and vessels. Disorders of the anterior mediastinum are generally thymic, thyroid (substernal goitre), teratoma (and other germ cell tumours) and lymphomas (Hodgkin disease, non-Hodgkin lymphoma).

INDEX

A

Abdominal aneurysms, 12, 22, 75, 86, 301, 341
Abdominal aorta, 13, 21, 77, 85
Abdominal aortic aneurysm, 22, 86
Abdominal compartment syndrome, 311, 352
Abdominal hernia, 20, 85
Abdominal pain, 225, 231, 238, 243, 251, 263, 271,
        276, 285, 311–312, 315–317, 352–353,
        356–358, 389, 417
Abdominal wall, 9, 16, 71, 80
Abdominal wall abscess, 369, 395
Abducens nerve, 48, 114
Abscesses, 221, 253, 369, 395
Acid–base balance, 151, 153, 195–198
Acid–base homeostasis, 154, 198–199
Acoustic meatus, 55, 57, 120, 122
Acoustic neuromas, 324, 364
Acromegaly, 306, 346–347
Actinomycosis, 249, 283
Action potentials, 164, 209–210, 384, 411
Acute inflammation, 222–223, 253–254, 378,
        379, 405, 407
Acute pancreatitis, 147, 189, 297, 312, 337, 353
Acute respiratory distress, 297, 337
Acute toxic colitis, 311, 352
Acute transfusion reaction, 376, 403
Acute urinary retention, 42, 106
Acute-phase protein, 384, 411
Addison's disease, 144, 186, 251, 285, 303, 305,
        343, 345
Adductor canal, 33, 37, 97, 100
Adenoidectomy, 52, 117
Adenolymphoma, 388, 416
Adenomas, 234, 266
Adenopathy, 306, 346
Adrenal cortex, 160, 204
Adrenal gland, 17, 81, 153, 159, 197, 203,
        379, 407
Adrenaline, 159, 203, 392, 421
Adrenocorticotropic hormone, 157–158, 162,
        202, 208, 251, 285, 305, 345
Ageing cells, 224, 229, 256, 261
Aldosterone, 156, 200
Alpha motor neurons, 377, 404–405
Alveolar nerve, 61, 126
Alveoli, 131, 171–172

Amyand hernia, 312, 353
Amyloidosis, 231, 263–264
Anaemia, 243, 245, 247, 276, 278, 280–281
Anal canal, 15, 79, 88
Anal carcinoma, 369, 370, 395, 397
Anal sphincter, 24, 88
Anaphylaxis, 242, 275
Anaplastic thyroid carcinoma, 306, 346
Anatomical dead space, 131, 171, 391, 420
Anatomical snuffbox, 28, 92, 378, 405
Anatomical triangle, 40, 42, 104, 107
Aneurysms, 12, 75, 228, 260, 301, 341
Angiotensin II, 161, 205
Anion gap, 152, 196, 383, 411
Ankle joint stability, 371, 397
Anterior mediastinum, 394, 424
Anterior triangle, 50, 381, 409
Antibody deficiency, 241, 273
Anticoagulants, 244, 246, 277, 279
Antidiuretic hormone, 152, 157, 197, 201, 371,
        388–389, 393, 397, 416, 423
Aorta, 3, 7, 66, 69
Aortic arches, 6, 68
Aortic dissection, 227, 259
Aortic stenosis, 301, 341
Apex beat, 3, 65
Apoptosis, 231, 264, 375–376, 379, 403, 406
Appendicectomy, 11, 23, 56, 73, 87, 121, 136, 176,
        379, 380, 407, 408
Appendicitis, 373, 400
Arm nerves, 30, 57, 95, 122
Arterial blood gas, 153, 154, 197, 198
Arterial blood supply, 392, 393, 421, 422
Arterial supply, 5, 20, 22, 23, 67, 84, 85, 86
Arterial ulcers, 227, 259
Arteritis, 377, 404
Arthritis, 293, 296, 333, 335–336;
        see also Rheumatoid arthritis
Asbestos exposure, 297, 337
Ascites, 228, 260
Atherosclerosis, 301, 341
Atrial natriuretic peptide, 152, 196
Auer rods, 243, 277, 390, 417
Auricle, 55, 120
Autoimmune thyroid disease, 303, 343
Autonomic nervous system, 54–63, 119–128,
        165, 211

Axillary artery, 26, 90, 92, 375, 377, 392, 402, 404, 420–421
Axillary dissection, 394, 423
Axillary lymph node clearance, 300, 339–340
Axillary lymph nodes, 27–28, 92
Axillary lymphadenopathy, 27, 92
Axillary nerve, 390, 417

B

β receptors, 142, 163, 183–184, 208
Back pain, 49, 58, 122, 238, 270–271, 384, 412
Back stab wound, 58, 122
Bacterial meningitis, 291, 329–330
Bacterial toxins, 249, 284
Baroreceptors, 144, 185
Basal cell carcinoma, 319, 360, 390, 417
Basal metabolic rate, 159, 203
Benign positional paroxysmal vertigo, 378, 405–406
Bile, 146, 149, 188, 192–193
Bilious vomiting, 317, 357
Bilirubin levels, 251, 285
Billroth I procedure, 12, 74–75
Bladder tumours, 308, 310, 349, 350
Blastomas, 230, 262
Blood flow disturbance, 138, 179
Blood groups, 247, 280
Blood loss, 139, 180
Blood pressure, 136, 142, 144, 176, 184, 185
Blood transfusion, 244, 247, 277, 280, 376, 403
Blood–brain barrier, 165, 211
Bochdalek hernias, 6, 68
Body site temperatures, 160, 204–205
Bone healing, 225, 257
Bone physiology, 378, 406
Bone tumours, 236, 268, 293, 295, 332, 335, 372, 399
Bowel infarction, 389, 417
Brachial plexus, 28, 29, 54, 62, 93, 94, 119, 126, 374, 401
Brachial plexus nervous damage, 56, 121
Brachioradialis weakness, 58, 123
Brainstem death test, 164, 210, 289, 327
Branchial arch, 48, 112
Breast anatomy, 28, 92
Breast cancer, 27–28, 92, 233, 238, 265, 270, 300, 340, 375, 402
Breast cancer, males, 234, 266
Breast cancer metastatic spread, 300, 340
Breast cancer presentation, 300, 340
Breast cancer risk factors, 299, 300, 339, 340
Breast cancer staging, 238, 270
Breast carcinoma sites, 300, 340
Breast concerns, 25–31, 89–95
Breast disorders, 299–300, 339–340
Breast lump, 237–238, 270, 299, 339
Breast sarcoma, 299, 339
Bronchial carcinoma, 297, 337

Bronchoscopy, 6, 69
Bronchus, 6, 69
Brown–Séquard syndrome, 289, 328
Buerger disease, 228, 260
Burn complications, 158, 202, 224, 256, 318, 359
Burn injuries, 318, 359

C

Ca^{2+} metabolism, 393, 423
Caecal carcinoma, 22, 86
Calcification, 294, 333
Calcitonin, 168–170, 215, 217, 393, 423
Calcium homeostasis, 385, 413
Calcium levels, 169–170, 216–217
Calcium metabolism, 393–394, 423–424
Calcium properties, 160, 205
Calot's triangle, 10, 73, 376, 404
Cancer screening programmes, 235, 267
Capillary fluid movement, 137, 177
Capillary pressure, 145, 187
Carbon dioxide, 132, 172
Carcinoembryonic antigen, 238, 271
Carcinogenesis, 236–237, 268–269
Carcinogenic viruses, 235, 267
Carcinoid tumours, 305, 345
Cardiac action potential, 371, 398
Cardiac cycle, 141, 182
Cardiac muscle cells, 141, 182
Cardiac output, 136, 137, 139, 143, 164–165, 177, 180, 185, 210
Cardiac physiology, 144, 186
Cardiac valve, 4, 66
Cardiovascular system, 136–145, 163, 176–187, 208, 301–302, 341–342
Carotid artery, 39, 43, 47, 48, 53, 103, 108, 112, 117–118
Carotid body tumour, 324, 364
Carotid endarterectomy, 162, 207
Carpal bone fractures, 27, 91
Carpal tunnel structures, 29, 93, 94
Carpal tunnel syndrome, 61, 125, 391, 420
Cast removal, 55, 121
Catabolic state, 160, 205
Cauda equina syndrome, 42, 106
Cavernous sinus thrombosis, 40, 105
Cavernous venous sinus, 47, 112
Cell cycle stages, 233, 265
Cell damage, 231, 263
Cell injury, irreversible, 224, 256
Cell injury, reversible, 222–223
Cell signaling, 385, 413
Cellular injury, 224, 256
Cellulitis, 242, 275
Central nervous system, 54–63, 119–128
Central venous catheter, 143, 185
Central venous pressure, 136, 143, 176, 185
Cerebral blood flow, 163–165, 209–210
Cerebral lesion, 291, 330

Cerebral perfusion pressure, 163, 208–209
Cerebral spinal flood, 164, 209
Cerebrospinal fluid, 165, 211, 376, 403
Cervical sympathetic trunk, 59, 124
Cervical vertebra, 48, 113
Chemical carcinogen, 233, 265
Chemical mediators, 222, 254
Chemical messengers, 222, 254
Chest drain, 6, 68
Chest pain, 4, 66, 227, 259, 392, 420
Chest wall, 8, 70
Cholecystectomy, 10, 22, 23, 73, 86, 225, 257,
        303, 343, 376, 388, 404, 416
Cholecystitis, 10, 73, 225, 257
Cholinergic receptors, 381, 408–409
Chondrocalcinosis, 296, 335
Christmas disease, 280, 387, 415
Chromosomal abnormalities, 230, 262
Chronic inflammation, 222, 254
Chronic obstructive pulmonary disease,
        249–250, 284
Cirrhosis, 9, 72, 161, 206, 314, 355
Clark's level, 320, 360–361
Clostridia bacteria, 249, 283
Clostridium perfringens, 370, 397
Clotting cascade, 142, 184
Clotting factors, 246–247, 280, 386, 414
Clotting function, 150, 194
Coagulation, 243, 276
Codman's triangle, 372, 399
Colles fracture, 225, 257
Colon, 22, 83, 86, 148, 190
Colonic dilatation, 311, 352
Colonic lymphatic drainage, 19, 83
Colorectal cancer, 236, 268
Colorectal cancer classification, 237, 269
Colorectal carcinoma, 237, 269
Compartment syndrome, 32, 34, 96, 98,
        374, 401
Complement cascade, 241, 273
Concussion, 328–329
Congenital hypertrophic pyloric stenosis,
        311, 352
Congestive cardiac failure, 156, 200
Constipation, 317, 358
Coronary artery, 4, 392, 393, 420, 421, 422
Coronary circulation, 138, 178
Coronary sinus, 5, 68
Coroner referral scenario, 325, 365
Cortisol, 156, 159–160, 200, 204
Costochondral joint, 3, 65
Cranial fossa, 48, 49, 51, 113, 114, 116
Cranial nerves, 39, 55, 62, 103, 120, 127, 149, 193,
        371, 398
Cremasteric reflex, 18, 60, 83, 125
Crohn disease, 311, 313, 316, 352, 354, 356
Cruciate ligament, 35, 100
Crystal arthropathy, 296, 335
C-spine injuries, 41, 106

Curling ulcer, 224, 256
Cushing syndrome, 304, 307, 344, 347
Cushing's ulcer, 162, 207
Cutaneous nerves, 47, 112
Cystic artery, 10, 73, 376, 404

D

De Garengeot hernia, 312, 353
Dead space, 131, 171, 391, 420
Death, 164, 210, 289, 325, 327, 365
Deep vein thrombosis, 228, 244, 259–260, 277,
        301, 341, 382, 387, 409, 415
Defecation reflex, 377, 404
Dermatological diseases, 318–320, 359–361
Di George syndrome, 241, 273
Diabetes mellitus, 303, 343
Diabetic ulcers, 227, 259
Diaphragm, 5, 67, 369, 389, 395, 417
Diaphragm levels, 3, 5, 66, 67, 68
Diaphragm paralysis, 5, 66–67
Diaphragmatic hernias, 6, 68
Diastolic murmur, 4, 66
Differentiation, 229–232, 261–264
Digestion, 149, 193, 370, 396
Disinfectants, 248, 282
Disseminated intravascular coagulation, 246, 247,
        279, 281
Distal fibula, 36, 100
Distal radius fracture, 294, 333
Distal tibia, 36, 100
Diverticular disease, 11, 73
Diverticulitis, 317, 358
Down syndrome, 230, 245, 263, 279, 317, 357
Dukes' classification, 237, 269, 383, 411
Duodenal ulcer, 9, 72, 153, 197, 223, 255
Duodenum, 21, 86
Dysphagia, 47, 237, 269
Dysplasia, 229, 261

E

Ear concerns, 46, 110, 324, 364
Ear nerves, 44, 109
Ear ossicles, 46, 110
Ectopic adrenocorticotropic
                hormonedrenocorticotropic
                hormone, 158, 202
Ectopic testicle, 18, 82
Edinger–Westphal nucleus, 60, 124
Ejection fraction, 144, 185
Elbow fractures, 26, 90
Electrocardiogram changes, 141, 182–183, 369,
        386, 395–396, 415
Embolism, 244, 278, 289, 292, 295, 327–328,
        331, 334
Endocrine functions, 156, 201
Endocrine neoplasia syndrome, 304, 305, 306,
        344, 345, 346

Endocrine system, 156–161, 200–206, 303–307, 343–348
Endogenous pyrogen, 242, 274
Endoneurium, 166, 212
Endothelial cells, 243, 276, 389, 417
Enzymes, 147, 149, 189, 193
Epidermal layers, 318, 319, 359, 360, 380, 407
Epididymitis, 310, 351
Epigastric artery, 16, 80, 370, 396
Epiploic formen, 15, 78
Epistaxis, 324, 364, 383, 410
Erythrocyte production, 142, 184
Evans syndrome, 245, 278
Ewing sarcoma, 293, 332
Exercise, vigorous, 143, 185
Expiratory reserve volume, 380, 408
External carotid artery, 43, 47, 53, 108, 112, 117–118
External jugular vein, 41, 106
Extracellular fluid, 152, 196
Extracerebral haemorrhage, 290, 328–329
Extradural haematoma, 291, 330
Extradural haemorrhage, 328

F

Facial nerves, 55, 57, 120, 122, 372, 398
Familial adenomatous polyposis, 315, 355
Familial cancer syndromes, 230, 235, 262, 267
Familial polyposis coli, 237, 269
Fascial layers, 39, 43, 104, 108
Fasciotomy, 32, 96
Fat embolism, 289, 292, 295, 327–328, 331, 334
Female pelvis, 20, 84
Femoral canal, 13, 76
Femoral head blood supply, 34, 98
Femoral hernia, 312, 353
Femoral nerve damage, 62, 126
Femoral nerve palsy, 60, 125
Femoral ring, 32, 96
Femoral sheath, 33, 37, 97, 101
Femoral triangle, 13, 36, 76, 100
Femoral vein, 33, 76, 97
Femur fracture, 33, 97
Fetal haemoglobin, 143, 185
Fight or flight response, 162, 208
Fine-needle aspiration cytology, 306, 346
Finger nerves, 57, 61, 121
Flexor digitorum brevis, 56, 121
Flexor retinaculum, 37, 101
Fluid distribution, 138, 178
Fluid secretions, 372–373, 400
Folate deficiency, 385–386, 414
Follicular thyroid cancer, 304, 344, 375, 402
Foot drop, 55, 119, 121
Foot muscles, 35, 37, 99, 101
Foot nerves, 35, 36, 99, 100
Foramen magnum, 39, 103–104
Fournier gangrene, 309, 350

Frank–Starling law, 136, 176
Free radicals, 221, 253
Fundus, 12, 74

G

Gag reflex, 162, 207
Gait abnormalities, 32, 34, 54, 96–98, 119
Gallstones, 146, 188, 314, 355
Ganglion, 60, 124, 125
Gangrene, 229, 248, 261, 282, 309, 350
Gas gangrene, 248, 282
Gastrectomy, 383, 411
Gastric acid, 146, 150, 188, 194
Gastric cancer, 237, 269
Gastric carcinoma, 238, 270, 380, 408
Gastric secretion, 373–374, 401
Gastric ulcer, 11, 12, 19, 73, 74, 84
Gastrin, 146, 149, 188, 192
Gastrointestinal carcinoids, 304, 344
Gastrointestinal haemorrhage, 376, 388, 403, 416
Gastrointestinal perforation, 315, 356
Gastrointestinal system, 146–150, 188–194, 311–317, 352–358
Gastrointestinal tract, 19, 83
Gastrointestinal tract fluid, 147, 189
Gastro-oesophageal reflux disease, 234–235, 266–267, 316–317, 357, 372, 399
Genitourinary system, 308–310, 349–351
Giant cell, 230–231, 263
Gilbert syndrome, 251, 285
Glasgow Coma Scale (GCS), 51, 116, 148, 163, 166, 191, 208, 212–213, 291, 316, 329, 356, 382, 410
Glial cells, 165, 211
Glomerular filtration rate, 153, 154, 155, 197, 199
Glucocorticoids, 159–160, 204
Glucose homeostasis, 156–161, 200–206
Goitre, 306, 346
Gram-negative bacillus, 248, 282
Gram-positive bacillus, 248, 282
Granulomatous chronic inflammation, 242, 274
Graves disease, 303, 343
Greater trochanter, 33, 37, 97, 101
Greenstick fractures, 294, 334
Groin pain, 293, 308, 309, 310, 332, 349, 350, 351, 374–375, 402
Growth disorders, 229–232, 261–264
Growth hormone, 156, 200
Growth stimulus, 231–232, 264
Gunshot wound, 162, 207, 224, 256
Gynaecomastia, 300, 340

H

H^+ concentration, 153, 197
Haematoma, 290, 328
Haemoglobin, 134, 143, 173–174, 185

Haemoglobin chain, 246, 280
Haemoglobin S, 243, 276
Haemolytic anaemia, 251, 285
Haemolytic transfusion reaction, 244, 277
Haemophilia B, 246–247, 280
Haemorrhage, 247, 281, 290, 324, 328–329, 364, 388, 416
Haemorrhagic shock, 313, 353
Haemothorax, 6, 68, 134–135, 175
Hamartomatous polyps, 311, 352
Hamstring muscles, 34, 98, 383, 411
Hand injuries, 26, 90
Hand muscles, 62, 127
Hand nerves, 29, 30, 57, 61, 93, 95, 122, 125
Hartmann's procedure, 11, 73
Hartmann's solution, 145, 187
Hashimoto thyroiditis, 305, 345
Hashimoto's disease, 303, 343
Head injury, 41–42, 48, 51, 106, 114, 116, 162–163, 166, 207–208, 212–213, 290–291, 328–329, 382, 410
Head veins, 44, 109
Headache, 290, 328
Heart, 3–6, 65–68
Heart anatomy, 393, 423
Heart block, 137, 177
Heart sounds, 136, 141, 177, 182
Helicobacter pylori, 248, 282, 388, 416
Hemicolectomy, 22, 86, 228, 260, 383, 411
Hemidiaphragm, 5, 66–67
Heparin, 243, 276, 384, 412–413
Hepatic artery, 393, 422
Hepatitis, 249, 283
Hepatocytes, 146, 188
Hepatosplenomegaly, 390, 417
Hering–Breuer reflex, 387, 415
Hernia repair, 226, 258
Herpes virus, 239, 271
Hesselbach's triangle, 10, 73
High altitude changes, 132, 172
High stepping gait, 54, 119
Hip fracture, 33, 97, 302, 341
Hip joint muscles, 38, 102
Hip replacement, 32, 33, 96, 97
Hirschsprung disease, 317, 358
Histamine, 160, 204
Hodgkin lymphoma, 322–323, 363
Hormone physiological effects, 157, 167, 202, 214, 389, 417
Hormone responses, 159, 204
Human leukocyte antigen, 305, 345
Human papilloma virus, 369, 395
Humerus fracture, 27, 30, 91, 95, 294–295, 334
Humerus muscles, 31, 95
Humerus rotation, 31, 95
Hunter's canal, 32, 96
Hydrocortisone, 159–160, 204
Hyperacute rejection, 241, 272–273
Hyperaldosteronism, 303, 343

Hypercalcaemia, 169, 216, 251, 285
Hypercapnia, 163, 208
Hypercoaguable state, 246, 279
Hyperkalaemia, 140, 181, 369, 395–396
Hypermagnesaemia, 158, 202
Hyperparathyroidism, 168, 215, 305, 345
Hypersensitivity, 240, 241, 242, 272, 274, 275, 376, 403
Hypertension, 311, 352
Hyperthyroidism, 307, 347
Hypertrophic pyloric stenosis, 311, 352
Hypertrophic scars, 225, 257
Hypertrophy, 232, 264
Hypocalcaemia, 169, 216
Hypokalaemia, 140, 159, 181, 203
Hypomagnesaemia, 158, 202–203
Hyponatraemia, 161, 206, 254, 285, 291, 329
Hypotension, 163, 208
Hypothyroidism, 307, 347–348
Hypoxia, 163, 208
Hysterectomy, 17, 82, 244, 277

I

Idiopathic thrombocytopenic purpura, 245, 278, 321, 362
IgA deficiency, 240, 272
Ileum, 13, 77
Iliac fossa pain, 313, 317, 354, 358
Iliopsoas muscle, 38, 102
Immune system, 240, 272
Immunodeficiencies, 241, 273
Immunoglobulins, 240, 272
Inferior alveolar nerve, 61, 126
Inferior epigastric artery, 16, 80, 370, 396
Inferior vena cava, 20, 84
Inflammation, 221–223, 242, 253–255, 274, 378, 405
Infrahyoid strap muscle, 46, 111
Infratemporal fossa, 43, 108
Inguinal canal, 9, 10, 15, 71, 73, 79, 385, 413
Inguinal hernia, 10, 14, 20, 73, 78, 85, 312, 353, 376, 379, 403, 407
Inhaled item, 6, 69
Injury response, 217
Innate immune system, 240, 272, 379, 407
Inotropes, 142, 183, 392, 421
Inspiration movements, 4, 66
Insulin, 157, 201
Insulin release, 149, 192
Internal carotid artery, 43, 48, 53, 108, 112, 117–118
Intestinal activity, 148, 191
Intestinal tumours, 315, 355
Intracranial pressure, 163, 208–209, 289, 327
Intravenous fluids composition, 145, 187
Iron deficiency anaemia, 243, 245, 246, 276, 278, 280
Irreversible cell injury, 224, 256

Irritable hip, 293, 332
Ischaemia, 25, 89, 231, 263, 377, 392, 404, 420

J

Jaundice, 148, 190
Jejunum, 13, 77
Jugular vein, 41, 106
Jugular venous pressure, 140–141, 181–182, 372,
        399–400

K

Kaposi sarcoma, 239, 271
Keloid scars, 226, 257
Ketoacidosis, 383, 411
Kidney anatomy, 13, 19, 76, 83
Kidney function, 151–154, 156, 195–199, 201
Knee joint muscles, 38, 102
Knee pain, 250, 284, 293, 332
Knife stab wound, 8, 11, 56, 58, 70, 74, 121–122,
        154, 165, 198, 210, 313, 353, 391, 419
Krukenberg tumour, 236, 268, 380, 408

L

Lanz incision, 11, 74
Laparotomy, 9, 72
Laryngeal nerve, 53, 116, 117, 118, 387, 416
Laryngopharynx, 44, 109
Larynx, 46, 52, 53, 111, 116, 117, 118
Lateral cord, 56, 121
Left coronary artery, 4, 66
Leg compartments, 32, 34, 56, 96, 98, 101, 120,
        121, 374, 401
Leg pain, 228, 260, 293, 332, 374, 401
Leg ulceration, 227, 259
Lesser omentum, 17, 81
Leukaemia, 243, 245, 277, 279
Levothyroxine absorption, 170, 217
Limb, lower, 32–38, 96–102
Limb, upper, 25–31, 89–95
Limb nerve injuries, 26, 90
Littre hernia, 376, 403
Liver cirrhosis, 9, 72, 161, 206, 314, 355
Liver disease, 230, 261
Liver function, 146, 150, 188, 194
Liver laceration, 9, 72
Lobar pneumonia, 297, 337
Longitudinal temporal bone fracture, 41, 106
Loop of Henle, 151, 195, 370, 375, 387, 397,
        402, 415–416
Low molecular weight heparin, 384, 412–413
Lower limb, 32–38, 96–102
Low-molecular-weight heparin, 243, 276
Lumbar plexus, 54, 119
Lumbar puncture, 40, 104–105
Lumbar vertebra, 48, 113
Lung carcinoma, 297–298, 338

Lung dead space, 131, 171
Lung pleurae, 3, 65
Lung volumes, 171, 221
Lungs, 7, 69, 131–135
Lymph nodes, 19, 27, 28, 83, 92
Lymphadenopathy, 27, 92
Lymphatic circulation, 145, 186
Lymphatic drainage, 28, 43, 92, 109
Lymphocytic leukaemia, 243, 277
Lymphoedema, 227, 259, 381, 409
Lymphoma, 322, 363
Lymphoreticular system, 321–323, 362–363

M

Macrolide antibiotics, 249, 282
Macrophages, 222, 254
Magnesium balance, 158–159, 203
Magnesium homeostasis, 375, 402
Male breast cancer, 234, 266
Male pelvis, 20, 84
Male urethra, 16, 80, 83
Malignancy paraneoplastic effect, 235, 267
Malignancy potential, 233–235, 265–267
Malignant bone tumours, 236, 268
Malignant melanoma, 319–320, 360–361,
        378, 406
Mandibular foramen, 61, 126
Mastectomy, 27, 28, 92, 300, 339–340, 375, 394,
        402, 423
Mastoid antrum, 46, 111
Maxillary nerve, 55, 120
Maximal plexus injury, 61, 125–126
Meckel's diverticulum, 14, 78, 313, 315, 354, 356,
        376, 403
Medial compartment, 56, 120, 121
Medial malleolus, 37, 101
Medial plantar nerve, 35, 99
Median nerve, 25, 59, 62, 89, 123–124, 127
Medullary carcinoma, 305–306, 345–346
Melanocytes, 266, 360, 380, 407
Melanoma, 319–320, 360–361, 378, 406
Membrane potential, 164, 209–210
Meningeal artery, 42, 106
Meningitis, 291, 329–330
Menorrhagia, 243, 276
Meralgia paraesthetica, 60, 125
Metabolic acidosis, 154, 198, 383, 411
Metaplasia, 229, 261, 372, 399
Microbial infection, 378, 405
Micturition, 151, 195
Middle cranial fossa, 48, 114
Middle ear, 46, 110
Milroy disease, 381, 409
Mineralocorticoid deficiency, 378, 406
Mitochondrion, 224, 256
Mitral valve prolapse, 227, 259
Monocytes, 242, 274
Morphogenesis, 229–232, 261–264

Morton's neuroma, 62, 126
Multiple adenomas, 305, 345
Multiple endocrine neoplasia, 304, 305, 306, 344, 345, 346
Multiple myeloma, 238, 270–271, 384, 412
Multiple trauma cases, 225, 257
Muscle physiology, 166, 211–212
Musculocutaneous nerve, 25, 89
Musculoskeletal system, 292–296, 331–336
Myelin degeneration, 245, 278
Myenteric plexus, 149, 193
Myocardial contraction, 137, 177
Myocardial infarction, 5, 67
Myocardial ischaemia, 392, 420
Myoglobin, 143, 184

N

Natal cleft discharge, 221, 253
Neck dissection, 40, 104
Neck injury, 41, 106
Neck laceration, 41, 106
Neck lump, 41, 106, 304, 306, 324, 344, 346, 364, 375, 381, 390, 402, 409, 417
Neck of femur fracture, 33, 97, 294, 333–334
Neck of fibula fracture, 382, 410
Neck stab would, 165, 210
Neck triangles, 47, 49, 50, 112, 114
Neck veins, 44, 109
Necrosis, 221, 232, 253, 264, 379, 406
Necrotizing fasciitis, 250, 284, 379, 407
Neoplasia, 233–239, 265–271
Nephron tubercle, 370, 387, 397, 415–416
Nerve fibres, 166, 213
Nervous systems, 54–63, 119–128, 162–166, 207–213, 289–291, 327–330
Neurofibromas, 289, 327
Neutrophils, 242, 274
Nitrosamines, 233, 265
Non-Hodgkin lymphoma, 322, 363
Noradrenaline, 142, 183
Nose concerns, 44, 110, 324, 364

O

Oedema, 145, 186
Oesophageal atresia, 317, 357
Oesophageal cancer, 234–236, 266–268
Oesophageal carcinoma, 4, 66
Oesophageal indentation, 7, 69
Oesophageal sphincter, 150, 193
Oesophageal swallowing, 149, 191, 193
Oesophagectomy, 4, 66
Oesophagitis, 316–317, 357
Oesophagogastroduodenoscopy, 388, 416
Oesophagus, 7, 69, 369, 395
Oesophagus carcinogen, 233, 265
Oesophagus constrictions, 7, 69
Olecranon fracture, 29, 94

Omental foramen, 17, 82, 393, 422
Oncogenic virus, 233, 265
Ophthalmic division, 47, 112
Ophthalmoplegia, 47, 112
Orbital blood supply, 45, 111
Orbital fissure, 45, 49, 110
Organelles, 224, 256
Ossicles, 46, 110
Osteoarthritis, 293, 294, 295, 333, 335
Osteochondromas, 292, 331
Osteoclasts, 168, 215
Osteomalacia, 295, 335
Osteosarcomas, 292, 295, 331, 335, 372, 399
Oxygen concentration, 390–391, 417–418
Oxygen consumption, 138, 178
Oxygen–haemoglobin dissociation, 133, 173
Oxyntic gland, 146, 189
Oxytocin, 161, 205

P

Paget's disease, 295, 334
Pain transmission, 374, 401
Pancreas, 21, 85
Pancreatic physiology, 148, 191
Pancreatic resection, 148, 190–191
Pancreatitis, 147, 170, 189, 216–217, 227, 259, 297, 312, 316, 337, 353, 356–357
Papillary adenocarcinoma, 305, 345
Papillary carcinoma, 304, 344
Papillary thyroid carcinoma, 306, 346
Paragangliomas, 291, 329
Paranasal sinuses, 44, 110
Paraneoplastic effect, 235, 267
Parasympathetic nervous supply, 62, 63, 127
Parathormone, 394, 423–424
Parathyroid carcinoma, 372, 399
Parathyroid glands, 45, 110, 167–170, 214–217, 394, 423–424
Parathyroid hormone, 167, 168, 214, 215
Parenteral nutrition, 150, 194
Paresthesia, 162, 207
Parietal cells, 146, 188, 189, 383, 411
Parotid gland, 42, 48, 51, 53, 63, 107, 113, 116, 118, 127, 324, 364, 371, 398
Parotid gland tumours, 388, 390, 416, 417
Parotidectomy, 48, 51, 113, 116
Pathology, 221–251, 253–286, 289–365
Pelvic inflammation, 308, 349
Pelvic injuries, 55, 62, 120, 126
Pelvis fracture, 33, 96–97
Pepsinogen, 370, 396
Perianal abscess, 221, 253
Perineal body, 24, 87, 88
Peripheral nerves, 57, 121, 166, 212, 374, 401
Peripheral nervous system, 54–63, 119–128
Peristalsis, 150, 193–194
Peritoneal dialysis, 311, 352
Peritonitis, 11, 73, 225, 257, 380, 408

Pernicious anaemia, 245, 278
Peroneal nerve, 32, 56, 63, 96, 121, 127
Peroneal nerve injury, 54, 119
Peroneal nerve palsy, 36, 100
Perthes disease, 293, 332
Peutz–Jeghers syndrome, 311, 312, 352, 353
Pharynx anatomy, 52, 117
Pheochromocytoma, 303, 343
Phrenic nerve, 59, 124
Phyllodes tumour, 299, 339
Physiological dead space, 391, 420
Physiology, 131–217
Pigments, 224, 229, 256, 261
Piriformis muscle, 15, 78
Pituitary adenoma, 49, 113, 306, 346
Pituitary gland, 49, 113, 156, 161, 200, 205
Platelets shelf life, 247, 281
Pleura, 3, 65
Pneumonia, 297, 337
Poland syndrome, 292, 293, 331, 332
Pons, 62, 127
Popliteal fossa, 34, 36, 37, 98, 100, 101, 381, 409
Portal hypertension, 311, 352
Portal vein, 15, 17, 79, 81, 384, 412
Portal venous system, 370, 396
Portosystemic anastomosis, 20, 84
Posterior coronary artery, 392, 420
Posterior cranial fossa, 48, 49, 113, 114
Posterior cruciate ligament, 35, 100
Posterior triangle, 47, 50, 112, 114–115, 381, 409
Potassium balance, 157, 201
Potassium levels, 151, 195
Practice papers, 369–424
Preganglionic parasympathetic fibres, 60, 124
Premalignant conditions, 239, 271
Primary antibody deficiency, 241, 273
Primary haemorrhage, 324, 364
Primary lymphoedema, 227, 259, 381, 409
Primary peristalsis, 150, 193–194
Pringle's manoeuvre, 9, 72
Prions, 248, 282
Projectile vomiting, 147, 190, 352
Prolactinomas, 306, 347
Prostate carcinoma, 234, 266
Prostate gland, 18, 82
Protein digestion, 149, 193
Prothrombotic effect, 243, 276
Psammoma bodies, 304, 344
Pseudogout, 296, 335
Psoas muscle, 35, 60, 100, 125
Pterion, 40, 41, 53, 104, 105, 117, 330
Pulmonary artery catheter, 381, 408
Pulmonary artery pressure, 136, 176
Pulmonary circulation, 132, 172
Pulmonary embolism, 228, 260, 388, 416
Pulmonary function tests, 131, 171
Pulse oximetry, 133, 173
Pulse pressure, 143, 184, 386, 414
Pyloric stenosis, 147, 190, 311, 352

Q

Quadrangular space, 27, 29, 92, 93

R

Radial nerve, 58, 63, 123, 127–128, 385, 413–414
Rectum anatomy, 23, 87
Rectum vasculature, 24, 87
Rectus abdominis muscle, 16, 80, 312, 353
Recurrent laryngeal nerve, 387, 416
Red blood cell formation, 138, 179
Reed–Sternberg cells, 322, 363
Renal calculi, 308, 349
Renal clearance, 153, 197
Renal colic, 17, 82
Renal failure, 168, 215
Renal injury, 310, 351
Renal physiology, 151, 155, 195, 199
Renal stones, 308–309, 349–350, 374–375, 402
Renal system, 151–155, 195–199
Renal transplant, 168, 215
Renal transplant rejection, 241, 272–273
Renal veins, 14, 20, 78, 84, 85
Renin, 152, 196
Renin–angiotensin–aldosterone system, 161, 205–206
Respiration regulation, 387, 415
Respiratory alkalosis, 153, 198, 388, 416
Respiratory control, 132, 133, 172, 173
Respiratory distress, 242, 275, 297, 337
Respiratory failure, 134, 175
Respiratory regulation, 132, 172
Respiratory system, 131–135, 171–175, 297–298, 337–338
Reticuloendothelial system, 321, 362
Retroperitoneal, 21, 85
Reversible cell injury, 222–223, 254
Rhabdomyosarcoma, 233, 265
Rheumatoid arthritis, 292, 296, 331–333, 335–336
Rhomboid major muscle, 25, 90
Rib anatomy, 8, 70
Rib fracture, 6, 68
Richter hernia, 314, 355
Right atrium, 393, 423
Rotator cuff muscles, 25, 89, 386, 414–415

S

Saliva, 376, 403
Saliva enzymes, 147, 189
Saphenous nerve, 54, 96, 97, 99, 100, 120
Saphenous vein, 35, 99, 100
Scalp structure, 39, 103
Scapula, 28, 93, 379, 407
Sciatic foramen, 24, 55, 87, 120
Sciatic nerve, 33, 55, 58, 96–97, 121, 122
Sciatic notch, 15, 78

Scrotal skin, 18, 83, 309, 350
Secondary haemorrhage, 324, 364
Sensory innervation, 52, 120
Sensory loss, 58, 123
Sensory nerves, 374, 401
Sepsis, 47, 112, 225, 257
Septic arthritis, 250, 284
Septic shock, 140, 181
Serum calcium levels, 169–170, 216–217
Serum potassium levels, 151, 195
Serum tumour marker, 310, 351
Shock, 139, 140, 179, 180, 313, 353, 391, 419
Shoulder abduction, 374, 391, 401, 419–420
Shoulder anatomy, 26, 90, 92
Shoulder dislocation, 30, 95
Shoulder injury, 374, 401
Shoulder nerves, 30, 95
Shoulder weakness, 61, 125
Sickle cell anaemia, 247, 280–281
Sickle cell disease, 243, 246, 276, 280
Sinoatrial node, 143, 185
Sinus discharge, 221, 253
Skeletal muscle fibres, 392, 421
Skeletal muscle tumour, 233, 265
Skull, 39, 40, 47, 55, 103, 104, 120
Skull fracture, 48, 112, 114, 115
Slipped upper femoral epiphysis, 293, 332
Smooth muscle tumour, 236, 268
Sodium–water balance, 151, 196
Spermatic cord, 9, 14, 23, 24, 71, 77, 87, 88, 385, 413
Spermatic fascia, 24, 88
Spigelian hernia, 16, 80, 312, 353
Spinal cord, 377, 404–405
Spinal cord injuries, 391, 419
Spinal cord lesion, 162, 207
Spinal nerve root, 57, 122
Spine injuries, 41, 106
Spirogram, 380, 408
Spleen, 16, 81, 382, 385, 409, 413
Splenectomy, 321–322, 362–363, 385, 413
Splenic flexure, 321, 362
Splenic rupture, 321, 362
Splenomegaly, 12, 75
Squamous cell carcinoma, 298, 318, 319, 338, 359, 360, 370, 397
Squamous temporal bone, 41, 106
Starling equilibrium, 137, 178
Starling forces, 137, 177
Stellate ganglion, 60, 125
Sternal angle, 4, 66
Sternum injury, 4, 66
Stomach arteries, 12, 75
Stomach carcinogen, 233, 265
Stomach secretions, 146, 188
Stratified squamous epithelium, 229, 261
Stretch reflexes, 393, 422
Stroke, 162, 207
Stroke volume, 141, 142, 183, 184

Stylomastoid foramen, 39, 103
Subarachnoid haemorrhage, 291, 328
Subclavian artery, 7, 40, 50, 53, 69, 105, 115, 118
Subclavian artery thrombectomy, 29, 94
Sublingual gland, 42, 107
Submandibular gland, 373, 400
Subscapular nerves, 8, 70
Sudden-onset headache, 290, 328
Superficial inguinal, 309, 350
Superior gluteal nerve injury, 377, 405
Superior orbital fissure, 45, 49, 110
Supracondylar fractures, 294–295, 334
Suprascapular nerve, 28, 93
Surfactant, 131, 132, 171–172
Surgery hormone response, 159, 204
Surgical anatomy, 3–63, 65–128
Surgical biochemistry, 251, 285–286
Surgical haematology, 243–247, 276–281
Surgical immunology, 240–242, 272–275
Surgical microbiology, 248–250, 282–284
Sutures, 225, 257
Swallowing, 149, 191, 193
Swinging pyrexia, 223, 255
Systemic venous system, 370, 396
System-specific pathology, 289–325, 327–365;
        see also Pathology
Systolic murmur, 301, 341

T

T_3/T_4 levels, 170, 217
Takayashu disease, 377, 404
Telomerase, 222, 254
Temperatures, body sites, 160, 204–205
Temporal bone, 41, 106
Temporal bone fracture, 41, 106
Temporomandibular joint, 45, 110
Tension pneumothorax, 134, 174, 175
Tentorial herniation, 290, 328
Teratogens, 230, 262
Testes vasculature, 24, 88
Testicles, 18, 82
Testicular lump, 310, 351
Testicular teratoma, 309, 350
Testicular torsion, 18, 60, 82, 125
Testicular tumours, 308, 310, 349, 351
Tetanus, 248, 250, 282, 284
Thigh lesion, 61, 125
Thigh stab wound, 56, 121
Thoracic aorta, 7, 69
Thoracic duct, 4, 6, 68, 380, 408
Thoracic nerves, 8, 70, 373, 400
Thoracic trachea, 6, 68
Thoracodorsal nerve, 54, 119
Thorax, 3–8, 65–70
Throat, 324, 364
Thrombectomy, 29, 94
Thrombocytopenia, 246, 279
Thrombomodulin, 389, 417

Thrombosis, 40, 105
Thymus gland, 394, 424
Thymus gland tumour, 241, 273
Thyroid, 167–170, 214–217
Thyroid carcinoma, 304–306, 344–346, 375, 402
Thyroid disease, 303, 343
Thyroid fine-needle aspiration cytology, 306, 346
Thyroid gland, 42, 43, 50, 51, 53, 107, 109, 115, 118, 167, 214
Thyroid receptors, 167–168, 215
Thyroid stimulating hormone, 169, 170, 216, 217
Thyroid surgery, 52, 114, 116
Thyroid tumour, 304, 344
Thyroidectomy, 50, 114, 169, 216
Thyrotropin, 169, 216
Tibial nerve, 35, 36, 99, 100
Tissue oedema, 162, 207
TNM classification, 238, 270, 351, 383, 411
Tongue, 43, 109
Tonsillectomy, 52, 117, 324, 364
Toxic megacolon, 311, 352
Trachea, 6, 68
Tracheostomy, 46, 48, 111, 113
Transcoelomic spread, 235, 267
Transpyloric plane, 10, 14, 72, 77, 384, 412
Transudate ascites, 228, 260
Transurethral resection of prostate, 152, 196
Transverse temporal bone fracture, 41, 106
Trauma cases, 225, 257
Trauma hormone response, 159, 204
Trauma response, 170
Trendelenburg gait, 32, 96
Trendelenburg test, 377, 405
Triangles of neck, 47, 49, 50, 112, 114, 381, 409
Triangular space, 29, 93
Trochanter, 33, 37, 97, 101
Trochlear nerve, 59, 124
Tuberculosis, 221, 253
Tumour, node, metastases classification, 238, 270, 351, 383, 411
Tumour markers, 234, 237, 238, 265–266, 269, 271, 310, 351, 372, 399
Tumour suppressor genes, 377, 405
Tumour/virus pairings, 234, 266
Tympanic cavity, 45, 111

U

Ulcerative colitis, 314, 354–355, 370, 397
Ulnar artery, 28, 92
Ulnar nerve, 25, 59, 89, 123, 382, 410
Umbilical fold, 14, 77
Unconjugated bilirubin, 251, 285
Upper limb, 25–31, 89–95
Upper limb pathology, 292, 331
Ureter anatomy, 18, 82

Ureter course, 13, 76
Urethra, 16, 19, 80, 83
Urinary bladder, 15, 19, 79, 83
Urinary calculi, 309, 350
Urinary concentrations, 154, 199
Urinary retention, 42, 106
Urinary tract calculus, 309, 350
Urinary tract infection, 308, 350

V

Vagus nerve, 58, 60, 62, 123–124, 126–127, 392, 421
Varicocele, 11, 74
Varicose veins, 35, 99
Vascular disorders, 227–228, 259–260
Vascular permeability, 222, 253, 378, 405
Venous drainage, 5, 67
Venous system, 370, 396
Venous thrombosis, 386–387, 415
Venous ulcers, 374, 402
Vermiform appendix, 312, 353
Vertebrae anatomy, 45, 48, 110, 113
Vertigo, 378, 405–406
Viral hepatitis, 249, 283
Viral meningitis, 291, 329–330
Virus carcinogens, 235, 267
Virus-laden cells, 240, 272
Virus/tumour pairings, 234, 266
Vitamin B_{12} deficiency, 245, 278
Vitamin D function, 157, 201
Vitamin E deficiency, 251, 285
Vocal cords, 52, 116, 117
Vomiting, bilious, 317, 357
Vomiting, projectile, 147, 190, 352
Von Recklinghausen's disease, 324, 364
Von Willebrand factor, 243, 276

W

Warfarin, 244, 277
Warthin tumour, 324, 364, 371, 398
Well's score, 302, 341–342
Wilson's disease, 230, 261
Wounds, 224–227, 256–258, 370, 373, 397, 400
Wounds, gunshot, 162, 207, 224, 256
Wounds, stab, 8, 11, 56, 58, 70, 74, 121–122, 154, 165, 198, 210, 313, 353, 391, 419
Wrist drop, 58, 123
Wrist tendons, 30, 95

Z

Zollinger–Ellison syndrome, 383, 411
Zona glomerulosa, 160, 204
Zygomatic arch, 40, 105